Molecular Pathology
of Nerve and Muscle

Experimental and Clinical Neuroscience

Molecular Pathology of Nerve and Muscle: Noxious Agents and Genetic Lesions, edited by **Antony D. Kidman, John K. Tomkins, Carol A. Morris,** and **Neil A. Cooper,** 1983

Neural Membranes, edited by **Grace Y. Sun, Nicolas Bazan, Jang-Yen Wu, Giuseppe Porcellati,** and **Albert Y. Sun,** 1983

Molecular Pathology of Nerve and Muscle

Noxious Agents and Genetic Lesions

Edited by

**Antony D. Kidman, John K. Tomkins,
Carol A. Morris, and Neil A. Cooper**

The Humana Press · Clifton, New Jersey

Library of Congress Cataloging in Publication Data

Foundation for Life Sciences (Australia). Symposium
   (3rd : 1983 : Sydney, N.S.W.)
   Molecular pathology of nerve and muscle.

   (Experimental and clinical neuroscience)
   "Proceedings of the Third Symposium of the Foundation
for Life Sciences, Sydney, February 9-11, 1983"--T.p.
verso.
   Includes index.
   1. Nervous system--Diseases--Congresses. 2. Neuro-
muscular diseases--Congresses. 3. Pathology, Molecular--
Congresses. I. Kidman, Antony D. II. Title.
III. Series. [DNLM: 1. Neuromuscular diseases--Pathology
--Congresses. 2. Muscles--Pathology--Congresses.
3. Neurons--Pathology--Congresses. W3 F076 3rd
1983m / WE 550 F771 1983r]
RC347.F68 1983   616.8′047   83-22809
ISBN 0-89603-057-1

Printed in the United States of America

PREFACE

The third Symposium of the Foundation for Life Sciences was held in February 1983 at the Newport Inn Conference Centre in Sydney.

It was direced towards an understanding of the molecular neuropathology of muscle and nerve under a wide variety of conditions that may be induced by external agents or genetic lesions.

The first session on experimental neurology explored the processes involved in maintenance of nerve and muscle function. This included many papers on myelination, studies on immune reactions affecting nerves, on synapses, and on neuronal development. This section was expanded to explore the control of muscle function in nerves, including a discussion on cross reinnervation.

Toxic models of disease in the nervous system were then discussed, including pathological states induced by physical agents such as kainic acid, diphtheria toxin, and IDPN.

A new dimension was added to the Symposium when for the first time psychologists participated and contributed to the session on external stressors and their effects on behavior. Heavy metals, herbicides, repetitive work, anxiety, and their effects on behavior and health were all represented. The discussion in this session attracted much interest from the participants, particularly the basic scientists.

The biochemical and physiological properties of muscle in response to genetic lesions were discussed on the last day. Special emphasis was placed on protein turnover and a lively debate about the role of protein synthesis versus protein degradation in the pathogenesis of muscular dystrophy ensued. The abnormalities in plasma lipoproteins of Duchenne patients were mentioned in relation to the detection of carriers and the possible primary defect in this type of dystrophy. In addition, the muscle session devoted some time to the importance of myosin isoenzymes, denervation, and trophic factors on muscle function.

v

The value of this small, live-in, three-day workshop was that it provided an unparalleled opportunity for participants to exchange ideas across a wide spectrum of disciplines associated with the rapidly growing field of molecular neuropathology. Biochemists could talk with psychologists, physiologists with physicians, pathologists with immunologists. Young investigators and graduate students had the chance to seek out and meet with established international authorities, and the discussions and debates continued far into the night.

A. D. Kidman
J. K. Tomkins
C. A. Morris
N. A. Cooper

FOUNDATION FOR LIFE SCIENCES

Foundation Members

A. D. Kidman	Head, Neurobiology Unit School of Life Sciences The NSW Institute of Technology
J. Weingarth	Legal Counsel Citicorp Australis Ltd.
G. P. Short	Managing Director Geoffrey P. Short & Associates
G. Rorke	Manager, Graphic Products Asia & Pacififc Nashua Australia Pty Ltd
J. Picone	Solicitor J. Picone & Co.
J. K. Tomkins	Senior Research Offifcer Neurobiology Unit School of Life Sciences The NSW Institute of Technology
C. J. Sutton	Finance Director Caltex Oil(Aust) Pty Ltd
P. J. Dunstan	General Manager Information & Public Affairs Unilever Australia Pty Ltd
T. R. Buckmaster	Senior Finance Executive C.I.G. Ltd
S. G. Davis	Managing Director Davis Homes Pty Ltd
L. Stromland	Managing Director Atlantica Insurance Co.

CONTENTS

I. Experimental Neurology

The Regulation of Schwann Cell Function in
Degenerative Disorders of the Nervous System
**P. S. Spencer, R. G. Pellegrino, S. M. Ross, M. J.
Politis, and M. I. Sabri**   **3**

The Sympathetic Nervous System: A Novel Perspective
on the Control of Myelinating Schwann Cells
J. W. Heath   **21**

The Schmidt-Lanterman Cleft in the Myelin Sheath:
Studies in Chicken Nerves
N. A. Cooper and A. D. Kidman   **39**

Interaction Between Neuronal Sets During Brain
Development
P. P. Giorgi   **51**

Maturation of Post-Synaptic Densities in Chicken
Forebrain
J. A. P. Rostas, F. H. Güldner, and P. R. Dunkley   **67**

Immune Diseases of the Peripheral Nervous System
I. M. Roberts and C. C. A. Bernard   **81**

Factors Underlying Ascending Paralysis in Rodents
during Experimental Autoimmune Encephalomyelitis
(EAE)
**R. D. Simmons, C. C. A. Bernard, and P. R.
Carnegie**   **99**

The Influence of Upper Motor Neurones on Excitation-
Contraction Coupling in Mammalian Skeletal Muscle
P. W. Gage and A. F. Dulhunty   **113**

Effect of Electric Fields on Nerve Regeneration and
Functional Recovery in the Cat Hindlimb
**R. W. Zeigenbein, R. A. Westerman, R. Silberstein,
H. Kranz, J. Cassell, D. I. Finkelstein, and D.
Bettess**   **119**

Properties of Cross and Self-Reinnervating Motor Axons
in the Cat
    **R. A. Westerman, D. I. Finkelstein, and D.
    Sriratana**   135
Morphometric Assessment of Peripheral Nerve
    S. Allpress, M. Pollock, H. Nukada   151

II. Toxic Models of Disease

Selective Defects in Axonal Transport in
Neuropathological Processes
    **J. W. Griffin, J. C. Troncoso, I. M. Parhad, and D.
    L. Price**   165
Amyotrophic Lateral Sclerosis Toxic and Animal Models
    **A. D. Kidman, A. Gow, R. T. Johanson, N. A.
    Cooper, and C. A. Morris**   185
Excitotoxins
    G. A. R. Johnston   195
Toxic Effects of Glutamic Acid Analogues on Retinal
Neurons
    I.G. Morgan   203

III. Behavioral Neurology

Stress Hormones and Health
    G. Singer and W. Fibiger   219
Stress and Work Behaviour
    R. Spillane   237
Stress, Catecholamines and Ischaemic Heart Disease
    J. R. Bassett   251
Herbicides and the Development of Brain and
Behaviour a Study in Behavioural Toxicology
    L. Rogers   267
The Effects of Heavy Metal Exposure on Behaviour
    A. M. Williamson   283
The Effect of Stress on Central Nervous System Protein
Phosphorylation and Cyclic AMP
    **P. R. Dunkley, J. Cockburn, P. A. Power, and M.
    G. King**   297

IV. Neuromuscular Pathology

Physiological Mechanisms for the Regulation of Protein
Balance in Skeletal Muscle
**D. J. Millward, P. C. Bates, J. G. Brown, D.
Halliday, B. Odedra, P. W. Emery, and M. J.
Rennie**   315

Therapeutic Strategies for Protein Wasting States
**P. M. Stewart, M. Walser, D. G. Sapir, and D. B.
Drachman**   343

Skeletal Muscle Fiber Bundles for the Study of Protein
Turnover in Normal and Dystrophic Mouse Tissue
L. Butcher and J. K. Tomkins   355

The Effect of the Loss of Weight-Bearing Function on
the Isomyosin Profile and Contractile Properties of Rat
Skeletal Muscles
J. F. Y. Hoh and C. J. Chow   371

Lipoproteins in Plasma of Duchenne Muscular
Dystrophy Patients and Female Carriers
L. Austin, H. Arthur, R. Iannello, and P. L. Jeffrey   385

Trophic Influences of Nerve on Skeletal Muscle
Sarcolemma
**P. L. Jeffrey, J. A. P. Rostas, W. N. Leung, and N.
T. Shatin**   399

Index   413

Contributors

S. Allpress, Department of Medicine, University of Otago Medical School, Dunedin, New Zealand

H. L. Arthur, Department of Biochemistry, Monash University, Clayton, Victoria, Australia

L. Austin, Department of Biochemistry, Monash University, Clayton, Victoria, Australia

J. R. Bassett, Macquerie University, North Ryde, New South Wales, Australia

P. C. Bates, Department of Human Nutrition, London School of Hygiene and Tropical Medicine, London, England

C. C. A. Bernard, Neuroimmunology Laboratory, LaTrobe University, Bundoora, Victoria, Australia

D. Bettess, Department of Physiology, Monash University, Clayton, Victoria, Australia

J. G. Brown, Department of Human Nutrition, London School of Hygiene, and Tropical Medicine, London, England

L. Butcher, Neurobiology Unit, The NSW Institute of Technology, Gore Hill, New South Wales, Australia

P. R. Carnegie, School of Agriculture, LaTrobe University, Bundoora, Victoria, Australia

J. Cassell, Neurology and Clinical Neurophysiology Department, Alfred Hospital, Prahran, Victoria, Australia

C. J. Chow, Department of Physiology, University of Sydney, Sydney, New South Wales, Australia

J. Cockburn, The Neuroscience Group, Faculty of Medicine, University of Newcastle, New South Wales, Australia

N. A. Cooper, Neurobiology Unit, The NSW Institute of Technology, Gore Hill, New South Wales, Australia

D. B. Drachman, Department of Neurology, The Johns Hopkins University School of Medicine, Baltimore, Maryland

A. F. Dulhunty, School of Physiology and Pharmacology, University of NSW, Kensington, Australia

P. R. Dunkley, The Neuroscience Group, Faculty of Medicine, University of Newcastle, Australia

P. W. Emery, Department of Human Nutrition, London School of Hygiene and Tropical Medicine, London, England

W. Fibiger, LaTrobe University, Melbourne, Australia

D. I. Finkelstein, Department of Physiology, Monash University, Clayton, Victoria

P. W. GAGE, School of Physiology and Pharmacology, University of NSW, Kensington, New South Wales, Australia

P. P. GIORGI, Neuroembryology Laboratory, University of Queensland, St. Lucia, Queensland, Australia

F. A. GOW, Neurobiology Unit, The NSW Institute of Technology, Gore Hill, New South Wales, Australia

J. W. GRIFFIN, Departments of Neurology and Neuroscience, The Johns Hopkins University School of Medicine, Baltimore, Maryland

F. H. GÜLDNER, Department of Anatomy, Monash University, Clayton, Victoria, Australia

D. HALLIDAY, Department of Human Nutrition, London School of Hygiene and Tropical Medicine, London, England

J. W. HEATH, The Neuroscience Group, Faculty of Medicine, The University of Newcastle, New South Wales, Australia

J. F. Y. HOH, Department of Physiology, University of Sydney, Sydney, New South Wales, Australia

R. IANNELLO, Department of Biochemistry, Monash University, Clayton, Victoria, Australia

P. L. JEFFREY, Department of Biochemistry, Monash University, Clayton, Victoria, Australia

R. T. JOHANSON, Neurobiology Unit, The NSW Institute of Technology, Gore Hill, New South Wales, Australia

G. A. R. JOHNSTON, Department of Pharmacology, University of Sydney, New South Wales, Australia

A. D. KIDMAN, Neurobiology Unit, The NSW Institute of Technology, Gore Hill, New South Wales, Australia

M. G. KING, The Neuroscience Group, Faculty of Medicine, University of Newcastle, Australia

H. KRANZ, Neurology and Clinical Neurophysiology Department, Alfred Hospital, Prahran, Victoria, Australia

W. N. LEUNG, Biochemistry Department, Chinese University of Hong Kong, Hong Kong

D. J. MILLWARD, Department of Human Nutrition, London School of Hygiene and Tropical Medicine, London, England

I. G. MORGAN, Department of Behavioural Biology, Australian National University, Canberra ACT, Australia

C. A. MORRIS, Neurobiology Unit, The NSW Institute of Technology, Gore Hill, New South Wales, Australia

H. NUKADA, Department of Medicine, University of Otago Medical School, Dunedin, New Zealand

B. ODEDRA, Department of Human Nutrition, London School of Hygiene and Tropical Medicine, London, England

I. M. PARHARD, Departments of Neurology and Pathology, The Johns Hopkins School of Medicine, Baltimore, Maryland

G. PELLEGRINO, Institute of Neurotoxicology, Neuroscience, Neurology, and Pathology Departments, Albert Einstein College of Medicine, Bronx, New York

M. J. POLITIS, Institute of Neurotoxicology, Neuroscience, Neurology and Pathology Departments, Albert Einstein College of Medicine, Bronx, New York

M. POLLOCK, Department of Medicine, University of Otago Medical School, Dunedin, New Zealand

P. A. POWER, The Neuroscience Group, Faculty of Medicine, University of Newcastle, Australia

L. PRICE, Departments of Neurology and Pathology, The Johns Hopkins School of Medicine, Baltimore, Maryland

M. J. RENNIE, Department of Human Nutrition, London School of Hygiene and Tropical Medicine, London, England

I. M. ROBERTS, Neuroimmunology Laboratory, LaTrobe University, Bundoora, Victoria, Australia

L. ROGERS, Department of Pharmacology, Monash University, Clayton, Victoria, Australia

S. M. ROSS, Institute of Neurotoxicology, Neuroscience, Neurology, and Pathology Departments, Albert Einstein College of Medicine, Bronx, New York

J. A. P. ROSTAS, Neuroscience Group, Faculty of Medicine, University of Newcastle, New South Wales, Australia

I. SABRI, Institute of Neurotoxicology, Neuroscience, Neurology, and Pathology Departments, Albert Einstein College of Medicine, Bronx, New York

D. G. SAPIR, Department of Neurology, The Johns Hopkins University School of Medicine, Baltimore, Maryland

N. T. SHATIN, Biochemistry Department, Chinese University of Hong Kong, Hong Kong

R. SILBERSTEIN, Department of Physics, Swinburne Institute of Technology, Clatyon, Victoria, Australia

R. D. SIMMONS, Brain-Behaviour Research Institute, LaTrobe University, Bundoora, Victoria, Australia

G. SINGER, Department of Psychology, and Brain-Behavior Research Institute, LaTrobe University, Bundoora, Victoria, Australia

P. S. SPENCER, Institute of Neurotoxicology, Neuroscience, Neurology, and Pathology Departments, Albert Einstein College of Medicine, Bronx, New York

R. SPILLANE, Management Studies Centre, Macquerie University, North Ryde, New South Wales, Australia

D. SRIRATAMA, Department of Physiology, Monash University, Clayton, Victoria, Austarlia

P. M. STEWART, Royal Prince Alfred Hospital, Camperdown, New South Wales, Australia

J. K. TOMKINS, Neurobiology Unit, The NSW Institute of Technology, Gore Hill, New South Wales, Australia

J. C. TRONCOSO, Departments of Neurology and Pathology, The Johns Hopkins School of Medicine, Baltimore, Maryland

M. WALSER, Department of Neurology, The Johns Hopkins University School of Medicine, Baltimore, Maryland

R. A. WESTERMAN, Department of Physiology, Monash University, Clayton, Victoria, Australia

A. M. WILLIAMSON, Department of Industrial Relations, Division of Occupational Health, Lidcombe, New South wales, Australia

R. W. ZIEGENBEIN, Department of Physiology, Monash University, Clayton, Victoria, Australia

I. Experimental Neurobiology

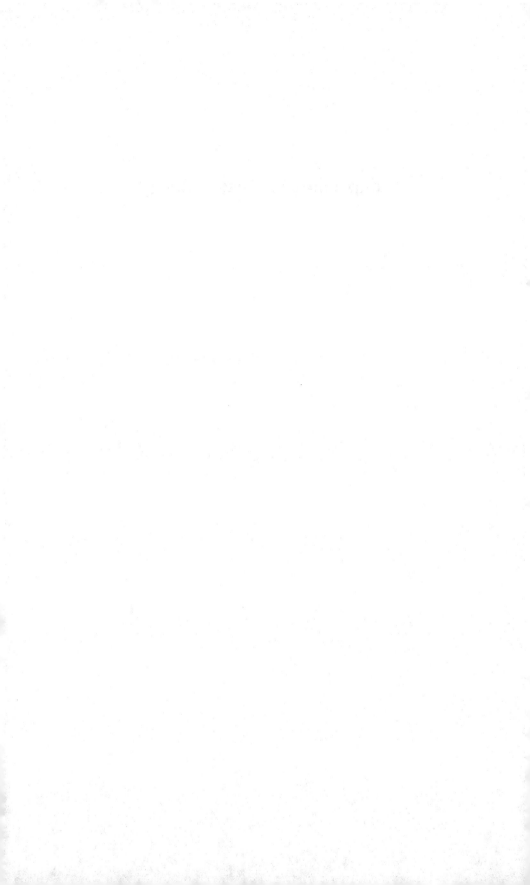

THE REGULATION OF SCHWANN-CELL FUNCTION IN

DEGENERATIVE DISORDERS OF THE NERVOUS SYSTEM

Peter S. Spencer, Richard G. Pellegrino, Stephen M. Ross, Michael J. Politis and Mohammad I. Sabri

Institute of Neurotoxicology, Neuroscience, Neurology and Pathology Departments, Albert Einstein College of Medicine, Bronx, N.Y. 10461.

ABSTRACT

Schwann cells are involved in all types of degenerative disorders of the peripheral nervous system, whether the primary lesion involves demyelination and remyelination, axonal degeneration and regeneration, or neuronal loss. The sequence of cellular changes in PNS disorders has been studied by examining the response of Schwann cells to loss and acquisition of axonal contact during Wallerian degeneration and nerve-fiber regeneration in the distal stumps of transected cat tibial nerves. Myelinating Schwann cells in distal stumps respond to axon degeneration by discarding and/or degrading their myelin sheaths, undergoing mitosis and adopting a quiescent state in which myelin-specific protein synthesis is suppressed. Myelin repair is activated by reassociation with regenerating axons destined to become myelinated: Schwann cells respond by undergoing cell division, expressing myelin-specific protein synthesis and elaborating a myelin sheath within a newly formed tube of basal lamina. The nature of the signalling mechanism from neuron to Schwann cell is unknown, although the interaction of specific ligands on the external surfaces of axon and Schwann cell is an attractive hypothesis. Since generally available methods have been developed to obtain fractions enriched in either the axolemma of myelinated fibers or the plasmalemma of quiescent Schwann cells free of neuronal regulation, the putative interactive properties of these surface membranes can now be explored.

3

SCHWANN-CELL CHANGES IN NEUROTOXIC DISEASES

Schwann cells are involved in all known types of peripheral nervous system degeneration, and myelin breakdown is the most obvious expression of a disturbance in cellular function. Experimental studies with neurotoxic chemicals have revealed a range of neurodegenerative diseases in which the Schwann cell is involved.

Primary Demyelination. Selective loss of myelin with preservation of axons can follow toxic-metabolic disturbances at many levels of cell function. Disruption of nucleic acids (ethidium bromide) or protein synthesis (diphtheria toxin) precipitates primary demyelination, with degeneration of affected myelinating cells (Pleasure et al., 1973; Yajima and Suzuki, 1979). However, most of the recognized Schwann-cell myelinotoxins (e.g. hexachlorophene, acetyl ethyl tetramethyl tetralin) seem to disrupt the integrity of the myelin sheath by mechanisms that do not impair the integrity of the Schwann-cell perikaryon. Fluid accumulation between myelin lamellae, the hallmark of these conditions, causes the myelin sheath to be transformed into a series of myelin blisters. This may reverse (Webster et al., 1974) or lead to phagocytosis and removal of altered myelin by cells of hematogenous origin (Spencer et al., 1979). Removal of myelin stimulates the appearance of large numbers of Schwann cells, some of which repopulate the denuded axon and elaborate shortened internodes of thin myelin (remyelination). The clinical consequences of exposure to a peripheral demyelinating agent, such as diphtheria toxin, consist of localized nerve dysfunction at the site of infection (pharyngeal neuropathy), with subsequent involvement of other cranial nerves and, many weeks after infection, a generalized sensory-motor neuropathy. The onset of weakness and sensory loss in affected nerves presumably correlates with the appearance of demyelination, while the rapid and usually complete recovery is a consequence of functionally effective remyelination (Schaumburg et al., 1983). Schwann cells may also participate in the remyelination of axons in the central nervous system following toxin-induced (e.g. ethidium bromide, sodium dichloroacetate, see Fig. 1) and other types of demyelination (Blakemore, 1982; Spencer and Bischoff, 1982).

Secondary Demyelination. Since Schwann cells appear to require an intact axon for the elaboration of a myelin sheath, neurotoxic agents that induce neuronal abnormalities also indirectly cause loss of myelin and concomitant changes in Schwann-cell structure and function. For example, demyelination and remyelination of paranodes or entire internodes commonly accompanies the focal axon swellings that herald the

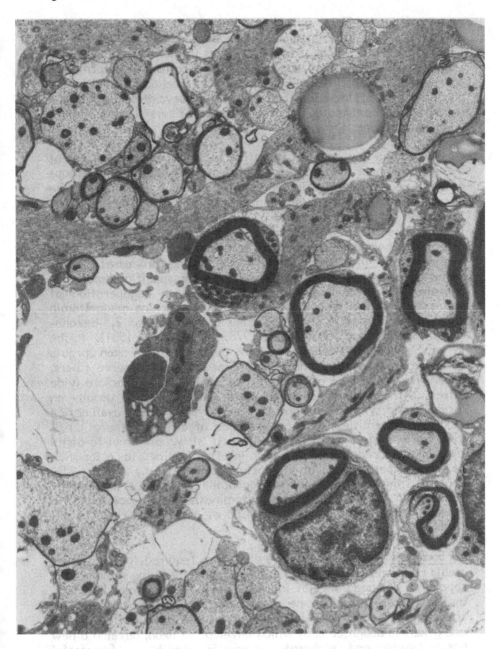

Figure 1. Remyelination of intrinsic CNS axons by Schwann cells that have invaded an area of spinal cord of a rat treated chronically with sodium dichloroacetate. X6,000.

onset of nerve-fiber pathology induced by agents such as acrylamide or 2,5-hexanedione (Spencer and Schaumburg, 1978). Chronic axonal swellings, found in animals treated with beta, beta'-iminodipropionitrile, can lead after many months to the formation of myelin bubbles, demyelination and remyelination, with the processes of proliferated Schwann cells devoid of axons and arranged concentrically around affected fibers ("onion bulb") (Griffin and Price, 1980).

<u>Axonal and Neuronal Degeneration.</u>   Schwann cells free of axons also appear as a consequence of axon degeneration. Groups of cells become aligned in longitudinal columns delimited by the basal lamina that surrounded the original nerve fiber.   The formation of these columns is a complex sequence of events that includes axon degeneration, removal of myelin debris, division of affected Schwann cells, and the adoption by daughter cells of a bipolar state with longitudinally overlapping processes.   This sequence of cellular changes is seen as a non-specific response in neurotoxic and other diseases associated with degeneration of nerve cell bodies (e.g. doxorubicin or pyridoxine-megavitamin sensory neuronopathy) or distal axons (acrylamide or 2,5-hexanedione) (Spencer and Schaumburg, 1978; Krinke et al., 1981). In the latter, Schwann-cell columns become associated with axon sprouts and form regenerating unmyelinated or myelinated nerve fibers, depending on the type of axon with which the cells associate (vide infra).   The clinical course of distal axonopathies is usually an insidious and symmetrical onset of sensory and motor dysfunction in distal extremities (as a consequence of distal degeneration of long peripheral axons), followed by a slow, proximal-to-distal recovery of strength and sensation in affected limbs (as a function of nerve-fiber regeneration) (Schaumburg et al., 1983).   By contrast, the experimental neuronopathy syndromes induced by doxorubicin or pyridoxine megavitaminosis are associated with sensory ataxia without weakness (Cho et al., 1979; Krinke et al., 1981).

<u>Summary.</u> Schwann cells are therefore required to sever their stable relationship with axons and to participate in the removal and repair of damaged myelin in many neurodegenerative disorders, including those caused by neurotoxic agents.   These pathological situations require that Schwann cells dispose of unwanted myelin and generate daughter cells which envelop the axon, develop a new basal lamina and elaborate a myelin sheath.   Successful completion of this sequence of events is required for the restoration of nerve conduction and recovery of normal neurological function.

The following account briefly covers recent progress in defining the mechanisms which regulate Schwann-cell behavior in neurodegenerative lesions. This updates earlier reviews (Weinberg and Spencer, 1978; Spencer, 1979; Spencer et al., 1981) and focuses on the responses of Schwann cells during axon degeneration and regeneration of adult cat tibial nerves.

AXON-SCHWANN CELL INTERDEPENDENCY DURING WALLERIAN DEGENERATION

Transecting or focally crushing a peripheral nerve initiates a sequence of cellular events distal to the lesion known as Wallerian degeneration. This subject has been reviewed extensively elsewhere (e.g. Allt, 1976) and only new data are presented here. The essential cellular changes in Wallerian degeneration appear indistinguishable from those that accompany nerve-fiber degeneration in toxic-metabolic states, and it is generally accepted that the stereotyped responses of Schwann cells in both situations are stimulated by loss of integrity and eventual breakdown of the axon. These Schwann-cell responses to axon loss are most readily studied in distal stumps of transected nerves because (unlike the situation in most toxic neurodegenerative diseases) all nerve fibers are simultaneously affected by processes that lead to complete degeneration. Nevertheless, an understanding of cellular interdependencies in Wallerian degeneration is likely to apply to all neurotoxic and other degenerative diseases characterized by severance of contact between axon and Schwann cell.

The Stimulus for Schwann-Cell Mitosis

Focal nerve injury induces a marked increase in the distal cell population, resulting mostly from the proliferation of Schwann cells associated with myelinated fibers (Abercrombie and Johnson, 1946; Abercrombie et al., 1959; Joseph, 1947, 1948, 1950; Thomas, 1948). After long periods of denervation, there is an attenuation of denervated Schwann-cell columns and the number of Schwann cells declines (Abercrombie and Johnson, 1946; Weinberg and Spencer, 1978). The factors controlling the initial increase and later decline in numbers of Schwann cells are unknown. Abercrombie and Johnson (1946) postulated a chemical stimulus for cell division prompted by nerve-fiber breakdown, and Salzer and Bunge (1980) have advanced the opinion that myelin breakdown, or turnover of myelin or of Schwann cell membranes, is the mitotic stimulus during Wallerian degeneration. However, these ideas are difficult to reconcile with evidence that cells also proliferate in

unmyelinated   nerves   undergoing   Wallerian   degeneration
(Abercrombie et al., 1959; Weinberg and Spencer, 1976).

These considerations stimulated a reexamination of the time-
course of Schwann-cell division during Wallerian degeneration of
myelinated nerves (Pellegrino et al., 1981a).   Cat tibial-nerve
distal stumps were used for this purpose. The uptake of tritiated
thymidine into distal stumps rose sevenfold above values for
normal nerves at 3 days post-transection and, by 4 days, had
increased approximately 40 times over baseline levels. By day 5,
incorporation had dropped sharply and was only 3-4-fold greater
than the uptake by normal nerves.   This value remained approximately constant for at least another 6 days. The monophasic peak
of cell division occurred simultaneously at 4 equal segments over
an 8-cm length of distal stump.   These findings are in general
agreement with previous studies of thymidine uptake during
Wallerian degeneration, although the peak of thymidine incorporation into murine sciatic nerve occurs at 3 days post-transection
(Bradley and Asbury, 1970; Weinberg and Spencer 1976).   Light-
microscope autoradiograms of cat tibial-nerve distal stumps at the
peak of thymidine incorporation demonstrated nuclear labeling
principally of Schwann cells and of relatively few endothelial cells
and endoneurial fibroblasts.   The peak of Schwann-cell division in
distal stumps of cat tibial nerves therefore occurs 4 days post-
transection.

Subsequent studies employed the mitotic inhibitor, Mitomycin
C, to inhibit Schwann-cell mitosis (Hall and Gregson, 1977).   The
drug was injected intraneurally (30-40 ul, 400 mg/ml) into cat
tibial-nerve distal stumps immediately following nerve transection,
and the temporal pattern of radiolabeled thymidine incorporation
was followed as before. Incorporation into Mitomycin-treated vs. -
untreated desheathed nerve stumps was reduced by 47%-73% (mean
-60%) at 4 days post-transection   and increased approximately
four-fold at 16 days.   The shape of the curve suggested that cell
division was taking place at much reduced levels over longer
periods of time.   This agrees favorably with the 60-90% (mean -
70%) reduction in thymidine incorporation in mouse sciatic nerves
treated with Mitomycin C (Hall and Gregson, 1975).

Morphological studies of tibial-nerve distal stumps revealed
similarities and differences between Mitomycin C-treated   and
untreated controls. Most nerves were largely normal at three days
post-transection, although a small number of myelinated fibers
displayed floccular axoplasm within an intact axolemma, and
others showed collapse of the myelin sheath into the axon compart-
ment. Formation of myelin ovoids was first evident in some fibers
at   4   days   post-transection,   with   similar   numbers   of

fibers showing this change in Mitomycin C-treated and -untreated nerves. Many nerve fibers in chemically-untreated nerves displayed large areas of Schwann-cell cytoplasm containing vacuolated mitochondria and myelin debris. Such fibers were rarely encountered in nerve stumps treated with Mitomycin C, suggesting that their appearance was associated with mitosis. By 16 days, uninjected nerves displayed a striking lack of myelin debris and many Schwann-cell columns surrounded by scalloped basal laminae. In contrast, nerves treated with Mitomycin C contained numerous collapsed myelin sheaths and a few Schwann cells containing myelin debris. When endoneurial tissue was dissolved in sodium dodecyl sulfate and electrophoresed on polyacrylamide gels (SDS-PAGE), a band of Coomassie blue-stained material comigrant with P_0, the major myelin glycoprotein, was found in nerves treated with Mitomycin C but was absent in chemically untreated nerves. In summary, the removal of degenerating myelin (including the P_0 component) was substantially delayed in distal stumps treated with the mitotic inhibitor.

These data challenge the suggestion that myelin debris is the stimulus for Schwann-cell mitosis during Wallerian degeneration for the following reasons. First, the peak of Schwann-cell division, which occurred in fibers of all diameters at 4 days, failed to correlate with the onset of ovoid formation in the large majority of fibers. Donat and Wisniewski (1973) have shown that nodal widening in denervated cat sciatic nerve (which takes place prior to ovoid formation; Lubińska, 1977) occurred progressively over 3-5 days. Furthermore, ovoid formation occurs first in smaller fibers and then progresses over a period of days to involve larger fibers (Lubińska, 1977). Second, there was no suggestion of a temporal, proximal-distal spread of mitosis that would correlate with the progressive, anterograde appearance of myelin ovoids during Wallerian degeneration (in the rat, the time between onset of ovoid formation in the smallest fibers in proximal segments and largest fibers in distal segments may span 2-3 days; Lubinska, 1977). Third, since the catabolism of myelin and of P_0 appear to be dependent on mitosis, it is unlikely that myelin degradation is the stimulus for mitosis. In our opinion, the synchronous wave of Schwann-cell division that invades the distal stump is more readily explained by turnover of a neuronal membrane component that is normally maintained by fast transport. Progressive loss of this component (which could interact with the Schwann-cell plasma membrane) may signal the Schwann cell to divide. The 4-day lag between loss of axonal transport and Schwann-cell division may reflect the half life of this component.

These ideas are consistent with the hypothesis that a mitogenic factor present on neuronal membranes stimulates apposed Schwann cells to divide during acquisition of axonal contact in vitro and in vivo (Wood and Bunge, 1975; Salzer et al., 1980; Pellegrino et al., 1980).

Loss of Functional Axolemma

Another series of studies with cat tibial-nerve distal stumps suggests that clearance of nodal axolemma from degenerating myelinated fibers is dependent upon Schwann-cell mitosis (Pellegrino et al., 1982). These investigations measured the binding of tritiated saxitoxin (STX), a marker of voltage-sensitive sodium channels which are predominantly located at nodes of Ranvier (Ritchie and Rogart, 1977), during the period of Wallerian degeneration and in the presence and absence of Mitomycin C. Saturable STX binding to chemically-untreated distal stumps three days post-transection was similar to values obtained from normal nerves. One day later, there was a precipitous loss of STX binding to approximately 20% of control values, and similar low levels were found for a further 7 weeks. This correlates with the loss of electrical conduction in degenerating myelinated fibers at 4-5 days post-transection (Erlanger and Schoepfle, 1946; Landau, 1953). Distal stumps injected with Mitomycin C immediately following nerve transection displayed approximately 80% of control STX binding at 5 days post-transection. By 16 days, STX binding to nerve stumps was similar to saline-injected controls. The blockade of mitosis induced by this drug therefore substantially delayed the loss of STX binding and possibly extended the time during which nerve fibers remained electrically excitable. The clearance of STX-binding sites from distal stumps therefore appears to be promoted by Schwann-cell mitosis.

Fate of Myelin-Protein Synthesis

The relationship between mitosis of Schwann cells and their metabolic status with respect to myelin-protein sythesis also has been examined. Previous studies have shown a temporally progressive loss of myelin-specific proteins during Wallerian degeneration (McDermott and Wisniewski, 1977), suggesting that Schwann cells lose their capacity to synthesize myelin proteins when deprived of axolemmal contact. Since many cells require a mitotic event to undergo dedifferentiation, was it possible that loss of myelin-protein synthesis occurred as a consequence of cell division?

This question was investigated by incubating desheathed cat tibial-nerve distal stumps with tritiated tryptophan, subjecting the tissue to SDS-PAGE, and counting radioactivity comigrant with P_0

after immunoprecipitation with antisera specific for this major myelin glycoprotein. Tritium incorporation into P_0 was variable at 3 days post-transection, had declined by 5 days and, by 7 days, accounted for less than one percent of total gel radioactivity. Synthesis of P_0 was undetectable at 70 days post-transection. Distal stumps treated with Mitomycin C at the time of transection showed no significant differences in the incorporation of ^{3}H-tryptophan into P_0 at 7 and 16 days post-transection, and P_0 synthesis appeared unaffected by Mitomycin C in unoperated nerves injected with the drug seven days earlier. Incorporation of ^{3}H-tryptophan into total protein of desheathed distal stumps was increased sevenfold over normal nerves at 3 and 16 days, with a peak value of 18X normal values at 5 days; similar values were obtained for nerve stumps treated with Mitomycin C (Pellegrino et al., 1981b). In summary, these data demonstrate that Mitomycin C does not significantly depress protein synthesis in distal stumps, nor does it delay the loss of P_0 synthesis that accompanies Wallerian degeneration. This suggests that the suppression of myelin-specific protein synthesis is unrelated to Schwann-cell mitosis and that another explanation (axonal factors?) must be sought to account for this phenomenon.

AXON-SCHWANN CELL INTERDEPENDENCY DURING NERVE-FIBER REGENERATION

The importance of axonal factors in the regulation of Schwann-cell function during regeneration has been well established (Aguayo et al., 1976a, b; Salzer et al., 1980; Weinberg and Spencer, 1975, 1976; Wood and Bunge, 1975). Studies in vivo have demonstrated that axons regenerating from a predominantly myelinated nerve into the distal stump of an unmyelinated nerve stimulate the indigenous population of Schwann cells in the latter to elaborate myelin sheaths around the foreign axons (Aguayo et al., 1976a, b; Weinberg and Spencer, 1975, 1976). The neuron and its axon therefore appear to regulate the presence or absence of myelin formation by Schwann cells (Spencer, 1979). In addition, studies conducted with neural elements grown in culture have shown that growing axons induce thymidine incorporation by Schwann cells when the two cellular elements approximate each other (Wood and Bunge, 1975). Moreover, Schwann cells in vitro can be stimulated to undergo mitosis by treatment with a neuritic membrane fraction. The mitogenic signal in the axolemma is inactivated by pretreatment with trypsin (Salzer et al., 1980; DeVries et al., 1982). In summary, these data suggest that regenerating neurons regulate Schwann-cell mitosis in vitro and myelinogenesis in vivo. Our recent experiments have sought to determine whether Schwann-cell mitosis occurs during axon regeneration in vivo and the

relationship between this event and onset and progress of myelinogenesis.

Addressing these questions required the development of a new
model of regeneration in which the temporal sequence of cellular
events during regeneration could be separated spatially to
facilitate their correlated morphological and biochemical analysis.
The model was established by a two-stage surgical manipulation of
cat tibial and peroneal nerves.   Initially, the tibial nerve was
transected to stimulate loss of axons and myelin from the distal
stump and the proliferation of Schwann cells (vide supra).   After
several weeks, Schwann cells in the fully denervated distal stump
were challenged with regenerating axons by coapting the tibial-
nerve distal stump to the proximal stump of a freshly transected,
neighboring peroneal nerve.   Three weeks later, the temporal
sequence of regenerative events associated with axon-Schwann cell
contact and myelinogenesis was separated reproducibly in a
proximal-distal gradient divisible into three well-defined regions:
(a) a proximalmost, myelinated zone, containing Schwann cells
elaborating myelin lamellae around small, regenerating axons; (b)
an intermediate, relatively immature, contact zone, exhibiting
Schwann cells enveloping axons prior to the formation of the first
myelin lamella, and (c) a distal, non-contact zone, where axons had
yet to advance and Schwann cells appeared dormant.   Precise
identification of the border between the contact and non-contact
zones was defined by the distal limit of movement of a
radiolabeled amino acid incorporated into the fast-transport
system of the regenerating axons.   The myelinated and contact
zones were defined respectively by the presence and absence of
myelin lamellae upon electron-microscope examination (Politis and
Spencer, 1981). Thus, with this new model of regeneration, it was
possible simultaneously to study tissue from each of the three
zones and thereby investigate the temporal sequence of events
during peripheral nerve regeneration.

Do Schwann Cells Divide During Regeneration In Vivo?

Analysis of the distribution of radioactivity along the reinnervated
tibial-nerve distal stump following incubation in tritiated
thymidine demonstrated marked differences between the three
zones defined above.   Thymidine incorporation into the non-
contact zone was similar to values obtained for uptake into control
denervated stumps; both of these values were somewhat higher
than those obtained for normal nerves.   In the regenerated stump,
thymidine incorporation first rose significantly above baseline
levels at the axon front in the contact zone, suggesting that
Schwann cells divide when in the proximity of the growing tips of

regenerating axons. Although a requirement for membrane-membrane contact cannot be established with this model, a diffusible mitogen active over millimeter distances can be ruled out since thymidine uptake did not rise distal to the axon front (Pellegrino et al., 1980). These data are therefore consistent with the tissue-culture studies of Salzer et al. (1980) demonstrating that regenerating axons stimulate Schwann-cell mitosis by close apposition.

Subsequent experiments utilized Mitomycin C to determine the role of Schwann-cell mitosis in the process of nerve-fiber regeneration. Injection of the mitotic inhibitor into the proximal limit of the denervated tibial-nerve distal stump (immediately prior to coaptation to the peroneal-nerve proximal stump) resulted in major changes in the pattern of reinnervation examined three weeks later. The position of the axon front in the reinnervated tibial nerve was found to be very variable, and the proximalmost zone that is normally myelinated showed little or no myelin. Although these results are difficult to interpret, they raise the possibility that axon regeneration is facilitated by Schwann-cell mitosis. Evidence from other studies suggests that a soluble molecule secreted from denervated stumps attracts and guides regenerating axons across gaps between nerves (Lundborg and Hansson, 1981; Politis et al., 1982a), but the role of such factors in the above experiment have not been assessed. In addition, further studies with Mitomycin C are needed to establish whether Schwann-cell mitosis during nerve regeneration is a prerequisite for myelin formation as has been suggested in other studies (Mukherjee et al., 1980).

Myelinogenesis and Myelin Formation During Regeneration

The cat tibial-nerve model of regeneration also proved useful in determining the sequence of events associated with the formation of myelin around regenerating peripheral axons. Several questions were examined: (a) When do Schwann cells in reinnervated stumps begin to synthesize myelin-specific proteins? (b) Do regenerating axons initiate changes in myelin-specific protein synthesis? (c) Can the synthesis of myelin proteins be detected prior to the elaboration of myelin lamellae? (d) In what sequence are specific myelin proteins synthesized?

These questions were addressed by conducting correlated bio-chemical, ultrastructural and light-microscope immunohisto-chemical studies of reinnervated tibial-nerve distal stumps (Politis et al., 1982b). Immunohistochemical studies utilized sections stained by the unlabeled antibody-enzyme (peroxidase-antiperoxidase) method for the localization of myelin antigens

(Sternberger et al., 1979). Examination of cross sections of the reinnervated tibial-nerve distal stump demonstrated the presence of specific staining of myelin sheaths in the myelinated zone, and an absence of detectable staining of nerve fibers in the contact and non-contact zone. Protein synthesis was assessed by incubating desheathed nerves in tritiated amino acids or fucose, subjecting the tissue to SDS-PAGE, and measuring radioactivity comigrant with myelin-specific proteins and immunoprecipitated by antisera raised against these myelin proteins. These studies demonstrated that the axon-free non-contact zone was indistinguishable from age-matched distal stumps in that there was no detectable myelin-specific proteins. Radioactive peaks corresponding to synthesis of P_0, P_1 and P_2 first appeared in the axon-Schwann cell contact zone indicating that proximity of axons to Schwann cells had stimulated myelin-protein synthesis and that the amount of each myelin-specific protein was insufficient to be detected immunohisto-chemically. Further examination of the proximal and distal portions of the contact zone demonstrated prominent synthesis of myelin basic proteins before the synthesis of P_0 had become optimal. This could represent either a longer latency for expression of P_0 synthesis (with the program for all myelin-specific protein synthesis being initiated at the same time) or temporal differences in the stimulation of their synthesis. Whatever the explanation, these data provide clear evidence of the sensitivity of this radiolabel-incorporation technique in dissecting the metabolic state of Schwann cells with respect to myelinogenesis. To our knowledge, this is the first demonstration of myelin-specific protein synthesis by Schwann cells that have yet to elaborate myelin lamellae. In summary, these data confirm earlier studies demonstrating the neuronal regulation of myelinogenesis. The absence of detectable synthesis of myelin proteins in regions free of axons demonstrates that Schwann cells are not signalled by axons to commence myelinogenesis by diffusible factors active over millimeter distances. These data would therefore favor the hypothesis that axons stimulate Schwann cells to commence myelinogenesis by cell-to-cell apposition, the stimulus being mediated perhaps by the interaction of specific ligands on apposed plasmalemmae of the two cells (Weinberg and Spencer, 1978).

The Surface Membrane of the Schwann Cell

The preceding studies firmly establish that cells resident in denervated distal nerve stumps are viable, dedifferentiated Schwann cells. Following nerve transection, Schwann cells in the distal stump appear to shut down myelin-specific protein synthesis, undergo cell division and align themselves in longitudinal columns in a quiescent state. They are maintained in this condition for long periods of time, although the columns gradually atrophy and Schwann cells eventually disappear (Weinberg and Spencer, 1978). However, if these dedifferentiated intratubal cells are challenged by axon sprouts from regenerating myelinated fibers, they undergo cell division, establish a unitary relationship with axons, develop a new basal lamina, commence myelin-specific protein synthesis and elaborate myelin lamellae. Dedifferentiated intratubal cells in distal stumps therefore represent a quiescent population of Schwann cells that are unregulated by neurons. They provide an opportunity to study surface receptors that may interact with axolemmal ligands in the initiation and control of mitosis and myelinogenesis. As a first step toward the realization of this goal, quiescent Schwann cells have been used to isolate and characterize a plasmalemmal fraction (Ross et al., 1982a, b, 1983).

The cat sciatic-nerve distal stump represents an almost ideal starting preparation for the isolation of Schwann-cell plasma-lemmae: Eight to ten weeks of sustained denervation leaves the nerve free of both axons and of intact myelin; systemic perfusion with isotonic saline prior to nerve excision removes all blood cells, and the connective-tissue sheath (epineurium plus perineurium) can be discarded after plucking out the tissue from individual fascicles (Brown et al., 1976). The cellular portion of the remaining intrafascicular tissue comprises approximately 90% Schwann cells and 10% endoneurial fibroblasts, endothelial cells and pericytes (Spencer et al., 1979; Ross et al., 1982a, b, 1983). Measurement of the length of plasmalemma on electron micrographs of cross sections of intrafascicular tissue demonstrate that Schwann cells contribute 90% of the total (Ross et al., 1982a, b, 1983). The starting tissue is therefore highly enriched in Schwann cells and their plasmalemmae.

Fractions enriched in plasma membranes (Fig. 2) have been prepared by mincing the intrafascicular tissue and homogenizing in sucrose. The crude homogenate is centrifuged to remove nuclei, unbroken cells and connective tissue. Pellets containing cell membranes are subjected to two osmotic shocks and layered over two discontinuous sucrose gradients. Biochemical and morpho-logical studies of the resulting fractions indicates that plasmalemmae are most enriched in material floating above the 0.85M sucrose phase. Ultrastructural examination of this fraction reveals an homogenous population of vesicular structures with single unit membranes, remarkably free of contaminating organelles and with no evidence of myelin debris. The fraction is enriched over the crude tissue homogenate 4.8-fold in the plasma-lemmal enzyme marker 5'-nucleotidase, 5.7-fold in specific ^{3}H-ouabain binding, and 3-fold in 2',3'-cyclic nucleotide 3'-phospho-hydrolase, a suggested marker for (human) Schwann cells (Reddy et

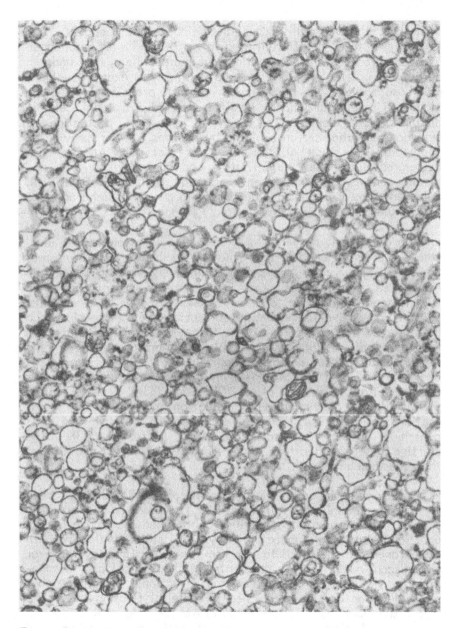

Figure 2. Typical field of homogenous unilaminar vesicles enriched in Schwann-cell plasmalemmae collected above 0.85M sucrose phase after two osmotic shocks and two discontinuous sucrose gradients. X26,600.

al., 1982).   In addition, the fraction is substantially low in the negative membrane markers succinic dehydrogenase, lactate dehydrogenase and glucose-6-phosphatase (9%, 13% and 15% of control values, respectively) (Ross et al., 1982a, b, 1983).

In summary, the intrafascicular contents of cat sciatic nerves denervated for 8-10 weeks have been used to isolate a fraction enriched in the plasmalemma of quiescent Schwann cells. Future studies will employ these fractions to analyze the molecular basis for axon-Schwann cell interactions and the mechanisms by which surface contact with axons can regulate Schwann-cell behavior.

Relevance to Neurodegenerative Diseases of Man

The experiments discussed in this chapter impact on all neurodegenerative diseases in which Schwann cells are involved. Although our studies have been restricted to highly controlled models of nerve degeneration and regeneration, it is likely that the principles governing Schwann-cell behavior gleaned from these studies apply to all conditions associated with loss of peripheral myelin. The challenge now is to learn how to use these principles to manipulate Schwann cells so that they can be utilized to promote nerve-fiber repair and recovery from human degenerative diseases. The ability of Schwann cells to remyelinate both central and peripheral axons broadens this therapeutic challenge to include CNS as well as PNS disorders of myelin.

ACKNOWLEDGEMENT

These studies were supported by NIH grant #13106.

REFERENCES

Abercrombie, M., and Johnson, M.L. (1946). J. Anat. 80, 37.
Abercrombie, M., Evans, D.H.L., and Murray, J.G. (1959). J. Anat. 93, 9.
Aguayo, A.J., Charron, L., and Bray, G.M. (1976a). J. Neurocytol. 5, 565.
Aguayo, A.J., Epps, J., Charron, L., and Bray, G.M. (1976b). Brain Res. 104, 120.
Allt, G. (1976). In "The Peripheral Nerve" (D.N. Landon, ed.), p. 666. Chapman and Hall, London.
Blakemore, W.F. (1982). Neuropathol. Appl. Neurobiol. 8, 365.
Bradley, W.G., and Asbury, A.K. (1970). Exp. Neurol. 26, 275.

Brown, M.J, Pleasure, D.E., and Asbury (1976). J. Neurol. Sci. 29, 361.

Cho, E.-S., Jortner, B.S., Schaumburg, H.H., and Spencer, P.S. (1979). Neurotoxicology 1, 583.

DeVries, G.H., Salzer, J.L., and Bunge, R.P. (1982). Dev. Br. Res. 3, 295.

Donat, J.R., and Wiśniewski, H.M. (1973). Br. Res. 53, 41.

Erlanger, and Schoepfle (1946). Am. J. Physiol. 147, 550.

Griffin, J.W., and Price, D.L. (1980). In "Experimental and Clinical Neurotoxicology" (P.S. Spencer, and H.H. Schaumburg, eds.), p. 161. Williams and Wilkins, Baltimore.

Hall, S.M., and Gregson, N.A. (1975). Neuropath. Appl. Neurobiol. 1, 149.

Hall, S.M., and Gregson, N.A. (1977). Neuropath. Appl. Neurobiol. 3, 65.

Joseph, J. (1947). J. Anat. 81, 135.

Joseph, J. (1948). J. Anat. 82, 146.

Joseph, J. (1950). Acta Anat. 9, 279.

Krinke, G., Schaumburg, H.H., Spencer, P.S., Suter, Y., Thomann, G., and Hess, R. (1981). Neurotoxicology 2, 13.

Landau, (1953). J. Neurosurg. 10, 64.

Lubińska, L. (1977) Brain Research 130, 47.

Lundborg, G., and Hansson, H.A. (1981). In "Posttraumatic Peripheral Nerve Regeneration" (A. Gorio, H. Millesi, and S. Mingrino, eds.), p. 229. Raven Press, New York.

McDermott, J.R., and Wiśniewski, H.M. (1977). J. Neurol. Sci. 33, 81.

Mukherjee, R., Mahadevon, P.R., and Antia, N.H. (1980). Int. J. Leprosy 48, 189.

Pellegrino, R.G., Politis, M.J., and Spencer, P.S. (1980). J. Cell Biol. 87, 76a.

Pellegrino, R.G., Politis, M.J., Ritchie, J.M., and Spencer, P.S. (1981a). Trans. Amer. Soc. Neurochem. 12, 96.

Pellegrino, R.G., Politis, M.J., and Spencer, P.S. (1981b). J. Cell Biol. 91, 93a.

Pellegrino, R.G., Ritchie, J.M., and Spencer, P.S. (1982). J. Physiol. in press.

Pleasure, D.E., Feldmann, B., and Prockop, D.J. (1973). J. Neurochem. 20, 81.

Politis, M.J., and Spencer, P.S. (1981). J. Neurocytol. 10, 221.

Politis, M.J., Ederle, K., and Spencer, P.S. (1982a). Brain Res. 253, 1.

Politis, M.J., Sternberger, N., Ederle, K., and Spencer, P.S. (1982b). J. Neurosci. 2, 1252.

Reddy, N.B., Askanas, V., and Engel, W.K. (1982). J. Neurochem. 39, 887.

Ross, S.M., Spencer, P.S., and Sabri, M.I. (1982a). Trans. Am. Soc. Neurochem. 13, 267.

Ross, S.M., Sabri, M.I., and Spencer, P.S. (1982b). Neurosci. Abstr. 8, 693.
Ross, S.M., Spencer, P.S., and Sabri, M.I. (1983). J. Neurochem., in press.
Ritchie, J.M., and Rogart, R.B. (1977). Proc. Natl. Acad. Sci. U.S.A. 74, 211.
Salzer, J.L., and Bunge, R.P. (1980). J. Cell Biol. 84, 739.
Salzer, J.L., Bunge, R.P., and Glaser, L. (1980). J. Cell Biol. 84, 767.
Schaumburg, H.H., Spencer, P.S., and Thomas, P.K. (1983). "Disorders of Peripheral Nerves." F.A. Davis, Philadelphia.
Spencer, P.S. (1979). In "Aspects of Developmental Neurobiology" (J.A. Ferrendelli, and G. Gurvitch, eds.), p. 275. Society for Neuroscience, Washington.
Spencer, P.S., and Bischoff, M.C. (1982). J. Neuropathol. Exp. Neurol. 41, 373.
Spencer, P.S., and Schaumburg, H.H. (1978). In "Physiology and Pathobiology of Axons" (S.G. Waxman, ed.), p. 265. Raven Press, New York.
Spencer, P.S., Sterman, A.B., Horoupian, D.S., and Foulds, M.M. (1979). Science 204, 633.
Spencer, P.S., Politis, M.J., Pellegrino, R.G., and Weinberg, H.J. (1981). In "Post-traumatic Peripheral Nerve Regeneration" (A. Gorio, H. Millesi, and S. Mingrino, eds.), p. 441. Raven Press, New York.
Sternberger, N.H., Quarles, R.H., Itoyama, Y., and Webster, H deF. (1979). Proc. Natl. Acad. Sci. 76, 1510.
Thomas, G.A. (1948). J. Anat. 82, 135.
Webster, H deF., Ulsamer, A.G., and O'Connell, M.F. (1974). J. Neuropathol Exp. Neurol. 33, 144.
Weinberg, H., and Spencer, P.S. (1975). J. Neurocytol. 4, 395.
Weinberg, H., and Spencer, P.S. (1976). Brain Research 113, 363.
Weinberg, H., and Spencer, P.S. (1978). J. Neurocytol. 7, 555.
Wood, P.M., and Bunge, R.P. (1975). Nature 256, 662.
Yajima, K., and Suzuki, K. (1979). Lab. Invest. 41, 385.

THE SYMPATHETIC NERVOUS SYSTEM: A NOVEL PERSPECTIVE ON THE CONTROL OF MYELINATING SCHWANN CELLS

J.W. HEATH

The Neuroscience Group, Faculty of Medicine

The University of Newcastle, N.S.W. 2308
Australia.

ABSTRACT

Several unusual phenomena of relevance to research into the control of Schwann cell myelination have recently been documented in sympathetic nerve of normal rats. Firstly, major increases occur in the population of myelinated axons in SCG of ageing male (but not female) rats. This finding may reconcile earlier differing reports on the prevalence of sympathetic myelination. Secondly, in the SCG myelination of many postganglionic sympathetic axons is apparently restricted to regions proximal to their nerve cell bodies. This might imply that the presumed neuronal signal initiating myelination differs even along the same axon, or perhaps a local change in the connective tissue environment at the transitional region. Thirdly, some regions of postganglionic myelinated axons are focally encircled by further myelinating Schwann cells, forming regions termed "double myelination". Though apparently lacking direct axonal contact, the outer Schwann cell and its myelin sheath apparently maintain structural integrity for some period. These observations on sympathetic nerve thus appear to afford novel perspectives and experimental opportunities with regard to possible hormonal influences, axon–Schwann cell communication, and the role of the local endoneurial environment in expression of the myelinating capability of the Schwann cell.

21

INTRODUCTION

Compelling evidence has emerged in recent years for a primary role of the axon in determining Schwann cell behaviour. Extending the earlier work of Simpson and Young (1945), two laboratories independently demonstrated that after cross-anastomosis, axons which had regenerated from a (normally) myelinated nerve trunk into a (normally) *un*-myelinated nerve trunk became myelinated, and that the converse also held (Aguayo *et al.*, 1976; Weinberg and Spencer, 1976). Further evidence suggests that the local endoneurial environment influences, perhaps in secondary fashion, the capability of the Schwann cell to realise its potential for myelination (Bunge and Bunge, 1978). Yet, the mechanisms which underpin these functional associations remain to be elucidated, and the view in the current literature is that further progress will be facilitated by the development of new experimental models (Aguayo *et al.*, 1980; Bunge, 1981; Spencer *et al.*, 1981).

Regarding the sympathetic nervous system, and in particular the postganglionic axons, the earlier literature indicates apparently conflicting views on the prevalence and even the presence of myelination (Langley, 1896; Forssman, 1964; Dunant, 1967). However, recent studies of sympathetic nerve in this author's laboratory have documented several unusual and previously unreported phenomena which appear to afford novel perspectives on the control of Schwann cell behaviour. The aim of this paper is to describe in brief several of these phenomena, in the context of research into the control of myelination in the peripheral nervous system.

METHODS

These studies were based on the superior cervical ganglion (SCG) of Sprague-Dawley rats. Techniques for light and electron microscopy have been previously described (Heath, 1982). Details of age, sex and numbers of animals are provided below, as appropriate.

INCREASED MYELINATION IN AGEING SYMPATHETIC NERVE

Postganglionic myelination of sympathetic nerve has

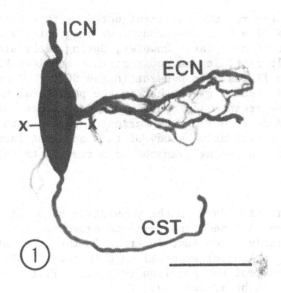

Figure 1. *Whole mount of rat SCG. The external carotid nerve (ECN) and internal carotid nerve (ICN) are post-ganglionic branches, while the cervical sympathetic trunk (CST) carries preganglionic axons to the ganglion. The standard level of section used for initial quantitation of the population of myelinated fibres is indicated by x - x. Bar = 2 mm.*

been reported in cat, rat, mouse, bird and amphibia (Langley, 1896, 1904; Bishop and Heinbecker, 1932; Koster-litz *et al.*, 1964; Dunant, 1967; Honma, 1970; Pick, 1970; Heath and Smith, 1981; Heath, 1982). In these reports the prevalence of myelination varies widely, and apparently not all such variation relates to species differences. For example, the reports by Dunant (1967) and Forssman (1964) were both based on the SCG of the rat. Dunant observed numerous small myelinated fibres (B fibres, both pre- and postganglionic). Forssman, however, found that myelinated fibres were rare, and indeed that the few fibres present were of large diameter, and concluded these were somatic fibres merely traversing the ganglion en route to cervical skeletal musculature.

The presence of substantial numbers of myelinated

fibres in the rat SCG was first noted by this author in
the course of a separate study involving animals aged
approximately one year. However, during later studies on
young adult rats, it was apparent that considerably fewer
myelinated fibres were present in the SCG. This was an
unexpected result, given that in the peripheral nervous
system, the great majority of axons destined to become
myelinated do so during the perinatal period (see Webster,
1975). A quantitative study of this apparent increased
myelination in ageing sympathetic nerve was therefore undertaken.

Quantitative data on the population of myelinated
fibres were obtained from complete cross sections of the
SCG, routinely taken just inferior to the level at which
the (postganglionic) external carotid nerve (ECN) branches
from the body of the ganglion (Fig. 1). Fibres were
counted by light microscopy.

Three age groups were examined (Fig.2). If an extrapolation was to be made from data available for somatic
peripheral nerve, it would be expected that in nerves
known to be myelinated in the adult, substantial myelination would be present following the perinatal period. One
group was therefore examined at 4 weeks of age. The second
group was examined at age 15 weeks, a stage following the
development of sexual maturity. The third group comprised
aged animals, ranging from 35-52 weeks. In the 4 week and
15 week groups, myelinated axons were consistently few in
the standard cross section, though there was a statistically significant difference in means ($p < 0.02$). In the
aged group, however, the mean number of myelinated axons
was greater by more than an order of magnitude ($p < 0.01$
and $p < 0.02$ when compared with the 4 week and 15 week
groups respectively).

In considering these results, three further points are
worthy of note. Firstly, by combinations of pre- and postganglionic lesions it was demonstrated that most of these
fibres arise from nerve cell bodies located within the
SCG itself, and that the contribution of preganglionic or
other myelinated fibres was small by comparison (Heath &
Smith, 1981). From inspection of the sections, most

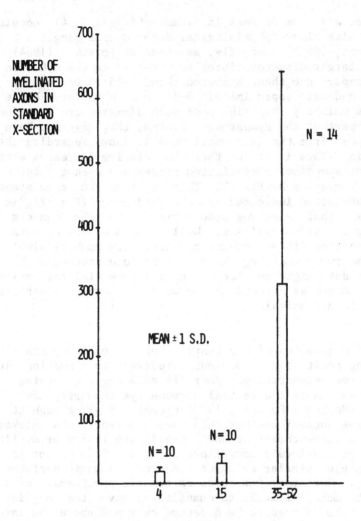

Figure 2. Quantitative analysis of age-related changes in the population of myelinated axons in the rat SCG. Fibre numbers refer to the standard level of section (Fig. 1). The means at 4 weeks, 15 weeks and 35-52 weeks were 18.0 ± 6.8 S.D, 31.5 ± 15.2 S.D. and 313 ± 327.9 S.D. respectively. Statistically significant difference was present between
    (a) 4 week and 15 week samples (p < 0.02)
    (b) 4 week and aged samples   (p < 0.01)
    (c) 15 week and aged samples   (p < 0.02)

fibres are 5 μm or less in diameter (Figs. 3, 4), consistent with electrophysiological data on this ganglion
(Dunant, 1967). Secondly, as noted by Forssman (1964)
some larger diameter fibres are present in the SCG. In
our experience these numbered about 5-15 regardless of
age, and were approximately 8-15 μm in diameter. While
it is unlikely that fibres of such diameter are functionally part of the sympathetic system, they have not been
excluded from the data until more is known regarding their
origin. Thus it may be that the relative increases with
age of *sympathetic* myelinated fibres are even greater
than suggested by Fig. 2. Thirdly, from the large standard deviation indicated for the aged group (Fig. 2), it is
evident that there was wide variation in fibre numbers
among individual animals. While specimens often contained
hundreds of fibres, others contained low numbers similar
to the two younger age groups. One interpretation of
these data might be that there is a potential for myelination in rat sympathetic nerve which, however, is not real-
ised in all animals.

The question of a potential for increased myelination
during adult life is obviously relevant to situations such
as nerve regeneration. There is evidence for ongoing
myelination in the central nervous system during adult
life (Norton & Poduslo, 1973; Giorgi, 1976), though it
remains unclear whether this increase represents thicker
myelin ensheathment around pre-existing fibres or myelination of previously unmyelinated axons. This author is
unaware of similar evidence concerning somatic peripheral
nerve. Certainly increases in somatic peripheral nerve
may be more difficult to quantitate, given that any increase would need to be detected over and above the large
population of myelinated fibres present from the perinatal
period. In the SCG, the mean increase (comparing the aged
group with the 4 week or 15 week groups) is greater than
an order of magnitude, thus facilitating study of factors
regulating age-related changes in myelination.

One experimental approach to this question is indicated
by the further recent finding (Heath and Jurd, 1983) that
there is a sex difference in sympathetic myelination,
myelin being largely absent in females, even in aged

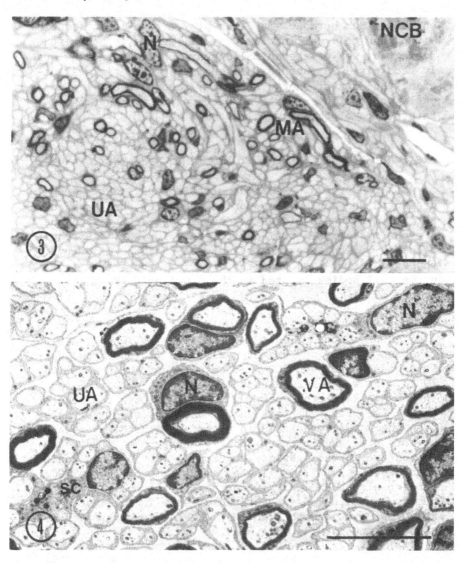

Figures 3, 4. Myelinated (MA) and unmyelinated axons(UA) in rat SCG. N, Schwann cell nucleus.

Figure 3. Light micrograph. NCB, nerve cell body. Bar = 10 μm.
Figure 4. Electronmicrograph. In contrast to the myelinated axons, multiple unmyelinated axons are frequently enclosed within the cytoplasm (SC) of a common Schwann cell. Bar = 5 μm.

animals. Sex hormones may thus play a role in the control
of Schwann cell myelination. At all events, since neither
ageing nor sex of the animal appear to have been previously recognised as factors influencing sympathetic myelination, the data presented above may reconcile earlier apparently conflicting reports on patterns of myelination in
this region of the nervous system.

PROXIMAL MYELINATION OF POSTGANGLIONIC SYMPATHETIC AXONS

In the preceding section of this paper, data were
presented and reviewed supporting the view that large numbers of myelinated fibres may be present in the sympathetic
nervous system of normal adult rats. Further, the results
of nerve lesion experiments indicate that the majority of
these fibres are postganglionic; i.e. they arise from
nerve cell bodies located in the SCG itself (Heath &
Smith, 1981).

An unexpected result emerged, however, when quantitative analyses of numbers of myelinated fibres in the various branches of the SCG were carried out (Heath & Smith,
1981). It was observed that whatever the number of fibres
in the standard cross-sectional level through the body of
a ganglion (Fig. 1), this number was consistently greater
than the *total* detectable in cross sections of all branch-
es(both pre- and postganglionic). Subsequent studies revealed two further aspects concerning the postganglionic
branches; firstly, myelinated axons arising in the SCG
project almost exclusively in the ECN. Secondly, while
numerous myelinated fibres were present in the most proximal cross-sections through the ECN, few were observed more
than 2-3 mm distally (Fig.5).

In considering the interpretation of these data, the
results of earlier nerve lesioning experiments may be recalled: the majority of myelinated axons associated with
the SCG survive various combinations of lesions to the
pre- and postganglionic branches (Heath & Smith, 1981).
Thus the progressive decrease in fibre numbers in the ECN
is unlikely to involve either preganglionic axons losing
myelin ensheathment close to their target cell, or retrograde entry of fibres (from unknown sources) into the gang-

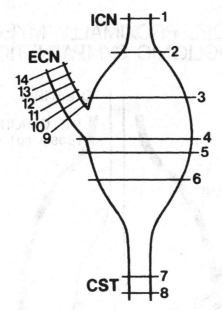

Figure 5. Quantitation of the population of myelinated axons in a single rat SCG (control specimen). In complete cross-sections at the indicated levels, the following numbers of fibres were counted:

(1)	*14*	*(2)*	*20*	*(3)*	*49*	*(4)*	*987*	*(5)*	*713*		
(6)	*445*	*(7)*	*107*	*(8)*	*70*	*(9)*	*878*	*(10)*	*511*		
(11)	*276*	*(12)*	*97*	*(13)*	*93*	*(14)*	*80*				

Fibres are most numerous in the body of the ganglion and in the proximal ECN (levels 9 and 14 were separated by approximately 2.5mm). Refer to Fig. 1 for abbreviations.

lion via the ECN. Rather, the interpretation favoured by this author is that in the rat SCG, only the proximal region of postganglionic axons is myelinated. This model is illustrated diagrammatically in Fig. 6.

A morphological correlate has been sought for this hypothesis of proximal myelination. Using tissue oriented in longitudinal section, transition in Schwann cell ensheathment from the myelinated to unmyelinated state was observed along the course of individual axons, both in the proximal ECN and in the body of the ganglion (Figs. 7, 8). At these regions, myelin ensheathment terminated

THE MODEL: PROXIMALLY MYELINATED POSTGANGLIONIC SYMPATHETIC AXONS

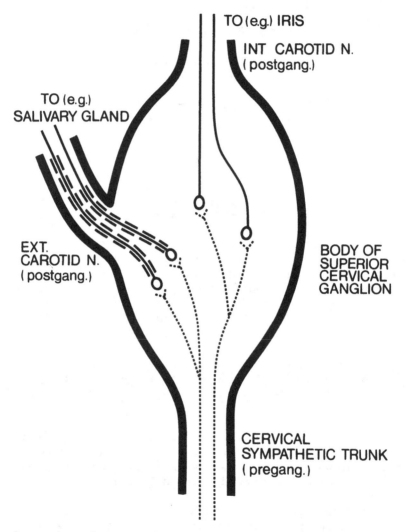

Figure 6. Diagrammatic summary of the proximal myelination model. Dotted lines = preganglionic axons (usually unmyelinated). Solid lines = postganglionic axons; many of those projecting in the ECN are myelinated, but only along regions proximal to the nerve cell body.

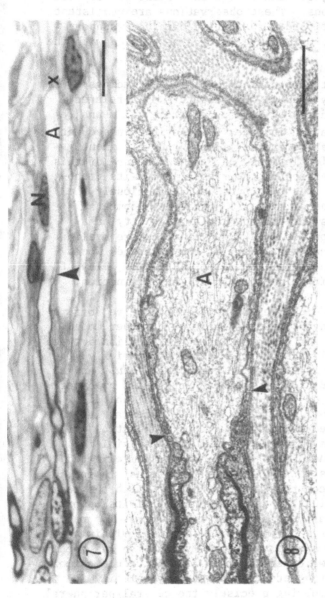

Figure 7. Light micrograph of apparent transition from the myelinated to unmyelinated state on an axon in rat SCG. The myelin sheath ends as a "hemi-node" (arrow). The axon (A) continues to the right, closely associated with a Schwann cell nucleus (N) but unmyelinated, and passes out of the plane of section at "x". Bar = 10 µm.

Figure 8. Electron micrograph of an apparent transitional region. A myelin "hemi-node" is present at left. The axon continues to the right, ensheathed by a non-myelinating Schwann cell. The small arrows indicate the region of apposition of the two contributing Schwann cells. Bar = 1 µm.

abruptly but in highly ordered fashion as a "heminode".
Immediately distal, Schwann cell ensheathment was typical
of unmyelinated axons. These observations are consistent
with the above-mentioned quantitative data, and support
the hypothesis of proximal myelination associated with the
rat SCG.

What might be the significance of these findings? One
approach frequently used to investigate myelin-related
problems is to produce, by various experimental means, a
region of demyelination in order to study the subsequent
events of remyelination in the affected nerve segment.
While providing valuable insights, the dependence of this
approach on an experimental intervention with its pathological sequelae raises the question of how closely the
regenerative response mimics the normal developmental
process. With this background, the availability of a
proximal myelination model (i.e. axons which are myelinated proximally but continue distally unmyelinated) would
appear to afford new experimental possibilities relevant
to questions of initiation and control of myelination.

The present model, based on sympathetic nerve, offers
a combination of advantages available in no other model
thus far developed for research into communication between
axons, Schwann cells and their environment. Briefly, the
region of interest is present in the *normal, adult* animal,
eliminating the additional variables introduced by experimental pathologies or dependence on perinatal animals.
Proximal myelination itself provides the important advantage of a myelinated region as an "internal control" (i.e.
the proximal region has demonstrated its potential for
myelination, yet the distal region remains unmyelinated).
Apparent *temporal stability* at the transitional region in
the present model contrasts with others in which the rapid
occurrence of myelination or remyelination limits opportunity for experimental modulation of the system. The region
of interest is *accessible,* and *well-localised* within the
peripheral nervous system. Partial myelination has been
reported at only two other sites in a normal adult animal;
the dorsal spinal rootlets of the cat, a physically in-
accessible site involving precisely the central/peripheral
transition (Carlstedt, 1977), and the vagus nerve of the
cat, where the transitions are by comparison poorly localised over a 6 cm length of the nerve trunk (Du Claux *et al.,*

1976). Finally, a significant *number* of fibres is available in the model. Presently, a fuller characterisation
of this model is being undertaken.

DOUBLE MYELINATION OF AXONS IN SYMPATHETIC NERVE

In addition to proximal myelination, a further phenomenon termed "double myelination" (Heath, 1982) has been
described in rat sympathetic nerve. The three-dimension-
al concept of double myelination is illustrated diagrammatically in Fig. 9. Briefly, these configurations com-
prise an apparently normal myelinated fibre focally encircled by an additional myelinating Schwann cell. In
some instances, several such "outer"Schwann cells are
arranged serially along the inner fibre. Serial section-
ing (Heath, 1982) and teased preparations (Fig. 10) indicate that the inner and outer myelin sheaths are the

Doubly Myelinated Axon (SCHEMATIC DIAGRAM)

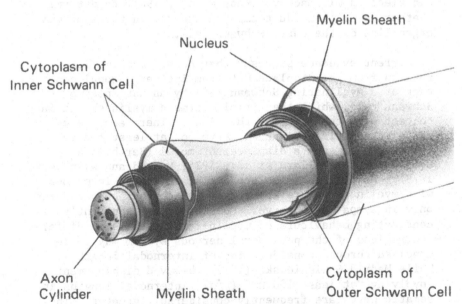

*Figure 9. Diagrammatic summary of double myelination. The
axon and inner (myelinating) Schwann cell are enclosed in
annular fashion by the outer (also myelinating) Schwann
cell. The separate nature of inner and outer Schwann
cells is emphasised by the presence of individual nuclei.*

product of separate Schwann cells. The most striking
feature of double myelination is, however, that the outer
Schwann cell apparently lacks direct axonal contact,
either with the centrally enclosed axon of the complex,
or with any neighbouring axon, since the inner Schwann
cell and endoneurial collagen fibrils intervene (Fig. 11).
Further, the structure of the outer Schwann cell, and in
particular its myelin sheath, appear largely if not completely intact.

Given the evidence for a primary axonal influence on
myelination by Schwann cells, it might have been expected
that the myelin sheath of the outer Schwann cell would
degenerate in the absence of direct axonal contact. The
question of how long the outer sheath may remain intact
is currently being investigated immunocytochemically:
using antisera directed against the specific myelin protein P_o, preliminary data show reaction product localised
both to inner and outer sheaths (Trapp & Heath, unpublished). Further work is in progress using correlated light
and electron microscopy (Trapp et al., 1981) to determine
whether reaction product can be detected in the synthetic
organelles of the outer Schwann cell.

Current evidence suggests that double myelination
results from the displacement from intimate axonal contact of a myelinating Schwann cell by an interposing
Schwann cell, which then itself forms a myelin sheath in
contact with the axon (Heath, 1982). There are prece-
dents in somatic peripheral nerve for at least the initial stages of such a displacement model (Berthold &
Sköglund 1968; Pollard et al., 1975; Madrid and Wiśniewski,
1978). However the displacement of an entire internode,
with myelin structure apparently intact, has been reported
only in sympathetic nerve. Possibly these apparently
contrasting behaviours of myelin-forming cells in different regions of the peripheral nervous system may be re-
conciled through consideration of internodal length.
While Madrid & Wiśniewski (1978) observed displacement
involving "at least 100 μm" (sic), internodal lengths in
somatic nerve are frequently considerably greater. In
contrast, internodal lengths in sympathetic nerve are
often as little as 15-20 μm (Heath, 1982) and thus in
physical terms might more readily be displaced entirely.

The phenomenon of double myelination, and in particular

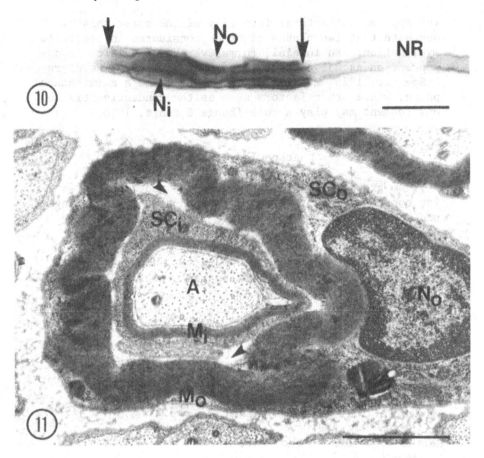

Figure 10. Doubly myelinated axon, teased fibre preparation.
From a node of Ranvier (NR), a myelin internode extends to
the left. Between the arrows, however, a double layer of
myelin is present. The nucleus (N_o) of the outer Schwann
cell is located external to the outer myelin sheath, and
that (N_i) of the inner Schwann cell between the two sheaths.
The infolding of the lateral extremities of the outer
sheath, particularly marked at right, is characteristic of
double myelination (Heath, 1982). Bar = 15 μm.

Figure 11. Electron micrograph of a doubly myelinated axon.
The axon (A) is apparently intact, as are both the inner
(M_i) and outer (M_o) myelin sheaths. Sc_i, inner Schwann
cell cytoplasm; SC_o, outer Schwann cell cytoplasm, N_o,
nucleus of outer Schwann cell. Arrows, endoneurial
collagen fibrils. Bar = 2 μm.

the apparent structural integrity of the outer sheath, suggests that two phases might be considered in regard to myelination: an initial, formative phase, critically dependent on axonal contact (Aguayo *et al.*, 1976; Weinberg & Spencer, 1976; Politis *et al.*, 1982), and a maintenance phase, where other factors such as the connective tissue environment may play a role (Bunge & Bunge, 1978).

Acknowledgements

I am grateful to Drs. Peter Dunkley and John Rostas for constructive criticism of the manuscript, John Single and Cheryl Grant for the artwork in Figures 6 and 9, Bruce Turnbull and Steve McInally for photographic assistance and to Lyndie Barrkman for particular care in typing this manuscript. This work was supported by the National Health and Medical Research Council of Australia and the Utah Foundation of Australia.

REFERENCES

Aguayo, A.J., Bray, G., Perkins, S. and Duncan, I. (1980). *In* "Neurological Mutations Affecting Myelination" (N. Baumann, ed.), p.87. Elsevier, Amsterdam.

Aguayo, A.J., Epps, J., Charron, L. and Bray, G.M. (1976). *Brain Res. 104*, 1.

Berthold, C.-H., and Sköglund, S. (1968). *Acta Soc. med. upsal. 73*, 127.

Bishop, G.H., and Heinbecker, P. (1932). *Amer. J. Physiol. 100*, 519.

Bunge, R.P.,(1981). *Trends in Neurosci. 4*, 175.

Bunge, R.P., and Bunge, M.B. (1978). *J. Cell Biol. 78*, 943.

Carlstedt, T. (1977). *Acta Physiol. Scand. Suppl. 446*, 61.

Duclaux, R., Mei, N., and Ranieri, F. (1976). *J.Physiol. (Lond.) 260*, 487.

Dunant, Y. (1967). *J. Physiol. (Paris) 59*, 17.

Forssman, von W.G. (1964). *Acta Anat. 59*, 106.

Giorgi, P.P. (1976). *Biochem. Soc. Trans. 4*, 742.

Heath, J.W. (1982). *J. Neurocytol. 11*, 249.

Heath, J.W., and Jurd, K. (1983) *J. Anat.*, in press.

Heath, J.W., and Smith, D. (1981). *J. Anat. 132*, 309A.

Honma, S. (1970). *Jap. J. Physiol. 20*, 281.

Kosterlitz, H.W., Thompson, J.W., and Wallis, D.I. (1964).

    J. Physiol. (Lond.) 136, 426.
Langley, J.N. (1896). *J. Physiol.20*, 55.
Langley, J.N. (1904). *J. Physiol. (Lond.) 30*, 221.
Madrid, R.E., and Wiśniewski, H.M. (1978). *J. Neurocytol.
    7*, 265.
Norton, W.T., and Poduslo, S.E. (1973). *J. Neurochem. 21*,
    759.
Pick, J. (1970). "The Autonomic Nervous System. Morpholo-
    gical, Comparative, Clinical and Surgical Aspects."
    Lippincott, Philadelphia.
Politis, M.J., Sternberger, N., Ederle, K., and
    Spencer, P.S. (1982). *J. Neurosci. 2*, 1252.
Pollard, J.D., King, R.H.M., and Thomas, P.K. (1975).
    J. Neurol. Sci. 24, 365.
Simpson, S.A., and Young, J.Z. (1945). *J. Anat. 79*, 48.
Spencer, P.S., Politis, M.J., Pellegrino, R.G., and
    Weinberg, H.J. (1981). *In* "Posttraumatic Peripheral
    Nerve Regeneration; Experimental Basis and Clinical
Implications", p. 411. Raven Press, New York.
Trapp, B.D., Itoyama, Y., Sternberger, N.H., Quarles, R.H.,
    and Webster, H. de F. (1981). *J. Cell Biol. 90*, 1.

THE SCHMIDT-LANTERMAN CLEFT IN THE MYELIN SHEATH:

STUDIES IN CHICKEN NERVES

NEIL A. COOPER and ANTONY D. KIDMAN

The N.S.W. Institute of Technology

GORE HILL   N.S.W.   2065   AUSTRALIA

ABSTRACT

Morphometric studies in the peripheral nervous system of the rat have shown that the relationship between the numbers of Schmidt-Lanterman clefts (incisures) per internode and the fibre diameter remains unaltered when nerve fibres undergo remyelination (Ghabriel and Allt 1981). However when nerve fibres remyelinate the internodal length is reduced and thus for each class of fibre diameter, the space between the incisures is reduced.

Hanwell *et al* (1982) had shown that the Schmidt-Lanterman incisures are far more numerous in the fibres of the chicken sciatic nerve than in the mammalian nervous system. Thus we decided to examine the relationship between fibre diameter, numbers of clefts in each internode and internodal length in juvenile, adult and remyelinated nerves of the chicken sciatic nerve. Our results show that as the nerve fibres mature the mean fibre diameter and internodal length increase. As the myelin sheath elongates and becomes thicker, the numbers of incisures also increase in each internode, but the distance between the clefts is reduced, and for each class of fibre diameter is fairly constant.

With remyelination, the Schwann cells multiply and consequently the internodal lengths are reduced, and are quite variable. Fibre diameter is reduced due to the

reduction of the thickness of the myelin sheath. Our
results show that the number of clefts per internode vary
with the length of the internode, such that the chicken
maintains a fairly constant distance between clefts of
approximately 20µm regardless of fibre diameter.

INTRODUCTION

      Schmidt-Lanterman incisures are conical compartments
of cytoplasm regularly interspersed in the myelin sheath
of central and peripheral nerves. Ultrastructural examination shows the cleft is in the form of a cytoplasmic
spiral where the myelin lamellae split to connect the inner
and outer Schwann cell cytoplasm. The clefts were originally described over a century ago, Schmidt (1874), Lanterman (1877), Boll (1877), when staining techniques indicated
their existence. There was later concern as to whether
they might be an artefact, with even Robertson (1958) in
the initial electron microscope examination of the clefts,
describing them as "shearing defects". However, the
classical light microscope study of Hall & Williams (1970)
clearly demonstrated their existence *in vivo*.

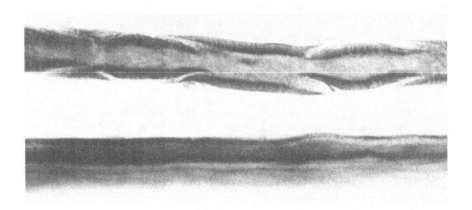

*Figure 1:   Prominent Schmidt-Lanterman incisures from the
             chicken sciatic nerve in a large diameter fibre
             under oil immersion, bright field, in the light
             microscope.*

Quantitative studies were first carried out by Boll
(1877). He showed there were 20-30 incisures per internode in the frog. Colasanti (1878) noted that the intervals between incisures were shorter in guinea pigs than in
frogs. Hiscoe (1947) studied the tibial nerve of the rat
and showed that the number of incisures per internode was
directly proportional to the fibre diameter in juvenile,
adult and regenerated nerves. Hiscoe (1947) developed the
concept of segment length, the mean distance between incisures for each internode. When the segment lengths were
related to fibre diameter, she was able to show that the
length of segment decreased as the fibre diameter increased
for juvenile, adult and regenerated fibres. This led
Hiscoe (1947) to propose that there is an upper limit to
the volume of myelin that can be maintained in a single
segmental unit. As the fibre diameter increases, additional incisures must be inserted into the myelin sheath.
Hiscoe (1947) postulated that new incisures are added when
the section of myelin sheath between existing incisures
comes to contain a certain critical volume of myelin.
Sotnikov (1965) studied segment length of frogs and cats.
He found that the mean segment length for cat sciatic
nerves was 37.6μm, two thirds that of the frog.

Recent interest in the Schmidt-Lanterman incisures
have been aroused by Ghabriel and Allt (1979, 1980, 1981)
who have used a quantitative light microscope technique to
study the clefts in Wallerian degeneration, remyelination
and regeneration in the rat. They have also stimulated
debate as to the mechanism of insertion of the clefts into
the sheath, and have reviewed their possible function.

This article describes some preliminary data for morphological relationships in the normal and remyelinated
chicken sciatic nerves, using techniques similar to those
described by Ghabriel and Allt (1979). Ultrastructural
examination has shown that the frequency of clefts in the
chicken sciatic nerve is greater than the mammalian
nervous system (Hanwell et al 1982).

MATERIALS AND METHODS
Four hens (White Leghorn and Australorp strain) aged
approximately eighteen weeks were used in these experiments.
Under nitrous oxide, oxygen and halothane anaesthesia,
diphtheria toxin (10μl of 10^{-5} Lf/μl toxin) was injected
on the contralateral side. The toxin was supplied by the

Commonwealth Serum Laboratories, Melbourne.

Paralysis of the toxin injected birds occurred after
7-10 days from the time of the injections, and lasted for
approximately three weeks. Saline injected limbs appeared
clinically normal. The birds were housed on sawdust,
singly in plastic crates. The birds had adequate room to
move, gained weight and appeared quite comfortable under
these conditions.

Two birds were anaethetised 100 days following the
injection of the toxin, and the remaining two birds anaesthetised after a further 100 days. Under general anaesthesia the heart was exposed and the animal euthanased by
rupture of one of the atria. The aorta was located by
elevation of the heart from the thorax and cannulated. The
vascular system was flushed using 0.9% sodium chloride to
which sodium nitrite (0.2%) and heparin (2,000 I.U./litre)
had been added. The birds were perfused using a freshly
prepared fixative containing 3% formaldehyde, 3% glutaraldehyde, and 0.1% picric acid in cacodylate buffer as described by Langford and Coggeshall (1979).

Perfusion lasted ½-1 hour *in situ* before the sciatic
nerves were removed and cut into 1 cm. lengths. Each
length was subsequently cut longitudinally and stored at
4°C overnight in fresh fixative. The following day the
specimens were washed in maleate buffer pH5.2, and post
fixed in osmium tetroxide for 48 hours at 4°C. The fibres
were again washed in maleate buffer pH5.2 and transferred
to 66% glycerine for 48 hours. The fibres were teased
using fine forceps under a dissecting microscope and
mounted in glycerine for examination under the light microscope using bright field and an oil immersion objective as
described by Ghabriel and Allt (1979). Five measurements
were made of the fibre diameter for each internode exclud-
ing the paranodal and Schwann cell nuclear regions using
an occular micrometer and the numbers of incisures were
counted in duplicate for each internode (Fig. 2). The
internodal lengths were measured using the occular micrometer and a 4x objective lens.

Fifty internodes were measured for each of the nerves
with the exception of the 200 day controls, where only 25
internodes were examined. A Hewlett-Packard HP85 computer
was used to plot the graphs relating internodal length and

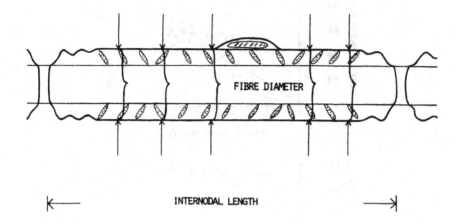

FIBRE DIAMETER

INTERNODAL LENGTH

SEGMENT LENGTH = MEAN INTER-INCISURAL DISTANCE

Figure 2:   Schematic representation of measurements in
             quantitative teased fibre study. Five meas-
             urements are made of the fibre diameter;
             duplicate counts are made of the numbers of
             clefts and a single measurement taken of the
             internodal length, using in each case an
             occular micrometer.

the number of clefts per internode to the fibre diameter
and to generate and plot the histograms relating mean interincisural distance to the fibre diameter.

RESULTS
     Figure 3 shows the relationship between the numbers of
clefts per internode and the fibre diameter for 100 day
control fibres, 100 and 200 day remyelinated fibres. The
regression coefficient for the controls is 0.8 and that
for the remyelinated nerves is 0.3 and 0.2 respectively.
Clearly the slopes of the regression lines for the normal
and remyelinated fibres are quite different and the variability of the relationship of the fibre diameter to the
numbers of incisures per internode is far greater in the
remyelinated nerve fibres.

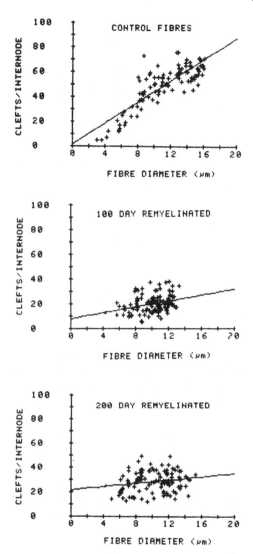

Figure 3:   *Relationship between the numbers of incisures*
and the mean diameter of the internode in the
chicken sciatic nerve. Each point represents
one internode for which the numbers of incis-
ures were counted and plotted against the mean
diameter, obtained from five measurements
along the internode.

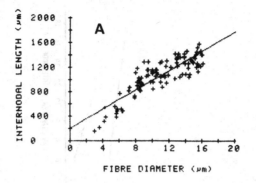

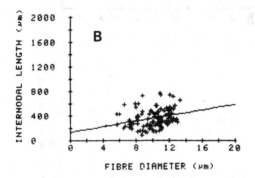

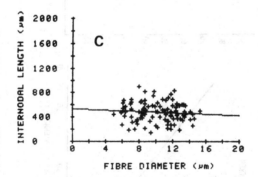

Figure 4: *Relationship between the internodal length and*
the mean diameter of the internode in the chick-
en sciatic nerve. A, Control fibres 100 days
following the injection of saline into the nerve.
B, Remyelinating fibres 100 days following the
injection of diphtheria toxin into the nerve.
C, Remyelinating fibres 200 days following the
injection of diphtheria toxin.

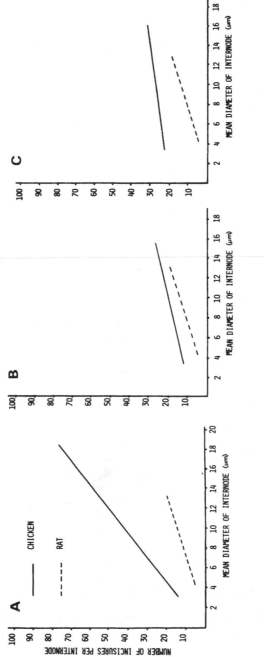

Figure 5 A-C: The three regression lines in Figure 3, shown with data for the rat from Ghabriel and Allt (1980). A, Normal rat and chicken nerve. B, Remyelinating nerve fibres 100 days following demyelinating agent. C, Remyelinating fibres 200 days following demyelinating agent.

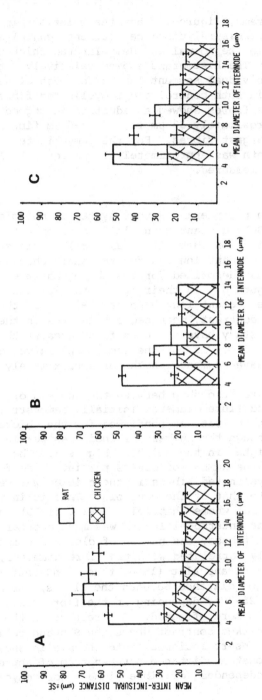

Figure 6 A-C: Histograms to show the mean interincisural distances for the fibre diameter classes 4-18 μm in the chicken sciatic and rat sural nerve. Standard errors are given where the population of internodes sampled was >4. A, Normal rat and chicken nerve. B, Remyelinating nerve fibres 100 days following demyelinating agent. C, Remyelinating nerve fibres 200 days following demyelinating agent. Rat data from Ghabriel and Allt (1980).

The histograms, Figure 6, show the relationship between mean interincisural distance (segment length) and
fibre diameter in the normal and demyelinated chicken
sciatic nerves. The histograms showed relatively little
variation in individual segment length for each class of
fibre diameter in both control and remyelinated fibres.
The normal nerve fibres showed a reduction in segment
length from approximately 33 µm for the 4-6 µm fibres to
20 µm for the largest fibres. For the remyelinated fibres
the segment length was approximately 20 µm for all classes
of nerve fibres measured.

DISCUSSION
        The chicken peripheral nervous system is notable for
the numbers of Schmidt-Lanterman clefts seen on ultrastructural examination (Hanwell et al 1982). This study
showed that the segment lengths for the adult chicken is
far less than that described for the rat by Ghabriel and
Allt (1980), Figure 6. In their study Ghabriel and Allt
(1980) found the segment length to be 65-83 µm in the
normal rat. In contrast, mean segment lengths in the
chicken in this study have not been found greater than
40 µm and the tendency is for the medium and larger diameter fibres to have segment lengths of approximately 20 µm.

        The linear relationship between the numbers of clefts
per internode and fibre diameter initially demonstrated by
Hiscoe (1947) in the rat was confirmed for the chicken in
this study, although the numbers of incisures per internode
was very much higher in the chicken, Figure 5. The relationship between the number of clefts per internode for 100
and 200 day remyelinated fibres in the chicken was very
much different to that of the controls. This is in marked
contrast to the rat where Ghabriel and Allt (1980) showed
that although the internodal length was much shorter in the
rat remyelinated fibres, the number of clefts per internode
was still closely correlated with the fibre diameter,
Figure 5. Ghabriel and Allt (1980) thus found that the
segment length (or distance between the clefts) was markedly reduced by 25-70%, depending on the fibre size, with
the larger fibres more affected. Our results in the
chicken are in marked contrast where the Schwann cell
would appear to insert incisures into the myelin sheath to
keep a fairly constant distance between them of approximately 20 µm, independent of fibre diameter or remyelination.

That there should be a difference in the incorporation of clefts between the chicken and rat is not surprising. Sotnikov (1965) reported the mean segment length of the cat at 37.6 μm which is far lower than that seen in the adult rat where the range is 65-83 μm (Ghabriel and Allt, 1979). In their teased fibre study of remyelination in the chicken sciatic nerve, Jacobs and Cavanagh (1969) showed that remyelinated internodes were not uniformly short, in marked contrast to the findings of Hiscoe (1947) for the rat. It was seen that the internode of a chicken nerve could reach a length of 800 μm for the larger diameter fibres after 200 days whereas those of the rat were about 400 μm irrespective of fibre diameter.

It would appear that the remyelinating Schwann cell inserts clefts into the meylin sheath to keep a fairly constant distance between them, but that the Schwann cell of the rat is programmed to insert a specified number of incisures into the myelin sheath dependent on fibre diameter rather than on internodal length. The question can be asked as to whether the organisation of the rat Schwann cell in regard to the insertion of incisures is typical for the mammalian nervous system.

Ghabriel and Allt (1981) reviewed the suggested functions of the incisures. Such proposed functions have included (a) transport of metabolic substances across the myelin sheath, (b) metabolic maintenance of the myelin sheath, (c) longitudinal growth of the sheath, (d) adjustment in myelin sheath geometry with limb movement, (e) peristaltic activity, (f) impulse conduction. The one function that has been clearly demonstrated is that of the cleft in Wallerian degeneration where it plays an active role in ovoid formation (Williams and Hall 1971).

Quantitative studies in the chicken show a regular insertion of the cleft into the myelin sheath. Such an observation would provide some support to hypothesis indicating a role for the cleft in the metabolic maintenance of the myelin sheath and/or axon, but as yet the biological function of this enzyme rich cytoplasmic cleft remains to be elucidated. The Schmidt-Lanterman incisures are potentially important features of the myelinated nerve fibre, and may play an important role in the pathophysiology of some myelin disorders (Ghabriel and Allt 1981).

ACKNOWLEDGEMENT

The authors wish to thank Hewlett Packard (Australia) for the generous donation of the HP85 computer used in this study.

REFERENCES

Boll, F. (1877). *Atti Accad. naz. Lincei Rc. Ser. 3, 1,* 75, cited by Hall, S.M. and Williams, P.L. (1970), *ibid.*

Colasanti, G. (1878). *Atti Accad. naz. Lincei 2,* cited by Sotnikov, O.S. (1965) *ibid.*

Ghabriel, M.N. and Allt, G. (1979). *Acta Neuropathol. (Berl.) 48,* 83.

Ghabriel, M.N. and Allt, G. (1980). *Acta Neuropathol. (Berl.) 54,* 85.

Ghabriel, M.N. and Allt, G. (1981). *Progress in Neurobiology 17,* 25.

Hall, S.M. and Williams, P.L. (1970). *J. Cell. Sci. 6,* 767.

Hanwell, M.A., Cooper, N.A. and Kidman, A.D. (1982). *Neurochemistry International 4,* 467.

Hiscoe, H.B. (1947). *Anat. Rec. 99,* 447.

Jacobs, J.M. and Cavanagh, J.B. (1969). *J. Anat. 105,* 295.

Langford, L.A. and Coggeshall, R.E. (1979). *J. Comp. Neurol. 184,* 193.

Lanterman, A.J. (1877). *Arch. mikrosk. Anat. Entw. Mech. 13,* 1 cited by Hall, S.M. and Williams, P.L. (1970) *ibid.*

Robertson, J.D. (1958). *J. Biophys. Biochem. Cytol 4,* 39.

Schmidt, H.D. (1874). *Mon. microsc. J. (London) 11,* 200 cited by Hall, S.M. and Williams, P.L. (1970) *ibid.*

Sotnikov, O.S. (1965). *Archiv. Anat. Gistol. Embriol. 43,* 31 (translated in *Fed. Proc. Fed. Am. Soc. Exp. Biol. (1966) 25,* T204.

Williams, P.L. and Hall, S.M. (1971). *J. Anat. 109,* 487.

INTERACTION BETWEEN NEURONAL SETS DURING BRAIN DEVELOPMENT

Piero P. Giorgi

Neuroembryology Laboratory, School of Anatomy,

University of Queensland, St. Lucia. 4067
Australia.

Abstract

The nervous system is very sensitive to perturbation by genetic and environmental factors due to the complexity of cellular interactions occurring during development. Basic mechanisms responsible for these interactions can be investigated in a simple experimental model like the visual system of Amphibia. The possible role of brain visual centres in promoting the growth of retinofugal axons was studied by grafting ectopic eyes above the spinal cord of *Xenopus* embryos. The reciprocal effect of ingrowing optic axons on the differentiation of visual centres in the brain was studied by removing both eye vesicles. A working hypothesis on reciprocal interactions between neuronal sets in the developing brain is proposed. Genetic information, morphogenetic characteristics of the embryonic environment, production of diffusable tropic substances and transynaptic induction, all seem to participate, at different stages, to the co-ordinated development of different regions of the brain.

Introduction

Several teratogenetic drugs and chemicals affect the development of the nervous system, which is particularly susceptible to toxic environmental factors and to congenital malformations (Clayton, 1973; Groff and Pitts,

1967; Kalter, 1968). For example, infants born to chronic alcoholic mothers (Golbus, 1980), or to mothers who ingested abnormally high levels of organic mercury (Bakir et al., 1973) are affected by mental retardation. About 10% of mothers who were exposed to lysergic acid diethylamide (LSD) before or during pregnancy gave birth to infants with nervous system defects (Jacobson and Berlin, 1972).

The high frequency of defects inducable during the development of the nervous system and the long period of sensitivity to environmental teratogens (3-38 weeks after conception) is probably related to a pattern of cellular interactions particularly complex. As during the development of other organs, four main events summarize the growth and maturation of the nervous system: cell multiplication, cell migration, cell differentiation and/or cell death. Each one of these events has features unique to the nervous system, the general feature being *the need to generate a high degree of regional segregation of neuronal sets as well as a precise pattern of connectivity among them*. The aim of this article is to discuss the nature of reciprocal influences during development between two regions destined to be linked together by synaptic connection (Jacobson, 1978; Lund, 1978). This concept will be illustrated by our work on the visual system of *Xenopus laevis* (Amphibia Anura) as an experimental model to investigate reciprocal influences between neuronal sets in the developing central nervous system.

Optic axons in the spinal cord: a model to study the influence of target organs upon growing afferent axons

Since the beginning of this century amphibian embryos have been used to investigate the ability of grafted optic vescicles to develop ectopically (Lewis, 1907b) and to grow retinofugal axons into regions of the central nervous system foreign to the visual system (Lewis, 1907a). This latter aspect could yield information on the mechanisms subserving axon guidance during brain development.

Originally concepts on axon guidance derived from regeneration experiments (Sperry, 1963) and tissue culture studies (Weiss, 1955). More recently the more difficult question of what happens in truly developing tissue has been asked with normal embryos (Rakic, 1971; Singer et al.,

1979) and grafted tissue (Giorgi and Van der Loos, 1978; Katz and Lasek, 1979; Constantine-Paton, 1978). The rationale for using ectopic eyes is the following. By testing the behaviour (i.e. choice of direction of growth) of ectopically growing axons in a variety of different situations, one hopes to induce the general principle guiding axons toward their correct target region in the brain.

After forcing optic axons to grow into the rhombo-encephalon (future medulla oblongata) of frog embryos and finding that they grew caudally, Constantine-Paton and Capranica (1976) suggested that dorso-caudal growth relative to the three major axes of the neural tube is an inherent property of optic nerve fibres. In order to test this hypothesis, we began (Giorgi and Van der Loos, 1977) a series of experiments involving optic axons forced to grow into the spinal cord of *Xenopus* embryos. This was obtained by grafting an eye vesicle upon the dorso-medial neurotube of an embryo. If the choice of direction of growth is dictated by the presence of orthogonally aligned gradients present throughout the central nervous system, the ectopic axons should grow toward the caudal end of the spinal cord. If, on the contrary, the critical factor regulating axon guidance is the reciprocal position between the eye and the target organ of retinofugal axons, then the ectopic axons should grow toward the rostral end of the spinal cord, where the optic tectum is located. The spinal cord is the ideal region of the central nervous system for this type of experiment, because long-axon neurons can grow their axon only in two directions.

Embryos of *Xenopus leavis* were operated at stages 23-24 (Nieukoop and Faber, 1956). Optic vesicles were removed from donor embryos and grafted on the dorsal region of host embryos. Particular care was taken in controlling the composition of the graft. The optic stalk was left behind the optic vesicle to allow a connection with the host's neurotube (which was split open). A careful elimination of the wall of the prosencephalon was done to avoid the development of part of the donor's brain between the graft and the spinal cord. This would have complicated the interpretation of results concerning axon guidance inside the spinal cord.

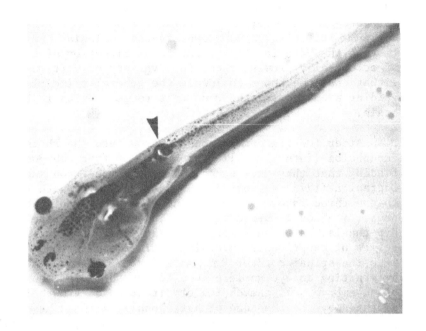

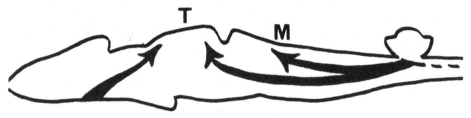

Fig. 1

*Xenopus larva at stage 53 with an eye grafted onto the
spinal cord (arrow). The diagram shows the direction of
growth of normal optic axons toward thr rostral optic
tectum (T) and of ectopic axons toward the medulla oblongata
(M) and the caudal optic tectum. Only a very small number
of ectopic axons grew caudad within the spinal cord.*

Morphologically normal eyes grew on the top of the spinal
cord of experimental animals, which were sacrificed at
midlarval stages (Fig. 1). Reduced silver staining of
sagittal sections showed that in about 30% of cases a
connection between the ectopic eye and the spinal cord
existed. Retinofugal axons were traced inside the spinal
cord by the method of suppressed silver staining of
degenerating axons (Giorgi and Van der Loos, 1978) and,
more recently, by the anterograde transport of horseradish
peroxidase. The vast majority of ectopic axons were found
to have grown toward the brain (Giorgi and Van der Loos,
1977, 1978). This result is in agreement with that
obtained by Katz and Lasek (1978, 1979), who also grafted
an eye on *Xenopus* spinal cord. However, the position of
their ectopic eye (at the caudal end of the spinal cord)
was not really suitable to test an alternative (rostrad v.
caudad) direction of growth. Results from both laboratories
refuted the suggestion put forward by Constantino-Paton
and Capranica (1976) that embryonic optic axons are
genetically programmed to grow caudally within the central
nervous system. This was later acknowledged by
Constantine-Paton (1978), leaving the problem of the
mechanism of guidance of optic axons open to the following
alternative. The tissue of the developing spinal cord
itself could have local cues designed to inform ingrowing
sensory axons on the correct direction toward higher
integration centres of the central nervous system, or,
alternatively, the target tissue (the optic tectum, for
example) could be able to affect the behaviour of growing
axons by producing a diffusable growth factor working at
distance. The proposal of Katz and Lasek (1979) of
guiding substrate pathways would seem to fit into the
first type of mechanism, although the physical nature of
such pathways was not made clear by these authors. Our
set of experiments involving eyeless host embryos (Giorgi
and Van der Loos, 1978) seems to favour the second type
of mechanism. When both eye vesicles of the host embryo
were removed soon after grafting an eye vesicle onto its
neurotube, the behaviour of ectopic retinofugal axons
changed. In tadpoles with eyes, ectopic axons terminated
in the medulla oblungata (in the nucleus of the solitary
tract and near the roots of cranial nerves V and IX-X).
In eyeless tadpoles ectopic axons also terminated in the
caudal part of the optic tectum (Fig. 1). Thus, the optic
tectum may release a diffusable factor which stimulates

growing afferent axons to reach their target organ;
perhaps it stops releasing this factor when invaded by
optic axons. This would explain why ectopic axons reach
only the medulla oblongata when the host retains its eyes.
The alternative interpretation of these results based on
competition for terminal space between normal host optic
axons and ectopic axons   is not likely, because at
larval stages normal optic terminations are present only
in the rostral part of the optic tectum (Steedman et al.,
1979), while ectopic terminations were found only in the
caudal part. Whether diffusable factors released by the
embryonic optic tectum would act at such a long distance
to affect the choice of direction along the spinal cord
(rostrad v. caudad growth), or only at short distances
to affect further growth from the medulla oblongata to the
optic tectum, it is not possible to speculate. The
possibility of an early growth toward both rostral and
caudal direction has been put forward (Giorgi et al., 1979).
The alternative idea that possible diffusable factors
released by the optic tectum act only at short distance
is favoured in the final discussion of this paper.

Experimental eyeless tadpoles: a model to study the effect
of growing axons on the differentiation of their target
organ.

When an embryo is deprived of both its eye vesicles
the diencephalon and the mesencephalon develop in the
absence of ingrowing retinofugal axons. What is the effect
of this alteration on their growth and differentiation?
Kollros (1953) already showed that removal of one eye
vesicle affects the growth of the contralateral optic
tectum in *Rana*. This phenomenon has been confirmed and
further analysed by Currie and Cowan, (1974). We have been
studying how the lack of ingrowing optic axons affects the
development of the diencephalon (future thalamus). The
diencephalon has several retinofugal terminations in
Amphibia (for a review see Fite and Scalia, 1976) and the
development of the related regions is only poorly
understood (Tay and Straznichy, 1982).

Both eye vesicles were removed from *Xenopus* embryos at
stages 25-26. All sets of operated embryos were kept
in the same container with an equal number of control
embryos and the two groups were reared together until
sacrifice.

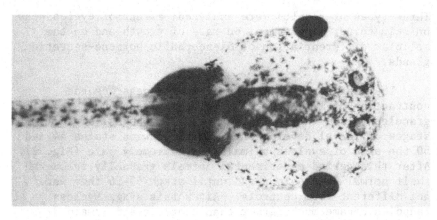

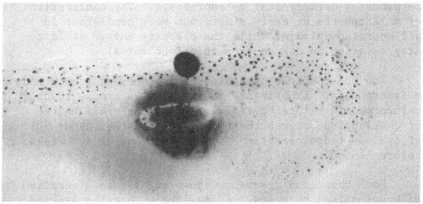

Fig 2

*Effect of embryonic eye removal on the regulation of skin
colour in Xenopus larvae. Top: normal tadpole (stage 45)
with star-shaped chromatophores which provide a normal
pigmentation. Bottom: experimental tadpole (eyeless) with
its chromatophores strongly contracted. Note that the
presence of an ectopic eye in the dorsal region does not
surrogate the absence of its normal eyes, as far as
pigmentation is concerned.*

Three types of results were analysed: effect of eyelessness
on skin colour regulation, on rate of growth and on the
cellular differentiation of diencephalic hormone-secreting
glands.

The most striking effect of eyelessness was the
contraction of melanophores (i.e. the migration of melanine
granules toward the perikaryon of melanophores) at early
stages of larval development. Thus, between stages 44 and
50 the skin of eyeless animals was extremely pale (Fig. 2).
After this period experimental animals gradually recovered
their normal skin colour and until stage 55-56 they were
not different from controls. After this stage eyeless
tadpoles became much darker than controls and remained
permanently darker after metamorphosis. The contraction
of melanophores at early stages was very consistent in
all operated animals, while the opposite change at later
stages varied in degree from animal to animal.

The other effect of eyelessness concerned growth and
metamorphosis. Experimental animals, as a group, reached
metamorphosis before controls. Although a small degree
of overlapping between the two groups existed, about 90%
of eyeless tadpoles metamorphosed about one or two weeks
before controls.

Both phenomena described above suggest an alteration
of hypophysisal hormones. It is likely that the lack of
retinfugal axons growing into the diencephalon causes a
retardation in the differentiation of the hypophysis (hence
lack of melanophore stimulating hormone -MSH- and the
paleness of skin). At later stages, when the
differentiation of a diencephalic inhibitory neuronal set
(Etkin, 1967) may also be affected by the lack of retinal
input, the production of MSH and of thyroid stimulating
hormone (TSH) would be higher than in control (hence the
darkness of skin and the acceleration of metamorphosis).
Obviously a chain of developmental events separates the
removal of optic vesicles from *Xenopus* embryos and the
physiological changes observed suggesting an alteration in
production of hormones. In order to investigate these
events two organs of the diencephalon known to produce
hormones involved in skin colour regulation were selected.
The pineal complex produces melatonin, which causes
lightening of the skin in lower vertebrates (Bagnara, 1960).
The pituitary gland produces MSH, which causes skin

darkening (Abe et al., 1969). A detailed analysis of both
organs was carried out by electron microscopy at stage 45,
when the effect of eyelessness first appears under the
form of a substantial degree of melanophore contraction.

In *Xenopus* at stage 45 the adenohypophysis is not
clearly divided, as yet,into anterior and intermedial lobes
(Nyholm, 1977), but MSH is already produced and released
since stage 38 (Nyholm and Doerr-Schott, 1977). Both
control and eyeless tadpoles had many neurons containing
secretory granules in their pituitary gland. Other cells
appeared to be undifferentiated neurons and glial cells.
After collating transverse sections of the whole gland at
15,000 magnifications (12 controls and 10 experimental
samples) it was found that eyeless tadpoles had 44%
($\pm$ 3 S.D) neurons containing secretory granules, compared
to 58% ($\pm$ 5 S.D.) in normal animals. The reduction of
24% in granule-bearing neurons in experimental animals
suggests that the lack of retinofugal input may cause an
inhibition or retardation in the differentiation of
hypothalamic nuclei which in turn regulate the development
of the pituitary gland. The identification of the nuclei
involved in this phenomenon will be the object of future
work. One logical target is the basal optic nucleus which
receivesdirect input from the eye (Fite and Scalia, 1976).

In Amphibia the pineal complex is composed of the
epiphysis proper, localised in the roof of the diencephalon,
and the frontal organ, localised between the brain and the
skin (Kelly and Smith, 1964). A preliminary histological
investigation showed that the frontal organ develops earlier
than the epiphysis and gradually shifts its position from
above the diencephalon to the tip of the telencephalon
(in between of the lateral eyes). The same ultrastructural
analysis described above for the pituitary gland was carried
out for the frontal organ. Six collages of frontal organs
from control tadpoles at stage 45 and six of eyeless
tadpoles were analysed. At this stage the frontal organ
already contains well differentiated photoreceptor cells,
neurons with a rich endoplasmic reticulum and Golgi apparatus
and glial cells. The lack of a morphological parameter to
identify the cell type possibly engaged in hormone
production, did not allow the same approach used for the
pituitary gland. In this case the percentage of each of
these three cell types was determined. No statistically
significant difference was found between control and

experimental animals. This seems to suggest that the lack
of retinofugal axons in the diencephalon may not affect
the differentiation of the frontal organ at least at early
stages of development. However, a similar analysis of the
epiphysis proper needs to be carried out at later
developmental stages, before assuming that the pineal
complex is not involved in the eyelessness syndrome. The
developmental stage 55-56, when eyeless tadpoles become
darker than control, is currently being investigated. In
this context it should be pointed out that possible
connections between diencephalic visual centres and the
pineal complex in Amphibia have not been described. However,
such a connection could exist through the habenular complex
(Kemali et al., 1980).

Discussion

        The two experimental models described in this paper
offer the possibility to analyse two modes of action with
which neuronal sets can influence each other: the effect
of the target neuronal set upon the afferent neuronal set
and viceversa. The use of the *Xenopus* visual system has
several advantages. A great deal of work on both normal
and experimental development has been done on this system
(Gaze, 1978). *Xenopus* is easily reared in laboratory as
an inexpensive and experimentally accessible animal (Gurdon,
1967). The eye is a convenient region of the central
nervous system for experimentation, because of its early
segregation into a peripheral and well defined vesicle.
Finally, the cellular basis of early interaction between
developing neuronal sets should be the same among
vertebrates, so that information obtained from Amphibia
should apply to Mammalia as well.

        The cellular events subserving phenomena observed in
both experimental models described in this paper are, as
yet, far from being elucidated. The following type of
information is, or will be, sought. Evidence is needed
to prove that a diffusable factor is produced by the
embryonic mesencephalon before being innervated by
retinofugal axons. We are currently checking this hypothesis
by studying the behaviour of axons issued from an eye
grafted upon the spinal cord of a Janus telobiont tadpole
(Swisher and Hibbard, 1967), with the optic tectum missing
on one side. We need to know what direction of growth
ectopic axons take at very early stages of development.

It is possible that axons issued from a grafted eye first grow equally well rostrad and caudad. Subsequently the retinal ganglion cells whose axon grew caudad may die because of a lack of suitable postsynaptic terminal sites. In this case the presence of ectopic axons in the medulla oblongata at later stages would represent preferential survival rather than preferential direction of growth.

Concerning the eyeless syndrome, we need to confirm the morphological evidence of a retarded differentiation of the hypophysis by a biochemical, or immunohistochemical, determination of MSH, or of MSH-producing cells in the gland. More information is also needed to rule out the involvement of the pineal complex in the eyelessness syndrome. The neural circuitry responsible for the possible effect of eyelessness on the basal and dorsal diencephalon also needs to be elucidated.

The study of reciprocal interactions between neuronal sets during brain development will be pursued in our laboratory on the basis of the following working hypothesis (Fig. 3).
a) *The initial outgrowth of axons* is initially conditioned by factors intrinsic to the neuron (Van der Loos, 1965). The intrinsic factors are probably genetically determined (like those responsible for the general shape of all cell types) so that the site of axon formation and its initial direction of growth are related to the morphology and orientation of the neuron. The extrinsic factors (those operating from the environment of the neuron) can be morphogenetic (Horder and Martin, 1978) or based on selective adhesiveness with pre-existing guiding pathways (Katz et al., 1980). Thus these factors specifying the initial outgrowth of axons (toward a close proximity with its target region) are specified by genetical information (through specific proteins related to the differentiation of neuronal and non neuronal cells) and by epigenetic information (spatio-temporal matching of events during embryonic development).
b) *The final outgrowth of axons* is guided by diffusable factors produced by target neuronal sets, which have both trophic (Bennett et al., 1980) and tropic (Levi-Montalcini et al., 1978) effects on growing neurons. As such effect is taking place at short distance (in the order of few millimeters) the target neuronal set needs to produce only

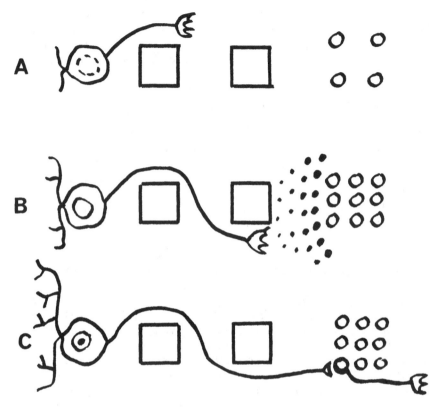

Fig. 3

Working hypothesis to explain reciprocal interactions
between neuronal sets during brain development. The neuron
on the left represents an afferent neuron growing its
axon through unrelated regions (square boxes), toward the
target set of neurons on the right. A) Initial outgrowth
of the axon. B) Final outgrowth of the axon. C) Synaptic
formation. The nature of cellular interactions is discussed
in the text.

minute amounts of factors characterized by a limited degree
of specificity.
c) *Synaptic formation* occurs when afferent axons have
established contacts with the target neuronal set. These
postsynaptic neurons undergo the final process of
differentiation as a consequence of receiving contacts,
with cell-cell interaction mechanisms (post-synaptic
induction) similar to those showed in the peripheral
nervous system (Jacobson, 1978; Lund, 1978).

The above working hypothesis implies a relatively
limited involvement of genetic information for neural
circuitry formation during brain development and it is in
general agreement with concepts derived from the development
of the peripheral nervous system and more recent
speculations on the development of the central nervous
system. However, interaction between neuronal sets during
development of the brain may differ from those between
peripheral and central nervous system during the development
of somatosensory and motor innervation. For this reason
the visual system represents a very convenient experimental
model, as it only involves central nervous system neurons.

Two main aspects of brain development are relevant to
teratology and brain pathology in general.
a) Critical events occur at a given stage of development
following a precise time table of regional maturation
within the brain. As a consequence, the effect of
teratogens can differ in type or degree according to the
time of exposure. b) Chains of interactions between
neuronal sets of the developing brain complicate the
understanding of both genetical and environmental causes of
malformations. The tangible effect of a teratogenetic
disturbance may become apparent at a later stage of
development and in a region different from the primary
target of the teratogen.

Acknowledgements

The author is grateful to G. Little, A. Hartshorn,
J. Macintosh and A. Trolliet for assistance and to
H. Van der Loos for discussion. This work is supported by
the Australian Research Grants Scheme and by a Special
Project Grant of the University of Queensland.

References

Abe, K., Butcher, R.W., Nicholson, W.E., Baird, C.E., Liddle, R.A. and Liddle, G.S. (1969). *Endocrinology*. 84, 362.

Bagnara, J.T. (1960). *Science*. 132, 1482.

Bakir, F., Damluji, S.F., Amin-Zaki, L., Murtadha, M., Khalidi, A., Al-Rawi, N.Y., Tikriti, S., Dhahir, H.I., Clarkson, T.W., Smith, J.C., Doherty, R.A. (1973). *Science*. 181, 320.

Bennett, M.R., Davey, D.F. and Uebel, K.E. (1980). *J. Comp. Neurol.* 189, 335.

Clayton, B.E. (1973). "Mental Retardation: Environmental Hazards". Butterworth & Co., London.

Constantine-Paton, M. (1978). *Brain Res.* 158, 31.

Constantine-Paton, M. and Capranica, R.R. (1976). *J. Comp. Neurol.* 170, 17.

Currie, J. and Cowan, W.M. (1974). *J. Comp. Neurol.* 156, 123.

Etkin, W. (1967). In "Neurosecretion", (L. Martini and W.F. Ganong, eds.). Vol. 2, p. 261. Academic Press, New York.

Fite, K.V. and Scalia, F. (1976). In "The Amphibian Visual System", (K.V. Fite, ed.), p. 87. Academic Press, New York.

Gaze, R.M. (1978). In "Specific Embryological Interactions" (D.R. Garrod, ed.), p. 53. Chapman and Hall, London.

Giorgi, P.P. and Van der Loos, H. (1977). *Acta Anatomica*. 99, 349.

Giorgi, P.P. and Van der Loos, H. (1978). *Nature* (Lon.). 275, 746.

Giorgi, P.P., Trolliet, A. and Van der Loos, H. (1979). *Neuroscience Lett.* Supp. 3, 21.

Golbus, M.S. (1980). *Obstet. Gynecol.* 55, 269.

Groff, R.A. and Pitts, F.W. (1967). In "Handbook of Congenital Malformations", (A. Rubin, ed.), p. 86. W.B. Saunders Co., Philadelphia.

Gurdon, J.B. (1967). In "Methods in Developmental Biology", (F.H. Wilt and N.K. Wessels, eds.), p. 75. Crowell, New York.

Horder, T.J. and Martin, K.A.C. (1978). In "Cell-Cell Recognition", (A.S.G. Curtis, ed.), Society for Experimental Biology Symposia Vol. 32, p. 275. Cambridge University Press, Cambridge.

Jacobson, M. (1978). "Developmental Neurobiology". Plenum Press, New York.

Jacobson, C.B. and Berlin, C.M. (1972). *J.A.M.A.* 222, 1367.

Kalter, H. (1968). "Teratology of the Central Nervous System", University of Chicago Press, Chicago.

Katz, M.J. and Lasek, R.J. (1978). *Science.* 199, 202.

Katz, M.J. and Lasek, R.J. (1979). *J. Comp. Neurol.* 183, 817.

Katz, M.J., Lasek, R.J. and Nauta, H.J.W. (1980). *Neuroscience.* 5, 821.

Kelly, D.E. and Smith, S.W. (1964). *J. Cell. Biol.* 22, 653.

Kemali, M., Guglielmotti, V., Gioffré, D. (1980). *Exp. Brain Res.* 38, 341.

Kollros, J.J. (1953). *J. Exp. Zool.* 123, 153.

Levi-Montalcini, R., Menesini-Chen, M.G. and Chen, J.S. (1978). *Zoon.* 6, 201.

Lewis, W.H. (1907a). *Amer. J. Anat.* 6, 461.

Lewis, W.H. (1907b). *Amer. J. Anat.* 7, 259.

Lund, R.D. (1978). "Development and plasticity of the brain", Oxford University Press, New York.

Nieuwkoop, P.D. and Faber, J. (1956). "Normal Table of *Xenopus laevis* (Daudin)". North-Holland, Amsterdam.

Nyholm, N.E.I. (1977). *Cell Tiss. Res.* 180, 223.

Nyholm, N.E.I. and Doerr-Schott, J. (1977). *Cell Tiss. Res.* 180, 231.

Rakic, P. (1971). *Brain Res.* 33, 471.

Singer, M., Nordlander, R.H. and Egar, M. (1979). *J. Comp. Neurol.* 185, 1.

Sperry, R.W. (1963). *Proc. Natn. Acad. Sci. U.S.A.* 50, 703.

Steedman, J.G., Stirling, R.V. and Gaze, R.M. (1979). *J. Embryol. Exp. Morhp.* 50, 199.

Swisher, J.E and Hibbard, E. (1967). *J. Exp. Zool.* 165, 433.

Tay, D. and Straznicky, C. (1982). *Anat. Embryol.* 163, 371.

Van der Loos, H. (1965). *Bull. Johns Hopkins Hosp.* 117, 228.

Weiss, P. (1955). In "Analysis of Development", (B.H. Willier, P. Weiss and V. Hamburger, eds.), p. 346. W.B. Saunders Co., Philadelphia.

MATURATION OF POST-SYNAPTIC DENSITIES IN CHICKEN

FOREBRAIN

John A.P. Rostas, Fritz H. Güldner* and
Peter R. Dunkley

The Neuroscience Group,
Faculty of Medicine
University of Newcastle
N.S.W. 2308 Australia

and*
Department of Anatomy
Monash University
Clayton, Victoria 3168, Australia

ABSTRACT

To study maturational events at CNS synapses we have
compared some morphological and biochemical properties
of synaptic junctions from 2 day and adult chicken forebrain. In this period the thickness of the average post
synaptic density (PSD) doubled while the length did not
change. In the same period the amount of the protein
which is the major component of mature PSDs (mPSDp)
increased almost 3 fold. These results suggest a direct
correlation between the thickness of a PSD and the amount
of mPSDp it contains. Cyclic AMP-and calcium plus
calmodulin-stimulated protein phosphorylation increased
in synaptic junctions during this period and the relative
incorporation into some protein species changed with
maturation. Except for the case of the mPSDp, whose
phosphorylation appears to be substrate limited, the
maturational changes in protein phosphorylation could
be explained by an increase in protein substrate or
protein kinase or both. These results suggest that the
PSD is first established as a basic protein structure
containing little or no mPSDp and that subsequent maturational events add specific structural (e.g. mPSDp) or

functional (e.g. kinases, phosphoproteins) to this basic
structure.

INTRODUCTION

The establishment of a mature synapse in the central
nervous system (CNS) depends on a complex series of molecular and cellular events. The process may be broadly
divided into two phases: synapse formation and synapse
maturation. Synapse formation covers the steps up to
the establishment of a functional synaptic contact
between two cells and includes the events related to
axon guidance, the mutual recognition of axon and target
cell and the cellular differentiation of the synaptic
site. Synapse maturation covers the little understood
events involved in changing a functional but immature
synapse into a mature synapse. Maturation includes
events related to synapse competition and validation and
morphological changes about which little or no biochemical information is available. In recent years it has
become clear that most mature CNS synapses possess a considerable degree of functional and morphological plasticity (Cotman et al, 1981; Reisine, 1981). Following
injury this plasticity may take the dramatic form of re-
active synaptogenesis (Cotman and Lynch, 1976) in which
case most of the events of synapse formation and maturation are presumably recapitulated. The less dramatic but
probably more common expressions of synaptic plasticity
involve changes in morphology and function of established
synapses. The mechanisms of these changes are not known
but are likely to involve reversals or extensions of the
changes involved in the original maturation process.

An elucidation of these mechanisms would have potential clinical significance. Future strategies for optimi-
zing the neurological recovery of patients following
acute nervous system trauma will need to be based on an
understanding of the various factors that promote the
plastic responses of synapses. Similarly, management of
the gradual nervous system impairment produced by senile
dementia and various degenerative disorders also requires
an appreciation of factors which, while not the cause of
the condition, may enhance the rate of recovery or slow
the rate of deterioration. As one way of obtaining some
insight into the events involved in plastic changes in

mature synapses we have been studying the changes involved in normal synapse maturation.

Although the distinction between synapse formation
and synapse maturation may be easy to make at any one
synapse, in developing CNS tissue as a whole, the two
phases largely overlap thereby complicating biochemical
studies in mixed synaptic populations unless an appropriate brain region or experimental animal can be found.
The newly hatched chicken is such an experimental animal
because its CNS is relatively mature at hatching (Corner
et al., 1977) and most of the maturational events at
synapses occur in the weeks following hatching. We have
been studying some biochemical changes that occur at
chicken forebrain synapses during maturation and concen-
trating on the post-synaptic density (PSD). The PSD is a
submembraneous protein assembly found on the cytoplasmic
side of the post-synaptic membrane and its function is
thought to be to regulate the properties of the overlying
membrane (Cotman and Kelly, 1980).

A number of laboratories have reported that during
maturation in the rat there is an increased incorporation
into the PSD of the protein, mPSDp, which forms the
major structural component of adult forebrain PSDs (Kelly
and Cotman, 1981; Fu et al., 1981). We have reported a
similar maturational change in chicken forebrain synapses
in which the only major protein change in the post-hatch
period was the specific increase in the amount of mPSDp
(Rostas and Jeffrey, 1981). We also observed that the
immature synaptic junctions which contain relatively little
mPSDp are more susceptible to disruption by detergents
(Rostas and Jeffrey,1981). As PSDs from immature brain
have been reported to appear less electron dense and
thinner than those from adult brain (Kelly and Cotman,
1981) we have examined the possibility of a direct correlation between the thickness of a PSD and the amount of
mPSDp it contains. We have also examined the changes in
intrinsic protein phosphorylation that occur in isolated
synaptic junctions during maturation because the mPSDp
has been reported to be a phosphoprotein (Grab et al.,
1981) and because phosphorylation may be one mechanism
whereby the regulatory properties of the PSD may themselves be regulated.

METHODS

Male chickens (commercial breed from Steggles Pty. Ltd., Beresfield, N.S.W.) were used in all experiments. Synaptic plasma membrane (SPM) fractions were prepared from forebrain by the method of Cotman and Taylor (1972). Synaptic junction (SJ) fractions were isolated as the detergent insoluble material that sediments through 1.0 M sucrose after treatment of SPM fractions with Triton X-100 (Cotman and Taylor, 1972). Synaptosomes were prepared on an isotonic Ficoll gradient by a modification of the method of Abdell-Latiff (1966) and collected from the 7.5% /13.0% (w.v) interface. An aliquot was processed for electron microscopy and the remainder was osmotically lysed and an SPM fraction prepared from it by the method of Cotman and Taylor (1972).

The samples for electron microscopy were fixed overnight at 4°C in isotonic 4% glutaraldehyde, post-fixed for 1 hour at 4°C in isotonic 1% osmium tetroxide, dehydrated and embedded in resin according to standard procedures. Representative fields were photographed in the electron microscope and printed to a standard magnification of x30,000 for analysis. Measurements were made using a magnifying glass with a graticule (1/10mm units). Electrophoresis in sodium dodecyl sulphate (SDS)polyacrylamide gels was carried out as previously described (Rostas et al, 1979); the stained gels were photographed and the amount of mPSDp was measured by scanning the negatives with a Helena Laboratories scanning densitometer.

Subcellular fractions were phosphorylated by incubation with $[\gamma^{32}-P]$ ATP under conditions which optimize either endogenous cyclic AMP-(Dunkley and Robinson, 1981a) or calcium- (Dunkley and Robinson, 1981b) stimulated protein kinases. Tissue was added to the standard incubation mixture (final volume 100μl) to initiate phosphorylation and reactions were terminated after 30 seconds. Calmodulin was purified by the method of Watterson et al (1976) and added to the incubation mixture (30ng/ml) when required. Labelled proteins were fractionated on polyacrylamide gradient gels and visualized by autoradiography (Dunkley and Robinson, 1981b).

RESULTS

Our first aim was to examine a possible correlation
between the thickness of a PSD and the amount of mPSDp
it contains. The morphological measurements needed to
be made in a sample where the thin PSDs of immature synapses or mature Gray type II synapses could be identified.
The determination of mPSDp levels needed to be made on a
sample that was as enriched as possible for this protein.
Finally, for any correlation to be meaningful, the samples for the two measurements should be the same or as
comparable as possible. Three sources of forebrain
synapses were of potential use: intact tissue, synaptosomes and synaptic plasma membranes. Intact tissue was
not suitable because a specific region of forebrain would
have had to be arbitrarily chosen for the morphometry
while mPSDp was measured in disrupted tissue from a larger
heterogeneous population of synapses. Despite the fact
that synaptic plasma membranes would be prepared from all
synapses in the forebrain this fraction is also not suitable for morphometry because, without the attached pre-
synaptic bouton, thin PSDs would be very difficult to
recognize. On the other hand estimations of mPSDp levels
would be easiest in an SPM fraction. Isolated intact
synaptosomes offered the ideal compromise of retaining
the presynaptic bouton for the identification of the thin
PSDs as well as providing a representative sample of synapses from whole forebrain. Therefore we chose to perform the morphological measurements on intact synaptosomes
from whole forebrain and, in order to facilitate the quantitation of the mPSDp levels, SPM fractions were prepared
from the synaptosomes for the protein determinations.

Table I shows that between 2 days and full maturity
the thickness of the average PSD approximately doubled.
At 2 days only 35% of the PSDs had a maximum thickness of
greater than 20nm (Gray type I synapses) whereas in the
adult 68% of the synapses were in this class (not shown).
When the SPMs prepared from the synaptosomes were examined
by SDS polyacrylamide gel electrophoresis there was a
marked corresponding increase in the mPSDp content of the
membranes. In order to aid in the quantitation of this
increase in mPSDp several protein species of similar
molecular weight were removed by a detergent extraction.
The membranes were briefly extracted at room temperature
with 0.5% (w/v) sodium deoxycholate/10mM Tris, pH8, and

Table 1 MATURATION OF POST SYNAPTIC DENSITIES IN CHICKEN
        FOREBRAIN

	PSD thickness (nm)	mPSDp (arbitrary O.D. Units)
adult chicken	38.6 ± 5.5 (192/5)	9.8 ± 1.8 (6)
2 day chick	20.0 ± 5.3 (121/5)	3.4 ± 0.4 (6)
16 day embryo	8.3 ± 7.8 (55/5)	trace (6)

Values given are mean ± standard deviation. The numbers in brackets are the number of PSDs measured and the number of animals from which they came (PSD thickness) and the number of animals (mPSDp). The PSD thickness is the maximum thickness because this is much easier to measure than average thickness and gives results which are directly proportional to measurements of average thickness (Güldner, unpublished). The level of mPSDp was measured by densitometry of the deoxycholate insoluble fraction from SPM (see text and Figure 1).

the soluble and the insoluble fractions were separated by centrifugation in a Beckman Microfuge. Under these conditions apparently all of the mPSDp remained in the insoluble fraction and the maturational change in the mPSDp content appeared to be of the same magnitude as that visualized in the unextracted SPMs but it was now possible to accurately quantitate it using densitometry (Figure 1). Table I shows that in the same period the mPSDp level almost tripled. Surprisingly, the length of the post-synaptic density profile did not change at all during this period (adult: 298 ± 86nm; two day: 304 ± 39nm.)

That this increase in PSD thickness and mPSDp content is part of an overall trend can be seen from results obtained from the material prepared from the forebrains of 16 day old chicken embryos. This age was chosen because previous studies (Rostas, Gray and Brent - unpublished) had shown that the mPSDp was first detectable in SJ fractions at 16 to 17 days of embryonic incubation. At 16 days the yields of synaptosomes and SPM were considerably lower than for the older tissue and intact synaptic appositions were much more difficult to find. The thickness of

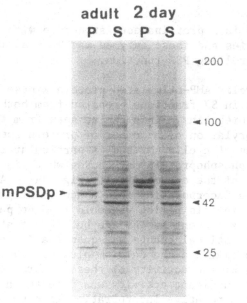

*Fig. 1 Protein composition of synaptic plasma membranes
from the forebrains of one 2 day and one adult chicken.
Apparent molecular weights are shown in daltons x 10⁻³.
P = pellet and S = supernatant obtained by deoxycholate
extraction; mPSDp = major post synaptic density protein.*

the average PSD was about half that of the newly hatched
animal with only 16% of the PSDs being greater than 20nm
thick at their thickest point. At this age the mPSDp is
barely detectable and not possible to quantitate. It is
not surprising that in the embryonic preparations the
average length of the PSD profile (170 ± 110nm.) was
considerably less than the two day value.

Apart from the mPSDp which is a major structural
component we also examined some quantitatively minor
components of SJ fractions which are likely to be functionally important: the membrane-bound intrinsic protein
kinases and their substrates. Protein phosphorylation is
an important and ubiquitous method of regulating protein
function and is the end point of many "second messenger"
systems including cyclic AMP and calcium   (Dunkley,1981).

The PSD is a proteinaceous structure with regulatory
properties and these enzymes may have an important role
in controlling PSD function.

Cyclic AMP-stimulated protein kinase activity was
present in SJ fractions prepared from both two day and
adult forebrains. This can be seen from the increase in
phosphorylation of a number of protein species after the
addition of cyclic AMP and in particular from the change
in the phosphoprotein marked Reg which is the regulatory
subunit of the enzyme itself (Fig. 2a). Although the
relative incorporation into a number of protein species
changed in this period we could find no phosphoprotein
which was present at one age but absent at the other i.e.
the maturational change was quantitative not qualitative.
We also examined the calcium plus calmodulin-stimulated
protein kinase activity of these membranes (Fig. 2b).
Again significant activity was detected at both ages and
while the relative incorporation into some proteins did
change during maturation the change was quantitative not
qualitative. The basal phosphorylation patterns in
Figs. 2a and 2b are not comparable because in Fig. 2a the
basal activity is that measured in the absence of any
additives whereas in Fig. 2b the basal activity is measured after the addition of EGTA to reduce the free calcium
concentration and inactivate the endogenous calmodulin.

The identity and function of most of the phosphoproteins is unknown (Dunkley, 1981) except for the ones
identified in Fig. 2. Of these myelin basic protein and
pyruvate dehdrogenase are known to be present in SJ
fractions as contaminants, and phosphoprotein I and the
cyclic AMP-stimulated protein kinase are regarded as components of the post-synaptic membrane but not specific to
it. Finally there is the calcium plus calmodulin-stimulated phosphoprotein which co-migrates with the mPSDp and
was identified as the mPSDp in dog brain (Grab et al,1981).
Our experiments in chicken brain are consistent with this
claim since the phosphoprotein is present in only those
particulate fractions known to contain PSDs and is present
in much lower levels in SJ fractions prepared from immature brain (Fig. 2b) or adult cerebellum both of which
are known to contain less mPSDp (Rostas, Brent & Dunkley,
unpublished). Fig. 2b. shows that the calcium plus calmodulin-stimulated phosphoprotein band co-migrating with
the mPSDp is also detectable in the

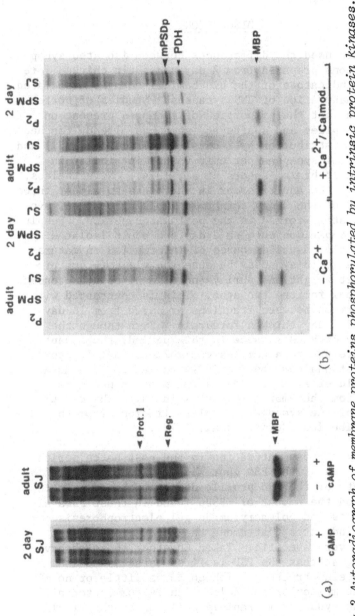

Fig.2.Autoradiograph of membrane proteins phosphorylated by intrinsic protein kinases. (a) cyclic AMP stimulated protein kinases;(b) calcium plus calmodulin stimulated protein kinases. MBP = myelin basic protein,19,000daltons; mPSDp= major postsynaptic density protein,51,000 daltons; PDH= pyruvate dehydrogenase, 42,000 daltons; Prot. I= phosphoprotein I,83,000 daltons;Reg.=regulatory subunit of cyclic AMP stimulated protein kinase, 55,000 daltons.

SPM and P_2 fractions both of which are precursor fractions of SJs in which the concentration of mPSDp is much
lower.

DISCUSSION

We have used the differences between isolated synaptic fractions prepared from 2 day and adult chicken forebrain as indicators of the biochemical changes associated
with the maturation of CNS synapses. Studies of cortex
have shown that the proportion of synapses present on
dendritic spines and shafts and soma has already reached
the adult distribution by 2 days (Corner et al, 1977) and
the number of synapses per unit volume is similar in 2
day and adult brain (Rogers et al, 1974). Nevertheless,
the size of the adult forebrain increases to almost three
times that of the 2 day forebrain implying that new synapses are still formed in the post hatch period. Despite
this the comparison between 2 day and adult isolated synapses is still a valid source of information on maturational change in synapses because the yield (4.4mg pro-
tein/g wet weight)and purity (not shown) of synaptosomes
is identical for the two ages. This is contrasted with
the comparison between fractions prepared from 16 day
embryo and 2 day chicken forebrain. Even though the
brain only doubles in size in this period, the synaptic
changes are due to a complex composite of developmental
and maturational events. This is reflected by a much
lower yield of synaptosomes (2.7mg protein per g wet
weight) from the embryonic tissue in which the cellular
location of the synapses is quite different from the mature distribution (Corner et al, 1977).

During synapse maturation in the post hatch period
the thickness of the PSD approximately doubles while the
mean length of the PSD profile does not change. In the
same period the amount of mPSDp found in these PSDs almost triples and polyacrylamide gel electrophoresis
analysis indicates that among the major proteins this
change is very specific. Taken together these observations suggest that the PSD is first established as a
basic protein structure which contains little or no mPSDp.
This basic molecular scaffold which is common for all
asymmetric synapses is rapidly built up to the final
length for that synapse. With maturation specific

functional (enzymes, receptors etc.) or structural (mPSDp)
components, are added to this structure as needed, altering its thickness but not its length. Of these changes
only the change in mPSDp is visible ultrastructurally
because the mPSDp is such a quantitatively major protein
component. Thus we propose that there is a direct correlation between the amount of mPSDp a PSD contains and its
thickness. This proposal is consistent with the findings
by Carlin et al, (1980) in dogs and confirmed by us in
chickens (Brent & Rostas - unpublished) that isolated
synaptic fractions from brain regions which on average
are known to contain synapses with thinner PSDs than those
from cortex also have less mPSDp. Furthermore, the elevation of circulating testosterone levels in 4 week old
male chickens for 7 days which increases the mPSDp level
of isolated SJs (Rostas and Jeffrey, 1981) also increases
the thickness of the PSD (Rostas and Güldner, unpublished).
Since these results were obtained with a mixed population
of synapses these observations are not based on one idio-
syncratic population and are probably applicable to most
if not all asymmetric synapses.

    Our observations on the changes in synaptic protein
phosphorylation during maturation in the post-hatch period
are also consistent with this model of specific components
being added into an existing framework. Because the isolated SJ fractions used in the phosphorylation experiments
are biased towards the post synaptic half of asymmetric
synapses most of the junctional enzymes and substrates
detected in these experiments are present in the post-synaptic membrane and/or PSD. Cyclic AMP- and calcium plus
calmodulin-stimulated kinase systems were all present in
SJ fractions from 2 day chicken forebrain but the amount
of phosphorylation increased with maturation. As both the
enzymes and their substrates are quantitatively minor protein constituents of SJs it is not possible to say from
these results whether the maturation involves an increase
in enzyme or substrate or both. Studies of the ontogeny
of protein phosphorylating systems in rat brain (Holmes
and Rodnight, 1981) have shown that the appearance of a
group of kinases usually precedes the appearance of its
substrates so the change during maturation is unlikely to
be due to an increase in enzyme level alone. The one exception to the maturational changes appears to be the increase
in phosphorylation of the protein which co-migrates with,

and is tentatively identified as, the mPSDp. As the
mPSDp is a major structural protein we can see that under
a variety of conditions, and from a number of brain regions, the amount of label incorporated into this band
appears to be directly proportional to the amount of
mPSDp detected by conventional protein stains (Fig. 2b.).
Therefore, in this case, the reaction appears to be substrate limited and maturation involves adding substrate
to the basic "molecular scaffold" or adding both substrate
and enzyme.

We also found that a major calcium plus calmodulin-
stimulated phosphoprotein co-migrating with the mPSDp
could be measured in SPM and P_2 membranes. These are the
fractions from which SJs are purified and in which the
level of mPSDp is at least one order of magnitude lower
than in SJs. If it can be shown that the phosphoprotein
in P_2 membranes is a single protein which is identical
to the one in SJs, because the incorporation of label is
substrate limited, it may be possible to measure the
amount of mPSDp in a crude fraction such as P_2 membranes
by measuring the incorporation of ^{32}P into this band.
This would enable mPSDp levels to be measured in small
discrete areas of the CNS where morphological studies
have reported maturational and plastic changes in the
PSDs of discrete neuronal populations (Güldner and Ingham
1979; Vrensen and Nunes Cardozo, 1981). This would permit a direct test of our proposal that a change in PSD
thickness is accompanied by a change in mPSDp content
(and vice versa) and provide a potentially useful tool
for investigating normal and pathological synaptic change.

ACKNOWLEDGEMENTS

We would like to thank Vicki Brent, Marion Gray,
Philip Robinson, Sue Rostas and Debbie Mills for technical
assistance, Bruce Turnbull and Steve McInally for photo-
graphy and Lyndie Barrkman for typing. This work was
supported by grants from the Research Committee of the
Faculty of Medicine and the NH & MRC.

REFERENCES

Abdell-Latif, A.A. (1966) Biochim. Biophys. Acta 121, 403

Carlin, R.K., Grab, D.J., Cohen R.S. and Siekevitz, P. (1980) J. Cell Biol. 86, 831.

Corner, M.A., Romijn, H.J. and Richter, A.P.J. (1977) Neurosci. Lett. 4, 15.

Cotman, C.W. and Kelly, P.T. (1980) In "Cell Surface Reviews" (C.W. Cotman, G. Poste and G.L. Nicolson, eds.), p. 505. Elsevier, Amsterdam.

Cotman, C.W. and Lynch, G.S. (1976) In "Neuronal Recognition" (S.H. Barondes, ed.) p. 69 Plenum Press, New York.

Cotman, C.W. and Taylor, D. (1972) J. Cell Biol. 55, 696.

Cotman, C.W., Nieto-Sampedro, M. and Harris E.W. (1981) Physiol. Rev. 61, 684.

Dunkley, P.R. (1981) In "New Approaches to Nerve and Muscle Disorders. Basic and Applied Contributions". (Kidman A.D., Tomkins, J.K. and Westerman R.A., eds) p.38. Excerpta Medica Amsterdam.

Dunkley, P.R. and Robinson, P.J. (1981a) Biochem. J. 199, 269.

Dunkley, P.R. and Robinson P.J. (1981b) Biochem. Biophys. Res. Comm. 102, 1196.

Fu, S.C., Cruz, T.F. and Gurd, J.W. (1981) J. Neurochem. 36, 1338.

Grab, D.J., Carlin, R.K. and Siekevitz, P. (1981) J. Cell Biol. 89, 440.

Güldner, F.H. and Ingham, C.A. (1979) Neurosci. Lett. 14, 235.

Holmes, H. and Rodnight, R. (1981) Dev. Neurosci. 4, 79.

Kelly, P.T. and Cotman, C.W. (1981) Brain Res. 206, 251.

Reisine, T. (1981) Neuroscience 6, 1471.

Rogers, L., Drennan,H.D. and Mark, R.F. (1974) Brain Res. 79, 213.

Rostas, J.A.P. and Jeffrey, P.L. (1981) Neurosci. Lett. 25, 299.

Rostas, J.A.P., Kelly, P.T., Pesin, R.H. and Cotman, C.W. (1979) Brain Res. 168, 151.

Vrensen, G. and Nunes Cardozo, J. (1981) Brain Res. 218, 79.

Watterson, D.M., Harrelson, W.G., Keller, P.M., Sharief, F. and Vanaman, T.C. (1976) J. Biol Chem. 251, 4501.

IMMUNE DISEASES OF THE PERIPHERAL NERVOUS SYSTEM

I.M. ROBERTS AND C.C.A. BERNARD

NEUROIMMUNOLOGY LABORATORY, LA TROBE

UNIVERSITY, BUNDOORA. AUSTRALIA.

I. INTRODUCTION

When considering the immunological mechanisms involved
in the pathogenesis of any disease of the peripheral
nervous system (PNS) three major questions must be asked:
1. What is the target antigen?
2. What causes the immune damage?
3. What triggers the immune response?

It is not surprising therefore that many investigators
have utilised various animal models to elucidate the
structure of the neuritogenic agent and its localisation
in the PNS and to study the role of cellular and humoral
immunity leading to the pathogenic damages.

Among the few models that have facilitated the
assessment of the immune mechanisms involved in demyelinating diseases of the PNS, experimental autoimmune neuritis
(EAN) has been the most widely studied. Because EAN bears
a close resemblance to the Guillain-Barré-Syndrome (GBS),
a human demyelinating disease of the PNS most researchers
accept that this experimental autoimmune disease is the
animal analogue of the human disease.

The pathological hallmark of both EAN and GBS is a
segmental demyelination with mononuclear infiltration of
peripheral nerve.

The characteristics of GBS are also mimicked in two
naturally occurring demyelinating viral diseases:

Mareks disease of chickens and coonhound paralysis of
hunting dogs.

II. PROTEINS OF PERIPHERAL NERVE MYELIN

Important for understanding the immunological
reactions in diseases of the PNS was the elucidation of
the protein composition of the peripheral nerve myelin.

Myelin produced in the CNS by oligodendrocytes and
in the periphery by Schwann cells share certain biochemical
characteristics. They are however distinct in terms of
overall protein composition, morphological localisation
of various proteins, and the type of disease experimentally induced by the myelin in adjuvant. Central myelin
lacks both Po and P2, two of the three major proteins
present in peripheral nerve myelin.

Po is a glycoprotein comprising over 50% of the total
protein in peripheral nerve myelin (Ishaque et al. 1980),
indicating it probably plays a structural role. Po has
an apparent molecular weight of 30,000 in SDS-polyacrylamide gels. Po minus its carbohydrate component, which
accounts for 6% of its total weight (Roomi et al. 1978),
migrates as an entity with a molecular weight of 23,000
(Roomi and Eylar 1980). Slight interspecies variations
exist in Po, but in all species there is a high percentage
(27-31%)of hydrophobic amino acids (Mezei and Verpoorte
1981).

Po, as detected by its carbohydrate moiety, is
located at the intraperiod lines of myelin which are a
continuation of the extracellular surface of the Schwann
cell plasma membrane (Wood and Mclaughlin, 1975).

P2, like Po, is restricted to peripheral nerve myelin.
It is a fully characterised basic protein, with 131 amino
acids and a MW of 14,800 (Ishaque et al. 1982; Kitamura
et al. 1980). Notable features of P2 are its high content
of β-pleated sheet conformation (Brostoff et al. 1972;
Uyemura et al. 1977), its lack of histidine, and its low
proline content (Ishaque et al. 1981). P2 is present in
the sciatic nerves of all species studied to date, but its
content varies widely, from less than 2% of total myelin
protein in rats and guinea pigs to 15-20% of that in bovine
intradural root (Greenfield et al. 1973). It is also

present in small amounts in spinal cord white matter
(De Armond et al. 1980). The immunocytochemical staining
of P2 in spinal cord was shown to be associated exclusively with nerve rootlets (Eylar et al. 1980) thus confirm-
ing its uniqueness to the PNS. Apparently not all PNS
myelin sheaths contain P2, it being conspicuously absent
from small ones (Winter et al. 1982; Schoeber et al.
1981).

P1 protein of PNS myelin is identical to the major
basic protein of CNS myelin, MBP (Brostoff and Eylar 1972).
It has a MW of 18,300 in its monomeric form and its 169
amino acid residues have been fully sequenced in a number
of species. The only difference between the two appears
to be in the location within the myelin sheath. P1 in the
PNS occurs in the intraperiod line (Mendell and Whitaker
1978) whereas in the CNS, MBP has been localised in the
major dense line of myelin (Poduslo and Braun 1975).
Myelin-associated glycoprotein (MAG), with a MW of
110,000, is also found in both PNS and CNS myelin. It
is present in the periaxonal portion of myelin sheaths of
both oligodendrocytes and Schwann cells and as such may
act as a marker for the cytoplasm of myelinating cells
(Trapp et al. 1979). Less than 1% of protein in CNS
myelin is MAG; its concentration in PNS myelin is
substantially less (Figlewicz et al. 1981).

III. MODELS OF PERIPHERAL DEMYELINATING DISEASES

Experimental Autoimmune Neuritis

Since Waksman and Adams (1955) first immunised
rabbits with heterologous or homologous peripheral nerve
tissue in Freund's complete adjuvant and induced the
disease experimental autoimmune neuritis (EAN), it has
proved to be a suitable and highly reproducible model for
the study of GBS. Clinical signs of EAN appear 10 to
20 days after immunisation, and include hind limb paralysis,
limp tail in rodents, loss of weight and, in more severe
cases, respiratory weakness and occasional forelimb
paralysis. Histological lesions are confined to the PNS
and show infiltration of the nerve roots, spinal ganglia
and peripheral nerves with lymphocytes and macrophages,
accompanied by demyelination and edema.

Neuritogenic antigens. Many studies have been undertaken
to determine the neuritogenic component(s) within the
peripheral nerve tissue. Human fetal peripheral nerve
and human adult vagus nerve, neither of which is significantly myelinated, did not induce EAN in rabbits while the
contrastingly heavily myelinated human adult sciatic nerve
did (Robinson et al. 1972). Sensitisation to bovine PNS
myelin produced EAN in rabbits and guinea pigs (Brostoff
et al. 1972 ; Uyemura et al. 1972). Lewis rats that were
immunised with human PNS myelin developed EAN, with no
involvement of the CNS (Smith et al. 1979; Suzuki et al.
1980). Subsequently, attempts to define the neuritogen
within the PNS myelin have met with inconsistencies.
Suzuki et al. (1980), using P2 purified from human PNS
myelin were able to induce only a mild form of EAN, while
human Po, total myelin lipids, gangliosides or
cerebrosides were ineffective.

Complexing of P2 protein with phospholipids, such as
phosphatidylserine, enhanced the neuritogenic activity
several fold when tested in Lewis rats (Ishaque et al.
1979; Ishaque et al. 1981). This suggests a particular
requirement for the conformation of P2 in the induction of
EAN. In support of this, Boggs et al. (1981) showed that
interaction of P2 with various lipids alters its antigenic
activity. They found that antibodies which reacted with
P2 in the aqueous phase recognised fewer determinants when
the P2 was complexed with lipids such as phosphatidic acid,
phosphatidylserine and cerebroside sulphate. P2 has been
shown to convert from a stable structure in aqueous
solution to a protein with increased α-helical structure in
the presence of lipid (Moore and James 1980). Immunisation
with peptide fragments of P2 have had different effects in
different species. Brostoff et al. (1977) found that the
amino terminal peptide (amino acids 1-20) induced EAN in
rabbits. This same peptide apparently induced EAE in
guinea pigs (Brostoff et al. 1977) and was inactive in rats
(Szymanska et al. 1981). The development of some histological lesions in rabbits immunised with the rest of the
molecule (amino acids 21-131) suggested there may be other
neuritogenic determinants (Brostoff et al. 1977). In
Lewis rats, residues 21-113 showed neuritogenic activity
equal to that of P2 complexed with phosphatidylserine
(Szymanska et al. 1981).

Rabbits immunised repeatedly with galactocerebroside,

a major glycosphingolipid found in both PNS and CNS myelin eventually developed lesions in the PNS but not the CNS (Saida et al. 1979a). However, no signs of EAN were observed in rats immunised with galactocerebroside (Hoffman et al. 1980).

Humoral immunity in EAN. The pathogenesis of EAN is accompanied by development of both a humoral and a cellular immune response. Waksman and Adams (1955) demonstrated complement-fixing antibodies to peripheral nerve in the sera of rabbits with EAN. Antibodies to P2, detected by RIA, were identified in Lewis rats at various times following induction of EAN (Hughes et al. 1981). In neither case did the clinical course of the disease correlate with the appearance or titre of antibodies. Zweiman et al. (1982) detected high levels of anti-P2 antibodies in Lewis rats in which EAN was induced with purified bovine P2 protein. In rats immunised with PNS myelin, they detected antibodies to both P2 and MBP, but only a PNS disease was noted. Hughes et al. (1981) could not detect complement-fixing antibodies to galactocerebroside in rats with EAN. Attempts to passively transfer EAN with serum have not been successful; however demyelinating activity has been demonstrated. Rabbit EAN serum injected into rat sciatic nerve caused extensive demyelination which was complement dependent (Hahn et al. 1980). Serum from rabbits with EAN when injected intraneurally also induced demyelination of rat peripheral nerves in vivo (Saida et al. 1979b). Rabbit antisera to galactocerebroside caused demyelination of both cultured PNS and CNS tissue in vitro (Fry et al. 1974; Saida et al. 1977). Antigalactocerebroside antibody can induce demyelination in vivo, as shown by intraneural injection of antibody (Saida et al. 1978).

Further evidence for the role of humoral immunity in EAN is suggested by a study by McLeod and his colleagues of rabbits with EAN. Plasmapheresis of a group of rabbits immunised with a homogenate of bovine peripheral nerve in FCA resulted in development of less severe symptoms of EAN compared with a non-plasmapheresed group (Antony et al. 1981).

Cellular immunity in EAN.   Most of the available evidence
suggests that EAN is primarily due to a cell-mediated
immune reaction.   In their extensive study, Waksman and
Adams (1955)demonstrated, by skin testing, delayed-type
hypersensitivity (DTH) to peripheral nerve tissue in
rabbits with EAN.   The disease was transferred with
lymphocyte suspensions from EAN animals (Astrom and
Waksman 1962; Hughes et al. 1981).   In vitro demyelination
of cultures of peripheral nerve has been obtained with
lymphocytes from animals with EAN (Winkler 1965).   This
was later confirmed in vivo by Arnason and Chelmicka-Szorc
(1972) who observed demyelination in sciatic nerves of
naive recipients of lymphoid cells from EAN animals.
Lymphocytes from monkeys with EAN transformed in vitro
in the presence of peripheral nerve antigens (Behan et al.
1972).   Lymphoid cells from animals sensitised to a complex
of the 21-113 amino acid residue of P2 and phosphatidylserine responded to P2 and the peptide in a mitogenic assay
(Brostoff et al. 1977).

    In lesions of sciatic nerves, only 9% of the infiltrat-
ing mononuclear cells were B cells, indicating a large
proportion are T cells (Brostoff et al. 1977).   Guinea pigs
immunised with rabbit PNS myelin developed DTH to both Po
and P2, as shown by positive skin tests (Carlo et al. 1975).

Suppression of EAN.   Suppression of EAN in rats can be
obtained by prior treatment with saline suspended nerve
antigens.   Such pretreatment inhibits drastically both
clinical signs and histological lesions of EAN (Lehrich
and Arnason, 1971).   More recently, McDermott and Keith
(1980) showed that when P2 protein is administered in
guinea pigs at the onset of clinical symptoms, the severity
of EAN induced by high doses of bovine PNS myelin is
greatly reduced.   In contrast MBP (P1) has no effect on the
progression of the disease and Po has only a marginal
suppressive activity (McDermott and Keith 1980).

Mareks Disease

    Mareks disease, as first described in Austria-Hungary
by Marek in 1907, is a demyelinating disease of the
peripheral nerve in chickens.   The disease affects birds
most commonly between the ages of three and eight months
and presents clinically as paresis of legs and wings.   The
causative agent has been identified as a herpes virus

(Churchill and Biggs 1967). The lesions which develop in
the peripheral nerve show lymphocytic infiltration and
demyelination, similar to that seen in Guillain-Barré
Syndrome (Borit and Altrocchi 1971).

Pepose et al. (1981) experimentally infected chickens
with Mareks disease virus and tested them seven weeks later,
a time at which there was active demyelination, for
cellular and humoral immunity to peripheral nerve antigens.
Eleven of thirteen birds developed classical delayed type
hypersensitivity reactions. When 5-7 week old chickens,
infected with Mareks disease virus at one day old, were
tested for humoral immunity, seven of nine had serum IgG
which reacted with myelin sheaths of normal chicken sciatic
nerves. Deposits of IgG were also detected in frozen
sections of sciatic nerve in three of the nine birds, as
shown by indirect immunofluorescence.

The importance of cell-mediated immunity in this
disease is borne out by the fact that thymectomy of
chickens reduced the incidence of the disease (Payne et al.
1976). Bursectomy did not influence the course of the
disease (Payne and Rennie 1970). Mareks disease virus can
be recovered from sciatic nerves at the same time as
infiltration of lymphocytes is observed histologically
(Pepose et al. 1981).

A hereditary basis has been observed in chickens, in
that different parentages have led to consistent differences
in degrees of susceptibility to infection with the virus.

Mareks disease virus can, later in the course of the
disease, cause development of neoplastic disease in
lymphoid cells. It is this form of the disease which has
received the most attention. The fact that Mareks disease
virus is a herpes virus, capable of inducing peripheral
nerve demyelination and lymphoid tumors in chickens are all
features shared with the Epstein-Barr virus, pathogenic for
man. Mareks disease of chickens thus appears to be a valid
model for the study of GBS in man.

Coonhound Paralysis

Coonhound paralysis is a naturally occurring neurological syndrome affecting hunting dogs. One to two weeks

after a bite from a raccoon, dogs may develop paralysis
and wasting of the hind limbs with occasional forelimb
paralysis and cranial nerve involvement. The histological
findings in the peripheral nerves correspond closely with
those observed in GBS (Cummings and Haas 1967).

Inoculation of a dog with saliva pooled from several
raccoons, including a known infectious animal, was
successful in inducing paralysis (Holmes et al. 1979).
The disease thus appears to be due to a virus which is
harboured naturally by raccoons and is transmitted in
their saliva. Again, differences in susceptibility to the
disease have been noted (Holmes and de Lahunta 1974), in
that closely related pairs of animals were susceptible.
Another interesting factor which should be investigated
further was the observation that offspring of dogs that
had recovered from coonhound paralysis appeared to be more
susceptible to induction of severe EAN than dogs selected
at random (Holmes and de Lahunta 1974).

IV.   HUMAN DEMYELINATING DISEASES OF THE PERIPHERAL

      NERVOUS SYSTEM.

                    Guillain-Barré-Syndrome

    The Guillain-Barré-Syndrome (GBS) is an acute
demyelinating disease of the peripheral nervous system in
man, first described by Landry in 1859 and subsequently
further defined by Guillain, Barré and Strohl (1916).
It typically, although not always manifests itself following viral infections, surgery, inoculation or mycoplasma
infections.

    No definite clinical or laboratory tests exist as yet
for the diagnosis of GBS. The onset of symptoms is acute
with involvement of the peripheral and in most cases
cranial nerves. Weakness of the respiratory muscles is
involved in 25% of the cases. Most patients recover
spontaneously but there may be residual motor weakness.
Occasionally, the acute form can become a chronic, non-
progressive or remitting polyneuritis. The usual criteria
for classification of GBS are progressive paralysis of
more than one limb, loss of tendon jerks, together with
an increased CSF protein level and evidence of a slowing
or block in nerve conduction. The pathological lesions

occur mainly in the peripheral nerves, with similar
changes in the cranial and autonomic nerves. A study by
Haymaker and Kernohan (1949) showed that the proximal
parts of the nerves were affected the most. The early
pathological changes include oedema and lymphocytic
infiltration, followed by demyelination without axon
damage.

Mechanism of Primary Demyelination. The diversity of
events preceding the onset of GBS suggests that nerve
injury results from manipulation of the immune system.
There is much experimental evidence to support this view.
Asbury et al. (1969) described the presence of inflammatory cells, mainly lymphoid cells with a few macrophages,
in the pathological lesions of fatal cases of GBS. In
another study, Whitaker et al. (1970) identified the cells
infiltrating the lesions as mostly macrophages together
with a few lymphocytes, plasma cells and lymphoblasts.
With the higher resolution of the electron microscope,
it was recognised that macrophages, in the presence of
lymphocytes, were essential for myelin breakdown
(Wisniewski et al. 1969; Carpenter 1972; Prineas 1972).

The important role played by macrophages in regulation
of the immune response has long been recognised. As
effector cells, macrophages can be stimulated either by
antibody or soluble factors released by T cells.

Humoral Immunity. IgA in CSF was found to be selectively
increased in patients with GBS (Asbury et al. 1969). Link
(1973) found increased amounts of IgG, IgA and IgM in
CSF. The presence of oligoclonal IgG bands in CSF has
been reported to occur occasionally (Link et al. 1979).

In 1963, Melnick was the first to find complement
fixing antibodies to peripheral and central nerve tissue
in sera of patients with GBS. These antibodies were
present in 50% of the cases studied, and were even found
at a high titre within 24 hours of the onset of symptoms.

F(ab')2 fragments of IgG reacting with peripheral
nerve were detected in an antiglobulin consumption test
(Nyland and Aarli 1978). Immunofluorescence studies by
Tse et al. (1971) found four out of six GBS sera reacted
with PNS and CNS tissue. All four had IgG antibodies,

three had IgM and two had IgA antibodies to myelin. Five
out of six GBS patients in another study had serum IgG
that reacted with rhesus monkey nerve by immunofluorescence
(Novak and Johnson 1973). Again using immunofluorescence,
Lisak et al. (1975) reported that antimyelin antibodies
were in significantly higher titre in GBS patients.

Primary demyelination of peripheral nerve tissue
in vitro, caused by a complement dependent 19S IgM, was
detected in 26 of 31 GBS sera tested (Cook et al. 1969).
Both Yonezawa et al. (1970) and Dubois-Daleq et al. (1971)
found that GBS sera caused complement-dependent demyelination of rat dorsal root ganglion cultures. Using a
microcomplement fixation assay, Latov et al. (1981) found
five sera reacting with peripheral nerve myelin out of 20
with acute or chronic forms of idiopathic polyneuritis.

Antineuronal antibodies, cytotoxic for mouse neuroblastoma cells were detected in each of six patients with
acute or chronic idiopathic polyneuritis (Rosenberg et al.
1975). This activity was attributed to both IgG and IgM.
Earlier, Dowling and Cook (1973) had detected nonmyelin
antineuronal antibodies in GBS sera. However, there is
virtually no evidence that these may play a role in vivo,
as neither axon nor Schwann cell damage is normally seen in
GBS.

In a study of ten patients afflicted with GBS for less
than 30 days duration, eight had cytotoxic serum activity
to neuroblastoma cells. The factor was shown to be heat
labile, seemingly not complement dependent, and thus not
likely to be an immunoglobulin (Tindall et al. 1980).

In an investigation of sensory peripheral nerve biopsies from six patients with GBS, Luitjen and de la Faille
Kuyper (1972), using indirect immunofluorescence, demonstrated the presence of IgM in a linear pattern along the
myelin sheath in three. Complement components were bound
in four of the biopsies; IgG and IgA could not be detected.
Similarly, Nyland, Matre and Mork (1980) detected immuno-
globulins along the myelin sheath in 4/8 patients.

The recent renewed interest in the role of humoral
immunity in GBS was stimulated by the rapid and remarkable
improvement after plasmapheresis of patients with GBS.

The apparent beneficial effect of plasmapheresis on the
clinical course of GBS (Asbury et al. 1980) could be due
to removal of antibody, immune complexes or other soluble
factors which regulate the immune response. The presence
of immune complexes was detected in 40% of GBS sera
subjected to analytical ultracentrifugation (Dowling et al.
1970). Using the Raji cell radioimmunoassay, Tachovsky
et al. (1976) determined that 5/11 sera from patients with
GBS contained immune complexes. Goust et al. (1978) found
that 15 out of 16 GBS sera tested had immune complexes,
by the $I^{125}Clq$ fluid phase assay. However, levels were
lower than those found in known immune-complex mediated
diseases. Of four GBS CSF samples, three were strongly
positive for immune complexes by a solid phase Clq-Protein
A binding assay (Glikmann et al. 1980). In the only study
in which the antigen in the immune complex has been identified, Penner et al.(1982) found immune complexes containing
hepatitis B surface antigen in serum and CSF during the
acute stage of a case of GBS. The patient developed the
neurological symptoms after an acute infection with hepatitis B virus. The immune complex material decreased with
recovery from GBS. The authors speculated that deposition
of these immune complexes along nerve structures may play
a role in pathogenesis of GBS in some instances.

GBS has also been reported in association with an immune
complex mediated glomerulonephritis (Behan et al. 1973;
Peters et al. 1973; Froelich et al. 1980).

Cell-mediated immunity. Classically, GBS is believed to
be due to a cell-mediated immune response to peripheral
nerve antigens, such as has been demonstrated for CNS
antigens in experimental allergic encephalomyelitis (EAE)
and possibly occurs in EAN (Arnason 1975). Support for this
hypothesis was obtained by Sheremata et al. (1974). They
detected circulating blood lymphocytes to P2 early in the
course of GBS. In a study of one patient with GBS, Berger
et al. (1981) using purified P2, showed an inhibition of
macrophage migration as well as stimulation of mitogenesis
of peripheral blood mononuclear cells, both in vitro
correlates of cell-mediated immunity.

Goust et al. (1978) suggested that a population of
suppressor T cells was reduced in GBS and there was also a
decrease in suppressor cell function. This depression of
suppressor cell function could be the common mechanism

through which the various precipitating factors in GBS
operate (Iqbal et al. 1981).

Lymphocytes from all of nine patients with GBS and
from all of four with chronic relapsing idiopathic polyneuritis were stimulated by P2 to transform in vitro
(Abramsky et al. 1975). In a later study, 18/30 GBS
patients showed cell mediated immune responses to both P2
and Pl in vitro (Abramsky et al. 1980). The role of cell
mediated immunity in GBS is further substantiated by
experiments in which circulating mononuclear cells from
patients with GBS caused demyelination of rat peripheral
nerves in tissue culture (Arnason et al. 1969).

Supernatants from leukocyte cultures from patients
with GBS also caused demyelination in vitro (Cook et al.
1969).

Genetics of GBS. Several autoimmune diseases have been
strongly correlated with HLA genotypes, in particular with
HLA B8 and DW3. Thus, the autoimmune features of GBS
suggest there could well be a genetic component in this
disease. Also consistent with this view is the fact that
only 5% of clinically apparent infections of humans with
Epstein-Barr virus result in neurological complications.

Stewart et al. (1978) found an association of chronic
relapsing polyneuritis with the antigens HLA-AW30 and AW31.
They considered that a larger study would probably point
to a significant association with the genes for HLA-B8 and
DW3 as well as the gene for the red cell enzyme glyoxalase
I. An increased frequency of these latter three were also
found in GBS, but significance was not attained. Adams
et al. (1977) also found a slight increase in HLA-B8 in
GBS patients.

Polyneuropathy and paraproteinemia

The association of polyneuropathy with an Ig-producing
tumor is rare (McLeod and Walsh 1975) but has nevertheless
been investigated with much interest. Julien et al.(1978)
detected, using immunofluorescence, immunoglobulin
deposited in peripheral nerve. Latov et al. (1980)
demonstrated that an IgMκ monoclonal protein, from a
patient with peripheral neuropathy, reacted with PNS myelin.
They subsequently, using an electroimmunoblot technique,
showed the antibody activity was against MAG (Latov et al.

1981).

V. CONCLUSION

At present the etiology and pathogenesis of GBS are
still an enigma. As exemplified by the studies performed in EAN, basic research in experimental animals is
extremely useful in providing a rationale for studies on
human demyelinating diseases such as GBS.

A clear understanding of the autoimmune processes and
regulatory events in models such as EAN will undoubtedly
provide better insight into the immunological events
leading to GBS with distinct possibilities for therapeutic
intervention.

Acknowledgements.

C.C.A. Bernard is a Senior Research Fellow of the
National Health and Medical Research Council of
Australia.

The authors wish to thank Mrs. P. Ciarma for excellent
secretarial assistance.

REFERENCES

Abramsky, O., D. Teitelbaum, C. Webb and R. Arnon (1975):
    J. Neuropath. Exp. Neurol. 34 36-45.
Abramsky, O., Korn-Lubetzky, D. Teitelbaum (1980)
    Ann. Neurol. 8 117
Adams, D., J.D. Gibson, P.K. Thomas, J.R. Batchelor,
R.A.C. Hughes, L Kennedy, H. Festenstein and J. Sachs
(1977):
    Lancet ii. 504-505
Antony, J.H., J.D. Pollard and J.G. McLeod (1981):
    J. Neurol. Neurosurg. Psych. 44 1124-1128
Arnason, B.G.W. (1975): In P.J. Dyck, P.K. Thomas,
E.H. Lambert (eds): Peripheral Neuropathy. Philadelphia
Saunders, p. 110-1148.
Arnason, B.G.W., and G.F. Winkler and N.M. Hadler (1969).
    Lab. Invest. 21 1-10
Arnason, B.G.W. and E. Chelmicka-Szorc (1972):
    Acta Neuropathol. (Berl.) 22 1-6
Asbury, A.K., B.G. Arnason and R.D. Adams (1969):
    Medicine (Baltimore) 48 173-215.
Asbury, A.K., R. Fisher, G.M. McKhann, W. Mobley, A. Server
(1980) Neurology 30 112
Astrom, K.E. and B.G. Waksman (1962):
    J. Path. Bact. 83 89-106.
Behan, P.D., W.M.H. Behan, R.G. Feldman and M.W. Kies
    (1972): Arch. Neurol. (Chicago) 27 145-152.
Behan, P.D., L.M. Lowenstein, M. Stilment and D.S. Sax
    (1973): Lancet i 850-854
Berger, J.R., D.R. Ayyar and W.A. Sheremata (1981):
    Arch. Neurol. 38 366-368
Boggs, J.M., I.R. Clement, M.A. Moscarello, E.H. Eylar
and G. Hashim (1981): J. Immunol. 126 1207-1211
Borit, A. and P.H. Altrocchi (1971): Arch. Neurol.
    24 40-49
Brostoff, S.W. and E.H. Eylar (1972): Arch. Biochem.
    Biophys. 153 590- 598
Brostoff, S., P. Burnett, P. Lampert and E.H. Eylar (1972):
    Nature New Biol. 235 210-212
Brostoff, S.W., S. Levit and J.M. Powers (1977):
    Nature 268 752-753
Brostoff, S.W. J.M. Powers and M.J. Weise (1980):
    Nature, 285 102-104
Carpenter, S. (1972): J. Neurol. Sci. 15 125-140
Churchill, A.E. and P.M. Whitaker and P. Dowling (1969):
    Nature 215 528-530

Cook, S., M.R. Murray, J.N. Whitaker and P. Dowling (1969)
    Neurology (Minneap.) 19 313–413
De Armond, S.J., G.E. Deibler, M. Bacon, M.W. Kies and
    L.F. Eng (1980): J. Histochem, Cytochem 28 1275–1285.
Dowling P.C. and S.D. Cook (1972): J. Neuropath. Exp.
    Neurol. 31 161
Dowling P.C., S.D. Cook (1973): Neurology (Minneap.)
    23 423
Dowling, P.C. J.N. Whitaker and S.D. Cook (1970):
    Neurology (Minneap.) 20 402
Dubois-Daleq, M., M. Buyse, G. Buyse and F. Gorce (1971);
    J. Neurol. Sci. 13 67–83
Eylar, E.H., I. Szymanska, A. Ishaque, J. Ramwani and
    S. Dubiski (1980): J. Immunol. 124 1086–1092
Figlewicz, D.A., R.H. Quartes, D. Johnson, G.R. Barbarash
    and N.H. Sternberger (1981): J. Neurochem. 37 749–758.
Froelich, C.J., R.P. Searles, L.E. Davis and J.S. Goodwin
    (1980): Ann. Int. Med. 93 563–565.
Fry, J.M. S. Weissbarth, G.M. Lehrer, M.B. Bornstein (1974):
    Science 183   540–542
Glickmann, G., S.E. Svehag, E. Hansen et al. (1980):
    Acta Neurol. Scand. 61 333–343
Goust, J.M. F. Cheais, J. Carnes et al. (1978):
    Neurology 28 421–425
Greenfield, S., S.W. Brostoff, E.H. Eylar and P. Morell
    (1973): J. Neurochem. 20 1207–1216
Guillain, G., J.A. Barré and A. Strohl (1916): Bull Soc.
    Med. Hop. Paris 40 1462–1470
Hahn, A.F., J.J. Gilbert and T.E. Feasby (1980): Acta
    Neuropathol. (Berl) 49 169–176.
Haymaker, W. and J.W. Kernohan (1949):   Medicine
    (Baltimore) 28 59–141
Hoffman, P.M., J.M. Powers, M.J. Weise and S.W. Brostoff
    (1980): Brain Res. 195 355–362
Hughes, R.A.C., M. Kodluboswki, I.A. Gray and S. Leibowitz
    (1981): J. Neurol. Neurosurg. Psych. 44 565–569.
Iqbal, A., J. J-F. Oger and B.G.W. Arsason (1981): Ann.
    Neurol. 9 (Suppl)   65–69
Ishaque, A., T. Hoffman and E.H. Eylar (1979): Fed. Proc.
    38 514.
Ishaque, A., M.W. Roomi, I. Szymanska, S. Kowalski and E.H.
    Eylar (1980): Can. J. Biochem. 58 913–921
Ishaque, A., T. Hoffman and E.H. Eylar (1982):
    J. Biol. Chem. 257 592–595

Julien, J., C. Vital, J-M. Vallat, A. Lagueny, C. Deminiere
    D. Darriet. Arch. Neurol. 35 423-425
Kitamura, K., M. Suzuki, A. Suzuki and K. Vyemura (1980):
    FERS Lett. 115 27-30
Latov, N., W.H. Sherman, R. Nemni, G. Galassi, J.S. Shyong,
    A.S. Penn, L. Chess, M.R. Olarte, L.P. Rowland and
    E.F. Osserman (1980): New Eng. J. Med. 303 618-621
Latov, N., P.E. Braun, R.B. Gross, W.H. Sherman, A.S. Penn
    and L. Chess (1981): Proc. Natl. Acad. Sci (USA)
    78 7139
Lehrich, J.R. and Arnason, B.G. (1971): Acta. Neuropath
    (Berl) 18 144-149
Link, H. (1973): J. Neurol. Sci. 18 11-23
Link, H. B. Wahren and E. Norrby (1979): J. Clin.
    Microbiol. 9 305-316.
Lisak, R.P., B.Zweiman and M. Norman (1975): Arch. Neurol.
    32 163-167
Luitjen, J.A.F.M. and E.H. Baart de la Faille Kuyper (1972):
    J. Neurol. Sci. 15 219-224
Marek, J. (1907): Dtsch. Tieraerztl Wochenschr 15 417-421
McDermott, J.R. and A.B. Keith (1980): J. Neurological
    Sci. 46 137-143.
McLeod, J.G., and J.C. Walsh (1975): In Dyck, P.J.,
    P.K. Thomas, E.H. Lambert, eds. Peripheral Neuropathy
    Vol.2 ch. 51, Philadelphia: W.B. Saunders 1975 p.1012.
Melnick, S.C. (1963): Brit. Med. J. i 368-373.
Mendell, J.R. and J.N. Whitaker (1978): J. Cell. Biol.
    76 502-511.
Mezei, C. and J.A. Verpoorte (1981): J. Neurochem.
    37 550-557.
Moore, W. and G. James (1980): Trans. Am. Soc. Neurochem.
    11 88
Novak, D.J. and K.P. Johnson (1973): Arch. Neurol.
    23 219-223
Nyland, H. and J.A. Aarli (1978): Acta Neurol. Scand.
    58 35-43
Nyland, H.R. Matre and S. Mork (1981): Ann. Neurol.
    9 (Suppl) 80-86
Payne, L.N. and M. Rennie (1970): J. Natl Cancer Inst.
    85 59-154.
Payne, L.N. J.A. Frazier and P.C. Powell (1976): Int.
    Rev. Exp. Pathol. 16 59-154.
Penner, E., E. Maida, B. Mamoli and A. Ganzl (1982):
    Gastroenterology 82 576-580.
Pepose, J.S. J.G. Stevens, M.L. Cook and P.W. Lampert (1981):

Am. J. Path. 103 309-320.

Peters, D.K. L.H. Sevitt, L.N. Direkze, S.G. Bayliss (1973) Lancet i 1183-4 Letter

Poduslo, J.F. and P.E. Braun (1975): J. Biol. Chem. 250 1099-1105

Prineas, J.W. (1972): Lab. Invest. 26 133-146

Robinson, H.C., G. All and D.H.L. Evans (1972): Acta Neuropath. (Berl.) 21 99-108

Roomi, M.W., A. Ishaque, N.R. Khan and E.H. Eylar (1978): Biochem. Biophys. Acta 536 112-121

Roomi, M.W. and E.H. Eylar (1980): Trans. Am. Soc. Neurochem. 11 87

Rosenberg, R.N., M.H. Aung, R.S.A. Tindall, et al. (1975) Neurology (Minneap.) 25 1101-1110.

Saida, T., D.H. Silberberg, J.M. Fry et al. (1977): J. Neuropathol. Exp. Neurol. 36 627

Saida, T., K. Saida, D.H. Silberberg and M.J. Brown (1978): Nature 272 639-641.

Saida, K., T. Saida, M.J. Brown and D.H. Silberberger (1979) Amer. J. Pathol. 95 99-116

Shoeker, R., Y. Itoyama, N.H. Sternberger, B.D.Trapp, E.P. Richardson, A.K. Asbury, R.H. Quarles and H. de Webster. Neuropath. App. Neurobiol. 7 421-434

Sheremata, W.A., R.E. Rocklin and J. David (1974): Can. Med. Ass. J. 110 1245-1247

Smith, M.E. L.S. Forno and W.W. Hoffman (1979): J. Neuropath. Exp. Neurol. 38 377-387

Stewart, G.J., J.D. Pollard, J.G. McLeod and C.M. Wolnizer. Ann. Neurol. 4 285-289.

Suzuki, M., K. Kitamura, K. Uyemura, Y. Ogawa, Y. Ishihara, H. Matsuyama (1980): Neurosci. Lett. 19 353-358.

Szymanska, I., A. Ishaque, J. Ramwani and E.H. Eylar (1981) J. Immunol. 126 1203-1206

Tachovsky, T.G., H. Koprowsky, R.P. lisak et al. (1976): Lancet 2 997-999.

Tindall, R.S.A. P. Zinn and R.N. Rosenberg (1980): Neurology 30 362-363.

Trapp, B.D. L.J. McIntyre, R.H. Quarles, N.H. Sternberger and H.D. Webster (1979): Proc. Natl. Acad. Sci. USA 76 3552-3556.

Tse, K.S., C.E. Arbesman, T.B. Tomasi, Jr. and D. Tourville (1971): Clin. Exp. Immunol. 8 881-887.

Uyemura, K., C. Tobar, S. Hirano, and Y. Tsukada (1972): J. Neurochem. 19 2607-2614.

Uyemura, K., T. Kato-Yamaneka and K. Kitamura (1977):

J. Neurochem. <u>29</u> 61–68
Waksman, B.H. and R.D. Adams (1955): J. Exp. Med.
    <u>102</u> 213–236.
Whitaker, J.N,. A. Hirano, S.D. Cook and P.C. Dowling
    (1970): Neurology (Minneap.) <u>20</u> 765–770.
Winkler, G.F. (1965): Ann. N.Y. Acad. Sci. <u>122</u> 287–296
Winter, J. R. Mirsky, M. Kadlubowski (1982): J. Neuropath.
    <u>11</u> 351
Wisniewski, H., R.D. Terry, J.N. Whitaker, S.D. Cook and
    P.C. Dowling (1969): Arch. Neurol. <u>21</u> 269–276.
Wood, J.G. and B.J. McLaughlin (1975): J. Neurochem.
    <u>24</u> 233–235.
Yonezawa, T., N. Robbins, Y. Ishihara et al. (1970):
    In Proceedings of the Sixth International Congress of
    Neuropathology, Paris, Aug. 31 – Sept. 4, 1970.
    Paris, Masson 688–690.
Zweiman, B., A.R. Moskovitz, A. Rostami, R.P. Lisak, D.E.
    Pleasure and M.J. Brown (1982): J. Neuroimmunol.
    <u>2</u>   331–336.

FACTORS UNDERLYING ASCENDING PARALYSIS IN RODENTS

DURING EXPERIMENTAL AUTOIMMUNE ENCEPHALOMYELITIS (EAE)

Rex D. Simmons[1] , Claude C.A. Bernard[1] and Patrick R. Carnegie[2]

[1] Brain-Behaviour Research Institute and [2] School of Agriculture

La Trobe University, Bundoora 3083 Australia

ABSTRACT

EAE in rodents has been the most widely-studied research analog of human demyelinating disease, especially multiple sclerosis. However, accumulating evidence indicates that classical, axon-sparing demyelination cannot be solely responsible for typical behavioral deficits during EAE. The puzzle of clinical pathologic correlation during EAE in rodents is reviewed, emphasizing the discrepancy between the consistent occurrence of "ascending" hind paralysis and the variability of histopathologic changes in the central nervous system (CNS). Several alternative hypotheses of the cause of paralysis during EAE are briefly discussed, including a recently-developed theory based on functional disturbance of peripheral nodes of Ranvier in nerve root myelinated fibers. It is argued that such a theory has definite advantages in explaining typical clinical signs of EAE in rodents.

I. INTRODUCTION

Experimental autoimmune encephalomyelitis (EAE) has been extensively studied as a putative analog of multiple sclerosis (MS). EAE is an inflammatory autoimmune disease of the central nervous system (CNS), readily induced in suscept- ible animal species by intradermal injection of homogenized CNS tissue, or purified myelin basic protein (MBP), in a suitable immunological adjuvant (Kabat et al, 1947; Kies and

99

Alvord, 1959). EAE has both clinical (behavioral) and
histopathologic manifestations which bear resemblance to
human demyelinating diseases, including MS (Raine and Stone,
1977; Wisniewski and Keith, 1977); however, EAE's status as
a viable research analog of MS remains equivocal after many
years of research (Levine, 1974a; Cuzner and Davison, 1979;
Poser, 1979).

An important theoretical difficulty for laboratory
simulation of pathogenic process during MS lies in the well-
known poor clinical pathologic correlation during the disease
(Poser, 1980; Waxman, 1981). During EAE in rodents, the most
widely-studied animal models, clinical pathologic correlation
is also poor (see Section II); in fact, the immediate
cause(s) of typical ascending paralysis during EAE is not yet
known (Carnegie, 1971; Paterson, 1976; Turecky et al, 1980;
Bieger and White, 1981; Simmons et al, 1981). Along with
others, we have recently attempted to elucidate some of the
underlying factors responsible for clinical signs of EAE in
rodents, in the belief that a clear understanding of such
factors would represent an important advance in the field of
research into human demyelinating disease.

II. DISSOCIATION OF CLINICAL SIGNS AND HISTOPATHOLOGIC CHANGES DURING EAE

Although EAE is classified as an immune-mediated demyelinating disease of the CNS (Ludwin, 1981), accumulating
evidence indicates that classical axon-sparing demyelination
cannot be solely responsible for the typical behavioral
deficits of EAE. The histopathologic hallmark of EAE is
perivenous infiltration of CNS tissue by mononuclear inflammatory cells, an event known to precede the occurrence of
demyelination (Waksman and Adams, 1962; Lampert, 1965; Levine,
1971; Lassmann et al, 1981). During acute EAE in rodents,
demyelination is relatively sparse or absent despite severe
hind paralysis (Freund et al, 1947; Bornstein and Crain,
1965; Paterson et al, 1970; Hoffman et al, 1973; Levine, 1974b;
Carnegie et al, 1976; Lassmann and Wisniewski, 1979a).
Analogously, in an initial attack of chronic relapsing EAE
(e.g., hindlimb paralysis occurring in inbred guinea pigs
2-3 weeks after inoculation with whole spinal cord tissue)
demyelination is minimal and appears some days after the onset
of paralysis (Lassmann and Wisniewski, 1978). Hence, there
is evidence that behavioral impairment during EAE is not

dependent on the occurrence of demyelination, a conclusion
supported by the findings of inoculum fractionation studies
which have shown that inoculation of rodents with purified
MBP or peptide fragments thereof, without lipid-containing
fractions of CNS white matter, does not lead to appreciable
demyelination or chronic relapsing disease, even though
clinical signs of hindlimb paralysis occur in all cases
(Hoffman et al, 1973; Raine et al, 1981; Schwerer et al,
1981). Although extensive demyelination is common in CNS
tissue during relapses of chronic EAE, a concomitant increase
in behavioral impairment with progressive demyelination is
frequently not found (Wisniewski et al, 1976; Lassmann and
Wisniewski, 1978; 1979b). Furthermore, the extent of
remyelination of axons during chronic relapsing EAE is
demonstrably too low to account for clinical remissions, as
recently pointed out during EAE in mice (Brown et al, 1982).
It is therefore open to question whether demyelination is
responsible for clinical signs during relapse (Simmons et al,
1981), though it must be borne in mind that recovery of
function in demyelinated axons is not necessarily dependent
on remyelination, but could occur via other mechanisms, e.g.
redistribution of ionic channels along the demyelinated axon
membrane (Ritchie and Rogart, 1977; Bostock and Sears, 1978).

The documented poor correlation between demyelination
and behavioral deficit during EAE in rodents is just one
salient aspect of a broader correlational problem. Despite
the use of many different inoculation procedures, producing
considerable histopathologic and focal variability of EAE
inflammatory lesions within and across rodent species,
*typical clinical signs of ascending paralysis remain the
major, if not only, reproducible impairment*. In guinea pigs
(Freund et al, 1947; Alvord, 1949; Stone et al, 1969;
Hoffman et al, 1973; Raine et al, 1974; Lassmann and Wisniewski, 1978; Bolton and Cuzner, 1980), rabbits (Kopeloff and
Kopeloff, 1947; Feldman et al, 1969), rats (Lipton and
Freund, 1953; Paterson et al, 1970; McFarlin et al, 1974)
and mice (Olitsky and Yager, 1949; Yasuda et al, 1975;
Lublin et al, 1981; Brown et al, 1982), atonia of the tail
(where one exists) and/or hindlimb weakness precedes
paraplegia, which usually precedes any observable forelimb
weakness. Paralysis of the forelimbs is rare (Paterson,
1976), despite focal variability of perivascular inflammatory
lesions within the neuraxis. For example, in rodents with
EAE, lesions have been reported to occur in forebrain and

midbrain (Waksman and Adams, 1962; Paterson et al, 1970;
Rain et al, 1974; Lassmann et al, 1980a), lower brainstem
and cerebellum (Levine, 1974b; Raine et al, 1974; Levine and
Sowinsky, 1980; Lublin et al 1981; Panitch and Ciccone, 1981;
Brown et al, 1982), nerve roots and spinal ganglia (Freund
et al, 1947; Piliero and Cremonese, 1973; Raine et al, 1974;
Paterson, 1976), and optic nerve (Raine et al, 1980) although
the "site of predilection" for EAE lesions in rodents is
spinal cord white matter (Lipton and Freund, 1953; Levine,
1974b; Raine et al, 1974; Lassmann et al, 1981). There is
some suggestion that lesion topography differs in acute and
chronic forms of EAE, in that acute inflammatory lesions
tend to occur randomly in CNS white matter whereas chronic
demyelinated "plaques" in rodents occur mostly in the
thoracic or lumbosacral spinal cord (Lassmann et al, 1980b;
1981).

    In summary, the basic puzzle of clinical pathologic
correlation during EAE in rodents has been to reconcile the
focal and histopathologic variability of EAE lesions with
the limited, strikingly similar clinical signs of ascending
paralysis. Although there is little evidence to suggest
that typical clinical signs of EAE occur in the absence of
perivascular inflammation (Levine et al, 1975 - but see
Paterson, 1982), this may simply indicate that clinical signs
and inflammatory lesions tend to occur together because both
rely for their occurrence on cells and substances coming into
neural tissue during breakdown of the blood-brain barrier
(see next Section).

        III. ALTERNATIVE HYPOTHESES OF NEURAL DYSFUNCTION
                UNDERLYING CLINICAL SIGNS OF EAE

    Having observed the poor clinical pathologic correlation
during MS and EAE, several authors have investigated the
possibility that factors other than demyelination may be
responsible for some of the behavioral manifestations of
these diseases, particularly *transient or fluctuating* changes
in symptoms. Bornstein and Crain (1965) initiated the search
for "neuroelectric blocking factors" i.e., antibodies or
other components of sera from MS patients or animals with
EAE which may interfere with synaptic function. (Limits on
space preclude a full discussion of this area: the reader
is referred to recent reviews by Seil (1981) and Schauf and
Davis (1981). In general, the case for neuroelectric block-

ing factors has been clouded by contrary findings with
respect to *specificity* (control sera have sometimes exhibited
"blocking" activity) and *demyelination-independence* (whether
blocking activity is purely synaptic or depends on disturbance of myelin in the in vitro test systems). Regarding
typical clinical signs of EAE in rodents it has yet to be
explained, even in theoretical terms, how blocking factors
interfering with synaptic function could plausibly result in
ascending hind paralysis. Assuming such blocking factors
enter neural tissue during breakdown of the blood-brain
barrier (Seil, 1981), which occurs throughout much of the
CNS in concert with perivascular lesion formation, why are
clinical signs usually limited to hindlimb paralysis?
Vulnerable sites to such blocking factors need to be postulated (e.g. specific neurotransmitter receptors and systems)
together with an explanation for the apparently greater
vulnerability of more caudal innervation. Perhaps it would
be easier to explain ascending paralysis in terms of *length
of fiber*, e.g. "blocking factors" which may temporarily
disturb adjacent nodes of Ranvier, or perhaps cause perturba-
tions in the electrical properties of the myelin sheath.

   Carnegie (1971) proposed that clinical signs of EAE in
guinea pigs may result from immunopharmacological blockade
of CNS serotonin receptor sites, since the region of MBP
which is encephalitogenic for guinea pigs (the "tryptophan
region" of MBP) bears a striking resemblance in structure to
that suggested for a serotonin receptor. Support for this
hypothesis included the finding that EAE in guinea pigs
could be ameliorated by feeding tryptophan (a serotonin
precursor) and tranylcypromine (a monoamine oxidase inhibitor),
thus increasing CNS levels of serotonin (Lennon, 1972).
Furthermore, guinea pigs with EAE were found to exhibit
impaired function of a peripheral serotonin receptor, since
low concentrations of serotonin added to an organ bath
containing ileum from guinea pigs with EAE failed to elicit
the normal tissue contraction response observed in controls
(Weinstock et al, 1977). This finding has been replicated
(Carnegie and Linthicum, 1979), however a similar failure of
contraction response did not occur when serotonin was added
to isolated jejunum from mice with EAE (Carnegie and Linthicum, 1979). A major problem with Carnegie's (1971) serotonin
hypothesis concerns *generality*: typical clinical signs of
ascending paralysis occur across all commonly-used rodent
species (see Section II) even though the encephalitogenic
determinant region of MBP varies across such species

(Carnegie and Linthicum, 1979). Nevertheless, impairment of
serotonergic function associated with behavioral and neuro-
physiologic events has been reported to occur in rats with
EAE (White et al, 1973; White, 1979; White and Bieger, 1980),
despite the fact that the encephalitogenic determinant for
the rat does not structurally resemble a serotonin receptor
(Carnegie et al, 1976).

Using fluorescence histochemistry, Bieger and White
(1981) have demonstrated monoaminergic axon damage in CNS
tissue of rats with acute EAE. Both catecholaminergic and
serotonergic axons were affected, particularly in bulbo-
spinal areas of perivascular inflammation. Bieger and White
suggested that the probability of axon damage increases with
fiber length, i.e. axons descending to more caudal regions
are likely to sustain more injury as they pass through more
foci of inflammation (Bieger and White, 1981). Such a
suggestion plausibly explains why hindlimb paralysis is far
more common than forelimb paralysis in rodents with EAE, and
in fact is conceptually similar to *implied* explanations of
paralysis based on areas of focal demyelination occurring
in the long tracts of the spinal cord. However, while it is
difficult to explain the *transience* of hindlimb impairment
during acute EAE in terms of demyelination (Simmons et al,
1981), it is even more difficult to explain how rapid recovery from paralysis could occur if the cause of such paralysis
were direct axon damage of the type demonstrated by Bieger
and White (1981). Disturbance of function in other neurotransmitter and putative neurotransmitter systems in the
spinal cord during EAE have been reported, including those
of γ-aminobutyric acid (GABA) (Gottesfeld et al, 1976) and
glycine (Turecky et al, 1980). It is possible that numerous
such effects occur and are secondary to metabolic disturbance
and lactacidosis occurring in the spinal cord during EAE
(see below).

Paterson (1976) observed fibrin deposition associated
with edema in the cauda equina of rats with EAE, and has
suggested that pressure on fibers of the cauda equina may
cause paralysis. Evidence supporting a role for fibrin in
the production of paralysis included the finding that rats
made hypofibrinogenemic by injections of ancrod exhibited a
marked reduction in clinical signs of EAE, without concomitant decrease in cellular infiltrates (Paterson, 1976). We
agree with Paterson that edema in nerve roots may well be
important during EAE in rodents, but have proposed a

different mechanism of paralysis (Simmons et al, 1982)
presently to be discussed. More recently, Paterson (1982)
has suggested that different populations of effector lymphocytes may be responsible for perivascular lesions and breakdown of the blood-brain barrier; further, that this could
explain some of the observed discordance between the occurrence of cellular infiltrates and clinical signs of EAE
(Paterson, 1982).

    Several studies of carbohydrate metabolism in CNS
tissue from rodents with EAE have been reported. Smith (1966)
found increased accumulation of lactate and decreased
production of $^{14}CO_2$ in spinal cord tissue slices (incubated
in vitro) from rats with EAE. These findings were interpreted as indicating possible malfunction of the TCA-cycle
(Smith, 1966). Saragea et al (1965) studied TCA-cycle
intermediates in CNS tissue slices from guinea pigs with EAE,
and found disturbances suggestive of uncoupled oxidative
phosphorylation. Wajda (1972) reviewed these and other early
findings of altered carbohydrate metabolism in CNS tissue
during EAE, and suggested that such disturbances may occur
because of tissue anoxia arising from vasogenic edema following breakdown of the blood-brain barrier (Wajda, 1972). The
wide variety of neurochemical disturbances reported to occur
in CNS tissue during EAE suggested to us that some basic
metabolic failure may underlie many such disturbances and
perhaps, ascending paralysis itself. Initial encouragement
for pursuing such an idea came from documented anatomical
differences in arterial supply to upper and lower regions of
the rat spinal cord (Woollam and Millen, 1955; Tokioka, 1973).
It seemed possible that vascular congestion, arising from
inflammation and increasing numbers of hematogenous cells
entering the CNS during EAE, may occur in the long, descending arterial supply to the lower cord; further, that this
may result in a temporary gradient of ischemia primarily
affecting more caudal regions. Seeking evidence of such
ischemia, we measured accumulation of lactic acid, soon
after decapitation, in three adjacent lower cord regions
during the clinical course of EAE in rats (Simmons et al,
1982). The rats had been inoculated with guinea pig MBP in
Freund's complete adjuvant (CFA). It was found that during
EAE, in correlation with the onset of paralysis of both
initial attack and short-term relapse, a gradient increase
in lactate accumulation occurred in rat spinal cord and
associated nerve roots compared with CFA controls, with

greater increase occurring in more caudal segments. The
maximum lactate increases (in sacrococcygeal regions) were
comparable in magnitude with those found in control cord
subjected to eight minutes of total ischemia at 37^0C,
indicating that considerable lactacidosis occurs in the
lowest cord regions during the onset of ascending paralysis
(Simmons et al, 1982). However, a ^{14}C-antipyrine method of
estimating relative spinal cord blood flow failed to find
evidence that the lactate accumulations were due to focal
ischemia; hence we rejected the hypothesis that anatomical
peculiarity of arterial supply to the lower cord may be related to the production of clinical signs. Subsequent measurements of tritiated water and total protein increases in the
same spinal cord regions indicated that a small but statistically significant increase in vasogenic edema occurred in
correlation with the increased lactate accumulation and the
onset of ascending paralysis. We interpreted these data as
lending support to a speculative, anatomically-based theory
of ascending paralysis during EAE in rodents, presented in
detail elsewhere (Simmons et al, 1982). Briefly, it is
proposed that breakdown of the blood-brain barrier during
EAE leads to accumulation of plasma transudates in high
compliance areas, including nerve root endoneurium which has
a large extracellular space. Due to anatomical ascensus of
the spinal cord in rodents, the length of nerve roots
increases dramatically for more caudal innervation (e.g.
coccygeal roots innervating the tail of adult rats are up to
100 times longer than cervical roots innervating the forelimbs). Hence, during EAE, axon segments innervating more
caudal regions of the body pass through longer regions of
edematous nerve root endoneurium. The peripheral node of
Ranvier's "paranodal apparatus", considered important for
maintaining the nodal sodium pump, contains an unusually
large accumulation of mitochondria within a restricted space
(the juxtanodal Schwann cell cytoplasm) which suggests that
peripheral nodes in nerve root axon segments may be vulnerable to decreased oxygen diffusion in edematous endoneurial
tissue. Critical conduction impairment occurs in the longest
(coccygeal) axon segments first, because more "low efficiency"
nodes in succession occur within the confines of edematous
endoneurium. Hence, in rodents with tails, the first clinical sign of EAE is tail atonia. As endoneurial edema
increases in the shorter roots innervating the hindlimbs,
fibers in these roots gradually develop conduction impairment,
leading to hindlimb paralysis. Frank paralysis of the fore-

limbs does not occur because the cervical roots are too
short for sufficient numbers of adjacent nodes to be affected.
Following initial conduction impairment through node disturbance, recovery from acute EAE may be delayed due to secondary
effects of the edematous insult to neural tissue (Simmons
et al, 1982). We have recently found some further evidence
in support of the above theory, in that when high concentrations of ouabain (a sodium pump inhibitor) were injected
into the lumbar subarachnoid space of normal rats, a flaccid
paraplegia quickly developed which was virtually indistinguishable from severe clinical signs of EAE. Control
injections of saline had no effect (unpublished observations).

While the above theory is certainly speculative, we
believe that it offers the following advantages:

(1)   The limited, ascending nature of typical clinical signs
       of acute EAE in rodents is explained on an anatomical
       basis without reference to variable, punctate neural
       damage occurring at perivascular lesion sites through-
       out much of the neuraxis. Hence, the documented poor
       correlation between clinical signs and demyelinating
       lesions is explained.

(2)   During acute EAE, severe hindlimb paralysis can be
       remarkably transient, as demonstrated by objective
       behavioral measure (Simmons et al, 1981). Rapid
       recovery from clinical signs is readily explained by
       our theory of edema-induced disturbance of neuro-
       physiologic function, because no major morphological
       changes to myelin sheaths or axons are postulated.

(3)   The explanation of clinical signs is not based on
       antibody "blocking factors" or other immunopharmacologi-
       cal events which may vary across different rodent species
       inoculated with different encephalitogenic emulsions.
       Hence, the generality of ascending paralysis during EAE
       in rodents is explained parsimoniously.

Finally, we would like to stress that no single theory
of neurophysiologic dysfunction during EAE is likely to
account for all behavioral permutations encountered during
the disease. For example, it is quite implausible that
chronic, unremitting paraplegia (e.g. Stone and Lerner, 1965)

occurs in the absence of major tissue damage, just as it is equally implausible that similar damage is responsible for fleeting attacks of paraplegia during acute EAE. Indeed, chronic relapsing models of EAE, despite the consistent re-occurrence of hindlimb impairment as the major clinical sign, may incur numerous, superimposed defects in neuro-physiologic function. In view of this real possibility, we believe that initial laboratory attempts to unravel the puzzle of clinical pathologic correlation during EAE should concentrate on elucidating the cause(s) of clinical signs in "simple" models, i.e. acute EAE induced with a well-defined antigen (e.g. purified MBP). As progress is made in the understanding of factors underlying behavioral impairment during "simple" EAE, hypotheses of neural dysfunction in the more complex, chronic relapsing models can be formulated and tested.

REFERENCES

Alvord, E.C. (1949). J. Immunol. 64, 355.

Bieger, D. and White, S.R. (1981). Neuroscience 6, 1745.

Bolton, C. and Cuzner, M.L. (1980). In "The suppression of experimental allergic encephalomyelitis and multiple sclerosis". (Davison, A.N. and Cuzner, M.L. Eds.) p. 189, Academic Press, New York.

Bornstein, M.B. and Crain, S.M. (1965). Science 148, 1242.

Bostock, H. and Sears, T.A. (1978). J. Physiol. (Lond). 280, 273.

Brown, A., McFarlin, D.E. and Raine, C.S. (1982). Lab. Invest. 46(2), 171.

Carnegie, P.R. (1971). Nature (Lond). 229, 25.

Carnegie, P.R. and Linthicum, D.S. (1979). In "The Menarini Series on immunopathology. Vol. 2" (Miescher, P.A. Ed.) p. 61, Schwabe and Co. Ltd., Basel.

Carnegie, P.R., Mackay, I.R. and Coates, A.S. (1976). In Int. Symp. on the aetiology and pathogenesis of the demyelinating diseases Sept. 1973 Kyoto (Shiraki, H. et al, Eds.) Jap. Soc. Neuropathol., p. 275, Japan Science Press, Tokyo.

Cuzner, M.L. and Davison, A.N. (1979). "The scientific basis of multiple sclerosis": Molec. Aspects Med. Vol. 2 p. 147, Pegamon Press Ltd. U.K.

Feldman, S., Tal, C. and Behar, A.J. (1969). J. Neurol. Sci. 8, 413.

Freund, J.,Stern, E.R. and Pisani, T.M. (1947). J. Immunol. 57, 179.

Gottesfeld, Z.,Teitelbaum, D., Webb, C. and Arnon, R. (1976). J. Neurochem. 27, 695.

Hoffman, P.M., Gaston, D.D. and Spitler, L.E. (1973). Clin. Immunol. Immunopathol. 1, 364.

Kabat, E.A., Wolf, A. and Bezer, A.E. (1947). J. exp. Med. 85, 117.

Kies, M.W. and Alvord, E.C. (1959) (Eds.) "Allergic encephalomyelitis", p. 293. Thomas, Springfield, Ill.

Kopeloff, L.M. and Kopeloff, N. (1947). J. Immunol. 57, 229.

Lampert, P.W. (1965). J. Neuropath exp. Neurol. 24, 371.

Lassmann, H. and Wisniewski, H.M. (1978). Acta Neuropathol. (Berl.) 43, 35.

Lassmann, H. and Wisniewski, H.M. (1979a). Brain Res. 169, 357.

Lassmann, H. and Wisniewski, H.M. (1979b). Arch. Neurol. 36, 490.

Lassman, H., Kitz, K. and Wisniewski, H.M. (1980a). In "Search for the cause of multiple sclerosis and other chronic diseases of the central nervous system: proc. 1st int. Hertie symp., Frankfurt, 1979". P. 96. Verlag Chemie, Weinheim.

Lassmann, H., Kitz, K. and Wisniewski, H.M. (1980b). Acta Neuropathol. (Berl.). 51, 191

Lassmann, H., Kitz, K. and Wisniewski, H.M. (1981). J. Neurol. Sci. 50, 109.

Lennon, V.A. (1972). Cellular humoral immune responses in experimental autoimmune encephalomyelitis. PhD Thesis, University of Melbourne (unpublished).

Levine, S. (1971). Res. Publ. Ass. nerv. ment. Dis. 49, 33.

Levine, S. (1974a). In Report and recommendations of the National Advisory Commission on multiple sclerosis (Vol. 2 p. 213) US Dept. of Health, Educ. Welfare Publ.

Levine, S. (1974b). Acta Neuropathol. (Berl.) 28, 179.

Levine, S. and Sowinsky, R. (1980). Am. J. Pathol. 101, 375.

Levine, S., Sowinsky, R., Shaw, C. and Alvord, E.C. (1975). J. Neuropathol. exp. Neurol. 34, 501.

Lipton, M.M. and Freund, (1953). J. Immunol. 71, 98.

Lublin, F.D., Maurer, P.H., Berry, R.G. and Tippett, D. (1981). J. Immunol. 126, 819.

Ludwin, S.K. (1981). In "Demyelinating disease: basic and clinical electrophysiology (Waxman, S.G. and Ritchie, J.M. Eds.) p. 123. Raven Press, New York

McFarlin, D.E., Blank, S.E. and Kibler, R.F. (1974). J. Immunol. 113(3) 712.

Olitsky, P.K. and Yager, R.H. (1949). Proc. Soc. exp. biol.
    Med. 70, 600.
Panitch, H. and Ciccone, C. (1981). Ann. Neurol. 9, 433.
Paterson, P.Y. (1976). Fed. Proc. 35, 2428.
Paterson, P.Y. (1982). Fed. Proc. 41, 2569.
Paterson, P.Y. Drobish, D.G., Hanson, M.A. and Jacobs, A.F.
    (1970). Int. Arch. Allergy 37, 26.
Piliero, S.J. and Cremonese, P. (1973). J. Reticuloendothel.
    Soc. 14, 100.
Poser, C.M. (1979). Med. Clin. North Am. 63, 729.
Poser, C.M. (1980). Arch. Neurol. 37, 471.
Raine, C.S. and Stone, S.H. (1977). N.Y. State J. Med. 77, 1693.
Raine, C.S., Snyder, D.H., Valsamis, M.P. and Stone, S.H.
    (1974). Lab. Invest. 31, 369.
Raine, C.S., Traugott, U., Nussenblatt, R.B. and Stone, S.H.
    (1980). Lab. Invest. 42, 327.
Raine, C.S., Traugott, U., Faroog, M., Bornstein, M.B. and
    Norton, W.T. (1981). Lab. Invest. 45, 174.
Ritchie, J.M. and Rogart, R.B. (1977). Proc. Natl. Acad. Sci.
    USA, 74, 211.
Saragea, M., Clopotaru, M., Sica, M. et al (1965). Med.
    Pharmacol. exp. 13, 74.
Schauf, C.L. and Davis, F.A. (1981). In "Demyelinating
    disease: basic and clinical electrophysiology" (Waxman,
    S.G. and Ritchie, J.M. Eds.) p. 267 Raven Press, New York.
Schwerer, B., Lassmann, H. Kitz, K. et al (1981). Acta
    Neuropathol. (Berl.) Suppl. 7, 165.
Seil, F.J. (1981). In "Demyelinating disease: basic and
    clinical electrophysiology" (Waxman, S.G. and Ritchie,
    J.M. Eds.) p. 281 Raven Press, New York.
Simmons, R.D., Bernard, C.C.A., Ng, K.T. and Carnegie, P.R.
    (1981). Brain Res. 215, 103.
Simmons, R.D., Bernard, C.C.A., Singer, G. and Carnegie, P.R.
    (1982). J. Neuroimmunol. 3, 307
Smith, M.E. (1966). Nature (Lond.) 209, 1031.
Stone, S.H. and Lerner, E.M. (1965). Ann. N.Y. Acad. Sci.
    122, 227.
Stone, S.H., Lerner, E.M. and Goode, J.H. (1969). Proc. Soc.
    exp. biol. Med. 132, 341.
Tokioka, T. (1973). Okajimas Fol. Anat. Jap. 50, 133.
Turecky, L., Liska, B. and Pechan, I. (1980). J. Neurochem.
    35, 735.
Wajda, I.J. (1972). In "Handbook of Neurochemistry Vol. 7"
    (Lajtha, A; Ed.) p. 221, Plenum Press, New York.
Waksman, B.H. and Adams, R.D. (1962). Am. J. Pathol. 41, 135.

Waxman, S.G. (1981). In "Demyelinating disease: basic and clinical electrophysiology (Waxman, S.G. and Ritchie, J.M. Eds.) p. 169, Raven Press, New York.

Weinstock, M., Shohan-Moshanov, S., Teitelbaum, D. and Arnon, R. (1977). Brain Res. 125, 192.

White, S.R. (1979). Brain Res. 177, 157.

White, S.R. and Bieger, D. (1980). Res. Comm. Chem. Pathol. Pharmac. 30, 269.

White, S.R., White, F.P., Barnes, C.D. and Albright, J.F. (1973). Brain Res. 58, 251.

Wisniewski, H.M. and Keith, A.B. (1977). Ann. Neurol. 1, 144.

Wisniewski, H.M., Oppenheimer, D. and McDonald, W.I. (1976). J. Neuropath. exp. Neurol. 35, 327 (Abstract).

Woollam, D.H.M. and Millen, J.W. (1955). J. Neurol. Neurosurg. Psychiat. 18, 97.

Yasuda, T., Tsumita, T., Nagai, Y., Mitsuzawa, E. and Ohtani, S. (1975). Jap. J. exp. Med. 45, 423.

THE INFLUENCE OF UPPER MOTOR NEURONES ON EXCITATION-CONTRACTION COUPLING IN MAMMALIAN SKELETAL MUSCLE

P.W. GAGE & A.F. DULHUNTY

NMRC, SCHOOL OF PHYSIOLOGY AND PHARMACOLOGY

UNIVERSITY OF N.S.W., KENSINGTON, AUSTRALIA

ABSTRACT

Asymmetrical charge movement was recorded in voltage-clamped muscle fibres in rat extensor digitorum longus and soleus fibres. Charge movement was significantly greater and occurred at more positive potentials in extensor digitorum longus fibres than in soleus fibres. A similar difference in voltage-dependence of contraction was recorded in the two types of muscle. There were more indentations in the terminal cisternae of extensor digitorum longus than in soleus fibres. Following spinal cord transection the amount and voltage-dependence of asymmetrical charge movement in soleus fibres became similar to values recorded in extensor digitorum longus. The number of indentations in soleus fibres increased to levels similar to those in extensor digitorum longus fibres. The results strongly support the idea that asymmetrical charge movement is intimately involved in excitation-contraction coupling. Indentations may also have a role in excitation-contraction coupling.

The electrical events leading to a twitch in a skeletal muscle fibre proceed as follows: an action potential, generated at the end-plate region, propagates along the surface membrane and down the transverse tubular system where, in some way, a signal transmitted to the

terminal cisternae of the sarcoplasmic reticulum
stimulates release of calcium. Very little is known about
the mechanism by which depolarisation of the transverse
tubular system causes calcium release from the terminal
cisternae. About 10 years ago, Schneider and Chandler
(1973) detected a small electrical signal in muscle,
generated during depolarization, that had a voltage-
dependence similar to that of contraction. This small
signal, essentially an asymmetrical capacity current, was
thought to represent movement of charge under the
influence of a change in electrical field and it was
suggested that this charge movement somehow increased
calcium conductance in the terminal cisternae.

The link between this asymmetrical charge movement
and excitation-contraction coupling is based on little
evidence apart from their similar voltage-dependence which
could be coincidental. We have exploited the different
voltage-dependence of tension in fast- and slow-twitch
mammalian skeletal muscles (Dulhunty, 1980) to test this
hypothesis. We have also recorded asymmetrical charge
movement in rats following spinal cord transection when
slow-twitch fibres have adopted the characteristics of
fast-twitch fibres. In addition to recording asymmetrical
charge movement, we have examined the morphology of the
terminal cisternae of fast- and slow-twitch fibres in
normal and paraplegic rats. Experiments were done in
extensor digitorum longus and soleus fibres. Paraplegia
was induced in weanling rats (21 to 24 days old) by
transecting the spinal chord in the mid-thoracic region in
anaesthetised animals. About 6-12 weeks post-operatively
the muscles of paraplegic rats were examined.

NORMAL RATS

Charge Movement

Capacity currents generated by imposed steps of
membrane potential were recorded in fibres voltage-clamped
using a three-microelectrode technique (Adrian, Chandler &
Hodgkin, 1970). Ionic currents were suppressed by using
solutions containing tetraethylammonium bromide
substituted for sodium chloride, rubidium chloride
substituted for potassium chloride, and tetrodotoxin.
Contraction was suppressed by adding tetracaine (2 mM).

When asymmetrical charge movement was measured in the
two types of fibre, it was found that the charge movement
was much greater in extensor digitorum longus fibres than
in soleus fibres. For example, in 11 extensor digitorum
longus fibres, the maximum charge was about 23
nanocoloumbs per microfarad whereas, in 11 soleus fibres
the maximum charge was about 4 nanocoloumbs per
microfarad. Half of the maximum charge was generated at a
potential of -19 mV in the extensor digitorum longus
fibres whereas half maximum charge was generated at a
potential of -37 mV in the soleus fibres. Thus there was
a difference both in the magnitude and the voltage-
dependence of charge movement in the two types of fibre.
The difference in the voltage-sensitivity of charge
movement is consistent with the difference in voltage-
sensitivity of contraction previously reported in mice
(Dulhunty, 1978).

Tension

Experiments were done to check the voltage-dependence
of tension in rat extensor digitorum longus and soleus
fibres. Two types of experiment were done. In the first,
two microelectrodes were used to point clamp part of the
surface of a muscle fibre and the threshold for
contraction detected for combinations of duration and
amplitude of depolarizing steps. For these experiments,
solutions contained tetrodotoxin to suppress action
potentials. It was found that, for long pulses (500 ms or
more), the threshold for contraction was, on average,
about 12 mV more negative in soleus than in extensor
digitorum longus fibres. This is similar to the previous
observations in mice. In the second type of experiment,
muscle fibres were depolarized by raising the
extracellular potassium concentration and the resulting
tension during the plateau of the potassium contracture
was recorded. Again it was found that less depolarization
was needed for half maximal contraction in soleus than in
extensor digitorum longus fibres. The difference, on
average, was of the order of 11 mV. These observations
strongly support the idea that the voltage-sensitivity of
contraction is related to the voltage-sensitivity of
asymmetrical charge movement.

Indentations

It has been found that there are more indentations in
the terminal cisternae in fast-twitch than in slow-twitch
fibres (Raynes et al., 1975; Beringer, 1976; Dulhunty et
al, 1981) and this was confirmed in the fibres used in
these experiments.

Freeze fracture techniques were used to visualise
indentations in extensor digitorum longus and soleus
muscles. The regular rows of indentations normally seen
in terminal cisternae of extensor digitorum longus fibres
were not seen in soleus fibres in which indentations
occurred singly or at distances greater than 100 nm from a
nearest neighbour. In five extensor digitorum longus
muscles, the average number of indentations per micron
length of terminal cisterna was 7.3. In contrast, the
average number of indentations in four soleus muscles was
0.9.

PARAPLEGIC RATS

Charge movement

The most obvious effect of chronic spinal cord
transection was an increase in the magnitude and a change
in the voltage-sensitivity of charge movement in soleus
fibres, both characteristics changing towards those of
extensor digitorum longus fibres. In 24 soleus fibres
from paraplegic rats, the average maximum charge movement
was 16 nanocoulombs per microfarad, four times larger than
in normal soleus fibres. Furthermore, half of the maximum
charge was seen with a depolarization of −14 mV (on
average) in contrast to the average value of −37 mV seen
in normal soleus fibres. There was little change in the
maximum charge movement or voltage-sensitivity of
contraction in extensor digitorum longus fibres following
spinal cord transection.

Tension

In soleus muscle fibres from paraplegic rats, the
twitch was much faster than normal. Furthermore the
voltage-sensitivity of contraction was shifted to more
positive levels. In two-electrode voltage clamp
experiments the threshold for contraction with long (more

than 500 ms) pulses was about 12 mV more positive than in soleus fibres in normal rats and was very similar to the level for extensor digitorum longus in paraplegic rats (which had not changed).

Similarly, the membrane potential for half maximal potassium contractures was shifted to more positive levels in soleus fibres from paraplegic rats. The tension-depolarization curves in soleus and extensor digitorum longus fibres from paraplegic rats were much the same as for extensor digitorum longus fibres from normal rats.

Indentations

There was a striking increase in the number of indentations in the terminal cisternae of soleus fibres from paraplegic rats. The terminal cisternae were broader and now contained rows of indentations. In nine soleus muscles from paraplegic rats there were, on average, 5 indentations per micron length of terminal cisterna compared with the 0.9 per micron in soleus fibres from normal rats. This is still less than the density in extensor digitorum longus fibres from normal rats (7.3 per micrometer).

These results point to a close correlation between charge movement and excitation-contraction coupling. Not only is there a parallel difference in these characteristics in normal extensor digitorum longus and soleus fibres but they also change together, and by an approximately equal amount, in soleus muscle fibres following spinal cord transection.

The reason for the difference in the amount of charge movement in the two types of fibre is not clear but presumably has some significance. It may be that in soleus fibres, less charge movement is required to produce calcium current from the terminal cisternae or that less calcium is required for contraction.

We do not know why spinal cord transection changes the characteristics of soleus fibres but think it most likely that it is related to a change in the activity of these fibres. It is known that impulse activity increases in lower motor neurones following upper motor neurone lesions and it could be that this increase in activity converts a slow-twitch fibre to a fast-twitch fibre.

CONCLUSIONS

It is tempting to speculate that there is a close
relationship between the density of indentations and the
magnitude of charge movement, especially as the two
increase by about the same factor in soleus fibres
following spinal cord transection. However, a close
correlation can also be shown between contraction time and
the density of indentations (Dulhunty & Valois, 1983).
Furthermore, it is difficult to devise a role for the
indentations in transferring a signal from transverse
tubule to terminal cisterna because they are located
rather far from the junction between the two. Thus their
role must remain the subject of speculation.

REFERENCES

Adrian, R.H. Chandler, W.K., and Hodgkin, A.L. (1970). *J.
    Physiol., 208,* 607-644.
Beringer, T. (1975). *Anat. Rec. 184,* 647-664.
Dulhunty, A.F. (1980). *J. Membrane Biol. 57,* 223-233.
Dulhunty, A.F. Gage, P.W., and Valois, A.A. (1981).
    Neurosci. Lett. 27, 277-283.
Dulhunty, A.F., and Valois, A.A. (1983). *J. Ultrastr.
    Res.* (submitted).
Rayns, D.G. Devine, C.E., and Sutherland, C.L. (1975). *J.
    Ultrastr. Res. 50,* 306-321.
Schneider, M.F., and Chandler, W.K. (1973). *Nature, Lond.
    42,* 244-246.

EFFECT OF ELECTRIC FIELDS ON NERVE REGENERATION AND FUNCTIONAL RECOVERY IN THE CAT HINDLIMB

R.W. Ziegenbein, R.A. Westerman,
R. Silberstein*, H. Kranz**, J. Cassell**
D.I. Finkelstein & D. Bettess
Department of Physiology,

Monash University, Clayton, Victoria, 3168.

INTRODUCTION, BACKGROUND, AIMS

Steady electric fields are known to affect development, growth and repair of various tissues in vivo and in vitro. Confirmed effects include accelerated repair and regeneration of articular cartilage and bone fractures (Norton, 1974; Baker et al., 1974; Bassett et al., 1974); the induction and control of morphogenesis in amputated forelimb regeneration in adult frogs (Smith, 1974); orientation and acceleration of neurite growth in chick dorsal root ganglia in tissue culture (Jaffe & Poo, 1979) and in differentiating frog embryonic neuroblasts (Patel & Poo, 1982) and myoblasts (Hinkle et al., 1981). Because there are few reports of electric fields influencing mammalian central and peripheral nerves (Wilson et al., 1974; Wilson, 1981), our aim was to examine the effects of such fields on peripheral nerve regeneration and functional recovery in the cat.

*   Department of Physics, Swinburne Institute of Technology

** Neurology and Clinical Neurophysiology Department, Alfred Hospital, Prahran, Victoria.

DC FIELD EFFECTS ON NERVE REGENERATION

METHODS AND EXPERIMENTAL STRATEGY

Operative Technique and Lesion

Symmetrical freeze lesions of the tibial and lateral gastrocnemius nerves were made below the branch to medial gastrocnemius in both hindlimbs of 11 anaesthetized cats. These lesions were equated in every possible way. A 20 mm segment of tibial nerve was exposed in the popliteal fossa and cleared of surrounding tissue, then a metal probe previously equilibrated in liquid N_2 was applied for 15 s to the middle of the exposed nerve segment. Common clinical nerve injuries include transections, avulsions, pressure injuries and contusions (Sunderland, 1978). The freeze lesion we chose produces more predictable bilateral nerve damage with faster regeneration (Samaras, 1981). Full aseptic surgical techniques were used and the incisions were closed in two layers. In the last 3 animals distal hindlimb deafferentation was achieved by L6, L7, S1 dorsal rhizotomy performed bilaterally at the time of the tibial nerve freeze lesions. Results from these animals were treated separately.

Histology

The effect and completeness of the 'standard' freeze lesion was assessed histologically after 11 and 32 d in two animals in which unilateral freezing of the tibial nerve was performed. At the completion of all experiments, after conventional aldehyde fixation and osmium treatment all nerves were embedded in araldite and toluidine blue stained thin sections (0.3 µm) were examined using a Leitz neopromar projecting microscope. The myelinated nerve fibres were counted and profiles were measured for axon diameter, total fibre diameter and myelin thickness with the aid of a Zeiss MOP Z80 image analyser. Figure 1 shows the microscopic appearance of the freeze lesion and the spectrum of regenerating nerve fibre diameters.

After the lesion and wound closure, an AC current was passed through the limb to determine the hindlimb resistance, which measured between 96-288 ohms in the 11 animals used. From this resistance we calculated the

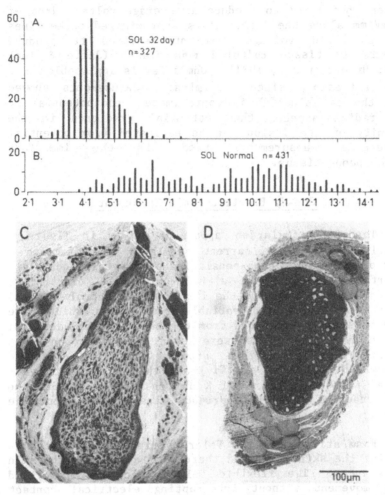

Figure 1.   Shows photomicrographs of soleus nerves
sectioned close to the muscle.   C = soleus nerve
regenerating 32 days after freeze lesion applied
unilaterally,   D = normal contralateral control.
Histograms A,B show the total soleus nerve fibre diameter
spectrum measured close to soleus muscle.   The normal
soleus nerve B shows a bimodal distribution of nerve
fibre diameters (μm) while the regenerating nerve A 32
days after freeze lesion, without electric field
treatment, shows a unimodal distribution of mainly small
diameter myelinated nerve fibres, reduced in total
number.

current necessary to produce an average voltage drop of
20 mV/mm along the limb. This approximated three times
the threshold voltage gradient required to produce
effects in tissue cultured neuroblasts (Jaffe & Poo,
1979; Hinkle et al., 1981). Ohm's law is applicable in
this situation, since preliminary measurements showed
that the cat hindlimb is approximately equipotential in
its radial aspect, thus potential gradients in the
vicinity of the lesion can be estimated from potential
difference measurements taken in the immediate
subcutaneous tissue.

Steady Electric Field Treatment

The DC stimulation apparatus shown in Figure 2
comprised a constant current generator 0-100 mA and a
pair of electrodes each consisting of a metal/electrolyte
interface contained in a half-cell with electrolyte
soaked wicks leading to the limb. The electrolyte/metal
interfaces represented variable resistances which have
been physically separated from the skin to preclude metal
ion transfer. Wicks were used to allow an even
distribution of current around the limb (carried
predominantly by Na^+ and Cl^-) and this electrolyte gel-
soaked wick also gave < 1 K ohm resistance against the
skin ensuring effective current transfer throughout the
limb.

Foam stitched to the Velcro strips also assisted in
keeping the skin moist and therefore in reducing the skin
resistance. The flexible Velcro electrodes permitted
limb movement without interrupting electrical contact
during the continuous 1 h stimulation. Eleven animals
(three with and eight without deafferentation, and all
with bilateral lesions) received 1 h daily unilateral
field stimulation 5 days per week for 32 days, giving an
average 18 h total treatment to one hindlimb of each cat
during this period. The limb treated was chosen at
random, with no restraint or sedation required during
daily stimulation and the electrodes were always
connected with the cathode at the ankle, that is, distal
to the lesion, as neurites grow toward cathode (Jaffe &
Poo, 1979; Hinkle et al., 1981).

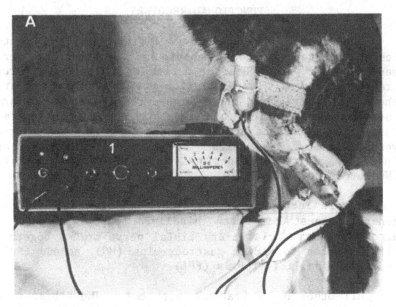

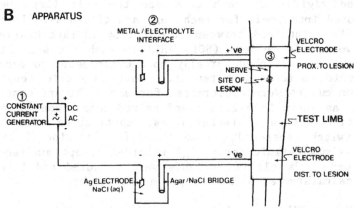

Figure 2. In A, the constant current device (1) is passing 13.0 mA through the half cell electrodes (2,3) and left hindlimb resistance of 139 ohms to achieve an average voltage gradient of 20 mV/mm along the stimulated hindlimb, with 6 cm interelectrode length.

In B the electric field stimulating circuit arrangement in diagrammatic form, using the same identifying numbers.

FUNCTIONAL RECOVERY

Behavioural Observations: During the 32 d post-lesion recovery period, behavioural observations were made of limb weight bearing during walking over a force transducer and of claw protrusion during climbing and are shown in Figure 3.   These manoeuvres tested ankle and knee extensor muscles, and long digit plantar flexors, respectively. Since nerves to both long toe extensors were lesioned, the first signs of claw protrusion indicate a degree of functional recovery of these muscles (Westerman et al., 1982).

Muscle Mechanical Properties: Under pentobarbitone general anaesthesia both hindlimbs were prepared to expose the main sciatic and tibial nerve trunks together with branches to medial gastrocnemius (MG), soleus (SOL) and flexor hallucis longus (FHL).

All other nerve branches were cut. The tibiae were clamped rigidly at both ends and the skin flaps were fashioned into pools for each leg, and filled with liquid paraffin maintained between 36°-37°C by radiant heating. The two muscle tendons (SOL, FHL) in each leg were tied to hooks and attached serially to a dynamometer to record isometric twitches and tetani.   Full isometric length: tension curves were constructed for each test and control muscle as shown in Figure 4 and paired comparisons of the isometric twitch characteristics, contraction time T_c, peak twitch tension P_t, time to half relaxation $(T \frac{1}{2} R)$ and maximum tetanic force (P_o) recorded at optimum length were made.   Muscle wet weights were measured and forces were calculated as N (or mN) per g wet weight.

Nerve Fibres: Using the histological techniques described, the number of regenerating nerve fibres, their axon diameter (d), total nerve fibre diameter (D), 'g ratio' (d/D), and myelin thickness (M) were calculated from the Zeiss MOP data.   Similarly from frozen sections of muscles stained with H & E or NADH the muscle fibre diameters were measured and oxidative enzyme capacity was qualitatively assessed.

RESULTS

Claw protrusion was first observed in electrically

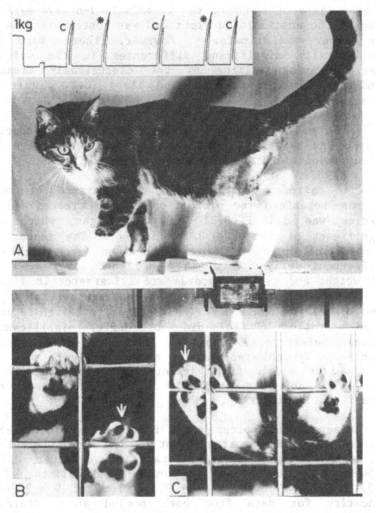

Figure 3.   A: cat walking on dynamometer with left
hindpaw.   Inset: records of 5 consecutive transits in
which limb thrusts (1 Kg calibration) are given by the
upward deflections, forelimb thrusts being almost
immediately followed by ipsilateral hindlimb thrusts;
responses from untreated (C) and stimulated (*) sides of
the animal. B: normal claw protrusion during climbing (R
hindpaw) and absence of claw protrusion after tenotomy of
FHL and FDL (arrow). C: shows claw protrusion more marked
on electrically treated side (arrow) during climbing than
on untreated side.

treated limbs of 6 out of the 11 animals 1-6 days earlier than in the unstimulated limbs and was contemporaneous in the other 5 animals. However, there were no statistically significant differences in the weight-bearing during walking by the electrically treated hindlimbs compared to untreated limbs (c.f. Figure 3, inset).

All nerve counting measurements were conducted blindly and by paired observers, but only the results of 9 soleus muscles and nerves are presently available.

In paired comparisons, the difference of mean maximum tetanic force production by the treated soleus muscles was 1.1 ± 0.32 N/g wet weight, which was significant at the $P < 0.01$; $n = 8$. The respective treated and untreated soleus P_o values from which the differences derived were 4.6 ± 0.55 and 3.5 ± 0.63 N/g wet weight and typical records are illustrated in Figure 4. The twitch characteristics of contraction time (T_c), time to half relaxation ($T \frac{1}{2} R$) and active twitch:tetanic tension ratios (Pt/Po) did not differ significantly between electrically treated and untreated soleus muscles. Typical records are shown in Figure 4. The mean soleus muscle fibre diameters from treated (51 ± 0.7 μm) and untreated (50 ± 0.8 μm) were not significantly different.

Regenerating soleus nerve fibres from electrically treated limbs showed significantly lower 'g ratio', that is, a smaller axon diameter/total fibre diameter, $d/D = 0.54 \pm 0.02$ than those from untreated hindlimbs $d/D = 0.57 \pm 0.12$ ($P < 0.04$; $n = 9$). Plots of D & M show linearity for data from both pooled and individual animals.

With distributions of the shape presently found for these fine regenerating myelinated fibres, neither the mean nor the modal diameter completely describes the population of small numbers of larger diameter fibres in the soleus nerves of treated hindlimbs.Therefore composite histograms of three nerve pairs are illustrated in Figure 5.

In the histogram distributions of regenerating soleus nerve fibres from the electrically treated limbs,

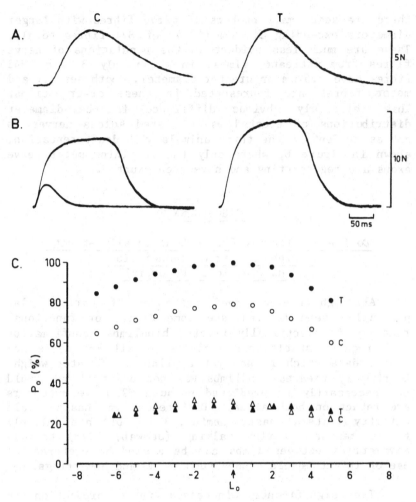

Figure 4. Isometric twitches (A) and tetani (B) are shown for soleus muscles from one animal. Responses from untreated soleus at left, treated hindlimb at right. Force calibrations in Newtons as marked. C. Composite length:tension curve for treated T and control C soleus twitch and tetanic responses. Lengths normalised to Lo ± mm and forces are expressed as % treated side P_o. The data from this one animal and the differences indicated in this figure are representative of the 8 undeafferented animals and correspond closely to the mean P_o differences for that group.

there are seen small numbers of nerve fibres with larger
diameters exceeding 5.5 μm (12.4% of 871 fibres total).
These are much less evident in the populations of nerve
fibres from untreated limbs, in which only 3.2% of 941
fibres have 5.5 μm or greater diameter. Both sensory and
motor fibres are represented in these distributions.
This relatively obvious difference in the diameter
distributions of treated vs untreated soleus nerves is
not as evident in the three animals with deafferentation,
shown in Figure 6, where only the remaining motor nerve
axons are regenerating and have been counted.

DISCUSSION

Do Steady Electric Fields Beneficially Affect
Peripheral Nerve Regeneration
and Functional Recovery?

Although the observed instances of earlier claw
protrusion seem to indicate some degree of functional
recovery in electrically treated hindlimbs, confirmation
will require statistical analysis of all FHL nerve and
muscle data which is not yet available. Greater weight
bearing by treated hindlimbs was not observed but would
not necessarily be predicted because MG ankle extensors
are intact on both sides. Differences in phasic muscle
activity (lateral gastrocnemius, FHL, FDL) are unlikely
to be measured during walking (Jedwab, 1978) because
asymmetries between limbs can be masked by preferential
use of intact muscle groups such as MG and hamstrings.

The significantly increased force production by
treated soleus may indicate a greater degree of
innervation or some increase in muscle functional
capacity such as degree of activation by nerve impulse,
muscle fibre cross sectional area, number of myofibrils,
content of oxidative enzymes etc; that is, a direct
action on muscle rather than its nerve supply.

The contractile characteristics of denervated muscle
have been well described (Lewis, 1972, 1973), but the
soleus twitch characteristics (T_c, P_t, $T \frac{1}{2} R$, P_t/P_o) did
not suggest a greater degree of reinnervation in treated
limbs, nor were the muscle fibre cross sectional areas
significantly greater for treated limbs. Electrical

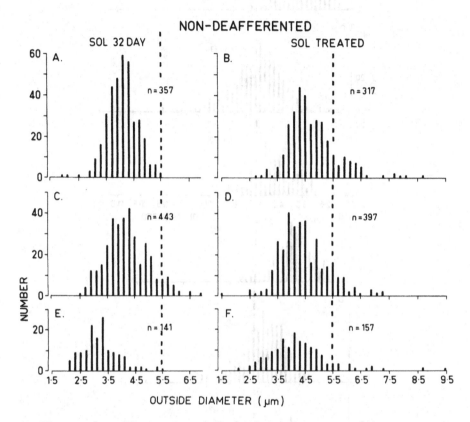

Figure 5.   Histograms A-F depict the nerve fibre counts
and outside fibre diameters for corresponding untreated
(left) and treated (right) soleus nerves from three
undeafferented animals.   The distributions B, D, F from
electrically treated limbs show some larger diameter
fibres (e.g. n=108 i.e. 12.4% above 5.5 μm). These are
not as evident in the nerve fibre diameter spectra A, C,
E from untreated hindlimbs, where only n=30 i.e. 3.2% of
nerve fibres have a diameter greater than 5.5μm.   For all
non deafferented animals, mean regenerating soleus nerve
fibre diameter for treated limbs is 4.5 ± 0.6μm and for
untreated limbs is 4.8 ± 1.3μm, n = 6.

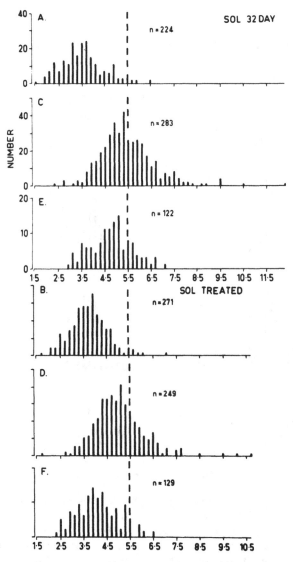

Figure 6. Histograms of counts and outside fibre diameters
for untreated (upper), treated (lower) soleus nerves from
3 deafferented animals. Motor nerve fibre diameters from
treated hindlimbs (B,D,F) show fewer, larger diameter fibre
(11%>5.5μm) than spectra from untreated nerves (A,C,E)
(22%>5.5μm) (Compare figures 5&6). For all deafferented
animals, mean regenerating soleus motor fibre diameter is
4.3±0.7μm for treated and 4.6±1.0μm for untreated nerves.

stimulation for one month after denervation was shown to increase the oxidative enzyme content of soleus muscle (Nemeth, 1982). This muscle in cat contains an almost homogeneous slow oxidative fibre population, but the NADH staining in the present study is more suitable for qualitative than quantitative comparisons, so no measures have yet been made. However, Nemeth's results argues for local effects on muscle contractility rather than innervation.

In contrast to Wilson et al's (1974) reported beneficial effects of RF pulsed electromagnetic treatment of nerve lesions, Hughes et al. (1981) describe myelin and axon degeneration following direct current peripheral nerve stimulation. The present results neither confirm nor refute this suggested deleterious action of DC electrical stimulation on motor nerves. The mean regenerating soleus nerve fibre diameter for treated limbs is smaller (4.5 ± 0.6 μm) than for untreated hindlimbs (4.8 ± 1.3 μm) in the 6 non deafferented, and in 3 deafferented animals (4.3 ± 0.7 μm; 4.6 ± 1.0 μm) respectively. These differences are not significant. However, in the 6 non deafferented animals, the regenerating soleus nerve fibres which may be presumed to be both motor and sensory (Hoffer et al., 1979) did show statistically significant reduction in the mean 'g ratio' for the treated limb nerves. This suggests a larger number of smaller diameter or more thinly myelinated axons in treated nerves. In the histograms of nerve fibre diameter spectra (Figure 5, 6) deafferentation was accompanied by reduction of larger diameter fibres > 5.5 μm in treated nerves but an increased number of such fibres in untreated nerves. This may represent random variation in regeneration and asymmetries in deafferentation (Boyd & Davey, 1968). These differences in fibre numbers between animals and between deafferented and non deafferented groups complicate interpretation of the present data.

The data argue against any beneficial effect of DC electrical stimulation on regenerating motor nerve fibres, but could suggest a contribution of the sensory nerves in the differences observed between electrically treated and untreated soleus nerves (see paper by Westerman et al., 1983). In support of this view the electric field stimulation effects shown in tissue

culture were obtained with sensory neuroblasts from
dorsal root ganglia (Jaffe & Poo, 1979). The persistence
of significant P_o tension differences between soleus
muscles of treated vs untreated hindlimb after
deafferentation suggests a direct effect of electric
field stimulation on the muscle, as discussed.

What Mechanisms Might Underlie the Effects of Electrical Stimulation?

Because the DC stimulation of hindlimbs in the
present study was applied between thigh and ankle, it
does not include neuronal cell bodies. It is therefore
more likely that axonal transport is affected by this
arrangement rather than protein synthesis which occurs in
neuronal cell bodies (Watson, 1974; Grafstein, 1975).
Cathodal accumulation of growth controlling axonal
membrane glycoproteins by the electric field may be
involved (Patel & Poo, 1982). The selective transport of
nerve growth factor (NGF) perhaps by sensory neurones,
has been suggesed (Varon, 1975; Hill et al., 1983) and
the present results of electric field stimulation and
deafferentation would be consistent with such a role for
the afferent connexions, but the small sample size (3
cats) demands cautious interpretation. The results of
deafferentation (Westerman et al., 1983) in a different
peripheral nerve regeneration situation are remarkably
consonant with the present findings, and also suggest
afferent involvement.

The present results are tantalising in several ways:
the number and distribution of total nerve fibre
diameters in histograms (Fig. 5,6) shows an effect of
electric field stimulation not observable in the simple
paired comparison of mean nerve diameters - which
are not significantly different. It is evident from
paired comparisons in deafferented animals that this
effect could be largely or even entirely restricted to
sensory fibres but requires deefferented animals to
confirm it, and this is ethically difficult. Asymmetries
in the number of regenerating nerve fibres within and
between groups complicates interpretation.

Of real concern is the possibility that DC
electrical stimulation may be detrimental to motor fibres

(Hughes et al., 1981). This is not refuted by our present data, apart from the increased force production by electrically treated soleus. In two deafferented animals so far analysed MG nerves show only small bilateral differences. Analysis of all MG data from the present study should provide a comparison between electrically treated and untreated muscles and nerves, which was proximal to and not involved in the freeze lesion. This should reveal any deleterious effects of DC electric field stimulation in the present study, and is being carried out.

REFERENCES

Baker, B., Spadaro, J., Marino, A., and Becker, R.O. (1974) *Ann. N.Y. Acad. Sci. 238*, 491-499

Bassett, C.A.L., Pawluk, R.J., and Pilla, A.A. (1974). *Ann. N.Y. Acad. Sci. 238*, 242-261.

Boyd, I.A. and Davey, M.R. (1968) Composition of peripheral nerves. Livingstone, Edinburgh.

Grafstein, B. (1975). *Exp. Neurol* , 32-51.

Hill, M.A., Nurcombe, V. and Bennett, M.R. (1983). *Neuroscience Letters,* Suppl.11, S52.

Hinkle, L., McCaig, C.D., and Robinson, K.R. (1981). *J.Physiol.314,* 121-135.

Hoffer, J.A., Stein, R.B., and Gordon, T. (1979). *Brain Res. 178*, 347-361.

Hughes, G.B., Bottomy, M.B., Jackson, C.G., Glasscock, M.E., and Sismanis, A. (1981) *Otolaryngol. Head Neck Surg. 89*, 767-775.

Jaffe, L.F., and Poo, M-M. (1979). *J. exp. Zool. 209*, 115-128.

Jedwab, D.J. (1977). *Unpublished B.Sc. Hons. Thesis,* Monash University.

Lewis, D.M. (1972). *J. Physiol. 222*, 51-57.

Lewis, D.M. (1973). *Nature, 241,* 285–286.

Nemeth, P. (1982). *Muscle & Nerve, 5,* 134–139.

Norton, L.A. (1974). *Ann. N.Y. Acad. Sci. 238,* 466–477.

Patel, N., and Poo, M-M. (1982). *J. Neurosci. 2,* 483–496.

Samaras, J. (1981). *Unpublished B.Sc. Hons. Thesis,* Monash University.

Smith, S.D. (1974). *Ann. N.Y. Acad. Sci. 238,* 500–507.

Sunderland, S. (1978). Nerves and Nerve Injuries. 2nd Edition, Churchill-Livingstone, Edinburgh.

Varon, S. (1975). *Exp. Neurol. 48,* 75–92.

Watson, W.E. (1974). *Brit. Med. Bull. 30,* 112–115.

Westerman, R.A., Sriratana, D., and Finkelstein, D.I. (1982). *Exper. Brain Res.* Suppl. 7, pp. 291–297.

Westerman, R.A., Finkelstein, D.I., and Sriratana, D. (1983). This volume.

Wilson, D.H., Jagadeesh, P., Newman, P.P., and Harriman, D.G.F. (1974). *Ann. N.Y. Acad. Sci. 238,* 575–580.

Wilson, D.H. (1981). In: Trans. 1st Ann. Meeting Bioelect. Repair & Growth Soc. Philadelphia, p. 54.

PROPERTIES OF CROSS AND SELF REINNERVATING MOTOR AXONS IN THE CAT.

R.A. Westerman*, D.I. Finkelstein and
D. Sriratana.
Department of Physiology,

Monash University, Clayton, Victoria, 3168.

INTRODUCTION, BACKGROUND, AIMS

Impulse conduction in normal and pathologically altered myelinated nerves has been extensively reviewed by many workers (Paintal, 1978; Sunderland, 1978; Waxman, 1978; 1980). Conduction velocity of nerve impulses is of particular clinical importance in demyelinating disorders (Rogart & Ritchie, 1977; Rasminsky & Sears, 1973). Notwithstanding these data, many aspects of nerve conduction velocity, particularly the underlying mechanisms that determine it, are incompletely understood (Paintal, 1978; Waxman, 1980).

Axotomy of a neurone is followed by a series of changes directed towards restablishing functional peripheral connexions (Watson, 1970; 1974; Grafstein, 1975). Cragg & Thomas (1961) showed that conduction velocity is slowed in nerve fibres regenerating after axotomy and this is associated with reduced axon diameter both proximal and distal to the neuroma at the lesion site (Sanders & Whitteridge, 1946). More recently the axon conduction velocity of reinnervating α-motoneurons above the neuroma was shown by Lewis, Bagust, Webb, Westerman & Finol (1977) to depend upon

*Partial support for this project has been provided by the Australian Research Grants Scheme and is gratefully acknowledged.

the type of muscle into which they regrow. They offered
explanations involving either a direct influence from
the muscle (Kuno, Miyata & Munoz-Martinez, 1974; Lewis
et al, 1977) or a change in the afferent information
sent from a muscle receiving a foreign innervation with
a different pattern of efferent and afferent activity
(Czeh, Gallego, Kudo & Kuno, 1978; Kuno et al, 1974;
Lewis et al, 1977; cf - Gregory, Luff & Proske, 1982).
     The present study further explores this effect of
muscle in determining some properties of reinnervating
motor axons.   It compares conduction velocity (CV) and
physical dimensions of soleus axons allowed to either
self-reinnervate   soleus   (SOL)   muscle   or   cross-
reinnervate the fast twitch muscle flexor digitorum
longus (FDL) or flexor hallucis longus (FHL), with or
without transection of the dorsal roots L6, L7, S1.
Similarly,   axon   dimensions   of   self   or   cross
reinnervating FDL axons were studied.   Thus, this study
is concerned with the effects of the target muscle upon
its innervating nerves and does not re-examine the well
known effects of nerve in determining muscle properties
(Buller, Eccles & Eccles, 1960).

METHODS AND EXPERIMENTAL STRATEGY

Operative and Recording Techniques

     At initial aseptic operations on 16 adult cats
under halothane anaesthesia, SOL and FDL nerves (9 cats)
or SOL and FHL nerves (3 cats) were divided and either
cross or self united to their distal cut stumps.   In 4
animals dorsal roots L6, L7, S1 were abalated at this
time (1 cat) or 3 months later (3 cats).   During
terminal experiments performed with pentobarbitone
anaesthesia six or twelve months after axotomy, single
reinnervated axons were isolated by splitting ventral
roots.   Identified by recording unitary antidromic
action potentials and isometric twitches, their
conduction velocity was calculated from latency and
distance measurements, and their peripheral connexions
to either SOL or FDL were determined.   Radiant heat
lamps maintained the hindlimb and back pool temperature
between 36-37°C.

Histological Methods

After each experiment, nerves were fixed with buffered paraformaldehyde-glutaraldehyde solution and post-fixed with osmium. Portions above and below the neuroma were embedded in araldite, thin sectioned at 0.2 μm and stained with toluidine blue. Other portions were teased (see Fig. 3B) in glycerine with ultrafine needles under a dissecting microscope. A Zeiss MOP measuring device controlled by a Z80 micro-processor was used to count, measure and calculate various physical dimensions. These include nerve fibre outside diameter (D), axon diameter (d), myelin thickness (M) and internode distance (L) from enlarged nerve profiles, microscopically projected onto the MOP measuring tablet by a front-silvered mirror (Finkelstein, 1982; Westerman, Finkelstein & Sriratana, 1983).

RESULTS

The CV findings of Lewis et al (1977) are confirmed by the present results summarized in Figure 1, namely that SOL axons cross reinnervating FDL muscle (Fig. 1A) exhibit a significantly faster CV (mean 73.6 ± 13.4 ms^{-1}, n=114) than axons self reinnervating soleus muscle (mean 65.8 ± 12.2 ms^{-1}, n=167) (Fig. 1B). The effect of deafferenting the hindlimb by dorsal roots (DR) ablation at the time of nerve union is indicated by filled bars in both the second and third histograms (Fig. 1B,C). There are no significant differences in the mean CV of DR ablated self reinnervating units (65.4 ± 14.1 ms^{-1}, n=71) compared to non-deafferented self reinnervating SOL units (65.8 ± 12.2, n=167). The mean CV of n=20 deafferented cross-reinnervating soleus units (DR ablated) was 66.0 ± 13.0 ms^{-1}, not significantly different from the n=71 self reinnervating units DR ablated. This is in marked contrast to the CV behaviour of SOL axons cross reinnervating FDL muscle or self reinnervating SOL muscle with intact DR connexions shown in Fig. 1A. The final CV comparison displayed in the lowest histogram (Fig. 1D) is that between self reinnervating SOL axons isolated from the self united soleus nerve (n=167) and a group of self reinnervating SOL axons, n=41, isolated from soleus nerves which were mainly cross reinnervating FDL muscle. These mean CV's (65.8 ± 12.1 ms^{-1} and 62.5 ± 11.2 ms^{-1} respectively) do not differ significantly.

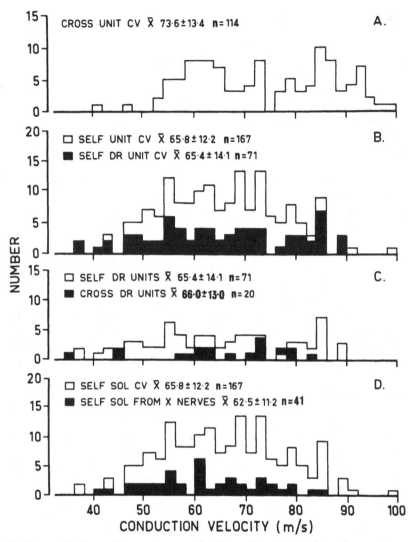

Figure 1A,B. Comparison of distribution of soleus axon
conduction velocity (CV) cross innervating FDL muscle,
A; with CV of self reinnervating SOL axons, B; self SOL
axons with dorsal root ganglia ablated shown as filled
bars in B. Fig. 1,C shows histograms of motor unit CV
from animals with DR ablated; self SOL open bars and SOL
cross reinnervating FDL muscle are filled bars. Fig.
1,D histograms of self SOL unit CV: axons isolated from
nerves which mainly cross reinnervated FDL are shown as
filled bars

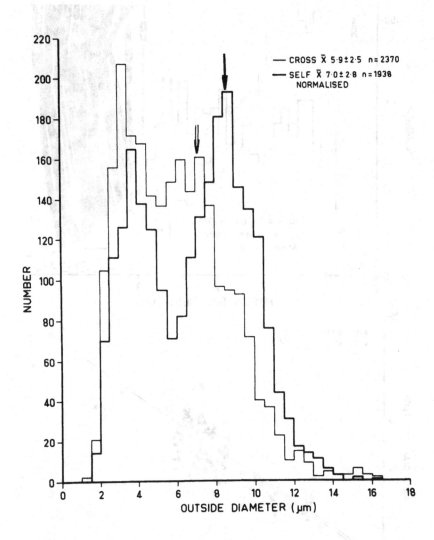

Figure 2. Shows the bimodal distribution of nerve fibre diameter (D) for all self-reinnervating soleus axons (thick histogram outline) and for all SOL axons cross reinnervating FDL (thin histogram outline). Crossed axons show a smaller mean diameter than self reinnervating SOL axons. The open arrow indicates the modal value of the larger diameter peak for SOLxFDL axons at 7μm, while a solid arrow indicates that for the S SOL axons the larger mode is about 8.5μm.

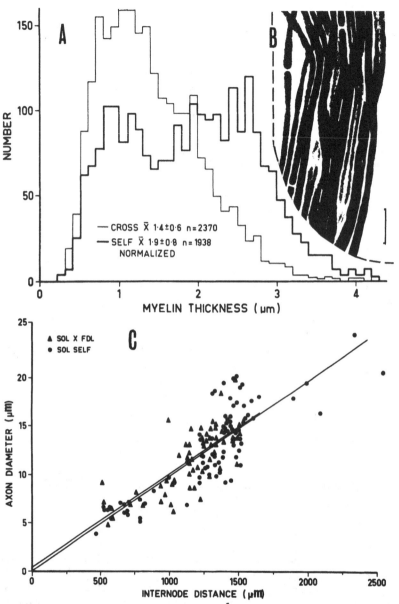

Figure 3.   A: Histograms of myelin thickness (M) for
all SOL self axons (thick outline) and SOL x FDL muscle
(thin outline).   Inset B illustrates individual teased
SOL axons (cal 25 μm) and 3C shows relationship between
internode length (L) and particular axon diameter (d).

The histograms for pooled data of fibre outside diameter (D) and myelin thickness (M) in Figure 2,3A show a smaller mean and mode for the large D or large M peak of the bimodal distribution (alpha modal value) for both D and M in cross reinnervating soleus axons compared to the self-reinnervating SOL axons. The latter distributions are more obviously bimodal. The larger modal peaks which includes alpha motor axons should be compared in these histograms and in Figures 4, 5. Figure 3B (inset) illustrates teased SOL axons and several nodes of Ranvier, and 3C shows the relationship between internodal length (L) and particular axon diameters (d). These linear regressions for internodal length of cross and self-reinnervating SOL axons are not significantly different.

A summary of the raw data distribution of outside diameters of soleus axons cross reinnervating FDL muscles is presented for three individual animals in Figure 4 and these three histograms show comparable distribution of diameters.

Similar data for self reinnervating SOL axons from 6 individual animals is presented in figure 5. No obvious difference is seen between the distribution for self SOL axons deafferented by DR ablation at the time of original operation (Fig. 5E) and the distributions for 5 non-deafferented animals (Fig. 5B,C,D,G,H.). The dimensional properties of regenerating SOL and FDL axons above the neuroma are summarized in Table 1.

The upper half presents the main features of the target muscles (SOL, FDL, FHL) including muscle size, fibre count, alpha axons numbers, innervation ratio and histochemical composition. The lower half table gives the values for pooled modal values in µm for D and M. The modal values given are those of the larger peak of the bimodal distributions becaused in mixed (motor and sensory) regenerating nerve this figure best indicates the alpha motor axons and can be correlated with their conduction velocity.

Figure 6A and Table 1 shows that myelin thickness (M) of both cross and self-reinnervating SOL axons are greater than that of normal soleus(NSOL)axons at any particular fibre diameter D. In turn, M for NSOL is greater than for NFDL. The M of FDL axons cross reinnervating SOL muscle and also self-reinnervating FDL axons is greater than that of normal axons. Comparison of these SOL and FDL results suggests that factors are

influencing SOL axons crossed to FDL muscle (SOL_n x
FDL_m) which are not acting on the FDL axons crossed to
SOL^m muscle (FDL_n x SOL_m)- compare with Lewis et al.,
(1977). Figure 6B depicts the SOL axon data points from
upper panel plotted onto the relationship for g ratio
(d/D) derived by Smith & Koles (1970). This attempts to
predict the effect of M on conduction velocity and
correctly suggests that SOL x FDL axon CV should be
faster than SSOL for any given fibre diameter D, however
it incorrectly predicts NSOL as being faster than SOL x
FDL. In Figure 6B the NFDL point (corresponding to d/D

TABLE 1.

Muscle	Mean Wet Wt.(g)	No.of alpha axons*	No.of fibres x 10^3	Inner- vation Ratio	Histochemical Fibre Types		
					S,	FF,	FR %
SOL.	3.0	155	$24^\dagger$	$155^\dagger$	S		$95\text{--}97^\dagger$
FDL.	1.5	155	23	148	FF	54	
					FR	25	
					S	22	
FHL.	4.5	255	85	333	FF	45	
					FR	47	
					S	8	

*Boyd & Davey, 1968
$\dagger$ Close, 1972.

Nerve type	no.	D(μm)	M(μm)	Nerve type	no.	D(μm)	M(μm)
Normal SOL	3	9.0	1.8	Normal FDL	2	11.5	2.2
Self SOL	6	7.5	2.6	Self FDL	6	11.5	2.8
$Sol_n xFDL_m$	6	7.0	1.8	$FDL_n xSOL_m$	3	11.5	2.9
$Sol_n xFHL_m$	3	9.5	2.5				

(Nerve type refers to operation: n = nerve, m = muscle).

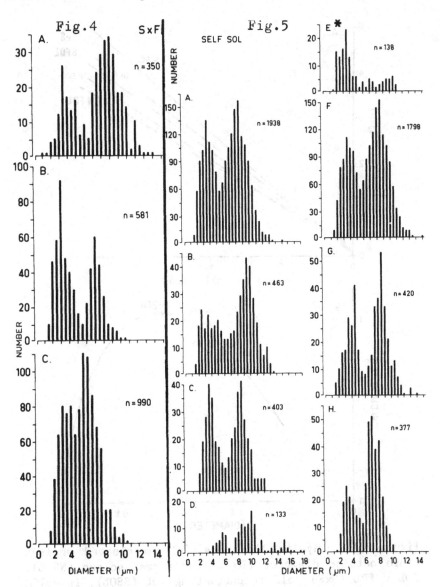

Figure 4. Histograms of fibre outside diameter of SOL axons cross reinnervating FDL muscles for 3 individual animals, A,B,C.

Figure 5. Histograms of fibre diameter of SOL axons self reinnervating SOL muscle. A = total of all SSOL diameters; B,C,D,G,H = SSOL diameters from individual animals SSOL 1-5 respectively. F = sum of SSOL cats 1-5 inclusive. E* = SSOL cat 6 with DR ablated.

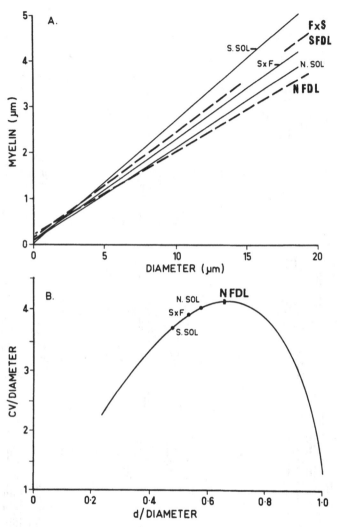

Figure 6A.   Myelin thickness (M) µm plotted against
fibre outside diameter (D) µm for normal soleus (NSOL),
SOL x FDL (SxF) self reinnervating SOL (SSOL), in solid
lines and NFDL, FDL x SOL (FxS), self reinnervating FDL
(SFDL) dotted lines.   Regression lines for FxS, SFDL are
indistinguishable at this scale.
Figure 6B.   SOL and FDL data points obtained from upper
panel are plotted onto the relationship derived by Smith
& Koles (1970) in which the effect of myelin thickness
on conduction velocity is predicted.   Ordinate CV for a
given D; Abscissa = g ratio of d/D.

values for normal FDL axons) is seen to lie close to the
theoretical maximum for g. Reinnervation decreases the
g ratio and the CV for any given FDL axon D (see FxS,
SFDL).

DISCUSSION

Axon Properties and Dimensions

Normally fast and slow motoneuronal properties
differ (Buller et al., 1960) and they show different
reactions to axotomy and following motor reinnervation
(Kuno et al., 1974; Lewis et al., 1977). Various other
experimental manipulations of the synaptic input or axon
termination of motoneurones results in alteration of
motoneuronal properties (Bagust, Lewis & Westerman,
1981) and altered axonal CV follows muscle tenotomy or
deafferentation during development in the rat. Factors
determining the axon CV of reinnervating nerve include
various structural parameters (Waxman, 1978; Westerman
et al., 1983) including fibre size, and contact with a
target organ – muscle – has the most powerful influence
on size of regenerating axons. After a high nerve crush
and either a self or cross-union near the muscle,
Aitken, Sharman & Young (1946) found that diameter of
the regenerating axons varied with the size of the
target organ. In the present study, crossed and self
reinnervating SOL and FDL axons above the neuroma were
compared, and internodal distance did not differ
significantly. Myelin thickness increased in all
reinnervated axons when compared to the normal axon
values with only the exception of SOL nerve
reinnervating FDL muscle. Furthermore, myelin thickness
(M) and axon diameter (d) did vary systematically but
the Smith & Koles (1970) plot of g ratio (d/D) could not
clearly indicate the importance of M as a variable.
Paintal (1978) suggests that for a 30% change in g
(between 0.47-0.74) CV would only vary by 5% so this
variable would contribute little to the observed CV
increase in cross-reinnervating SOL axons. If was found
that the diameter (d) of reinnervating SOL axons varied
with the weight or the innervation ratio of the target
muscle. The alpha mode (larger D peak) increased when
SOL axons reinnervated the larger FHL muscle, and fell
when they reinnervated the smaller FDL muscle (c.f.
Aitken et al., 1946). By contrast the FDL axon did not

exhibit this effect and the diameter of FDL axons did
not increase when they innervated the larger SOL muscle
(c.f. Lewis et al., 1977; Bagust, Lewis & Westerman,
1981). These results are in large part consistent with
the early observations of Aitken et al. (1946) on the
effect of peripheral target field on size of
regenerating axons. Because the D of SOL axons cross-
reinnervating FDL is smaller than D of SSOL axons,
diameter cannot be involved in the observed CV increase.

Of the other known determinants of CV the recording
conditions would exclude temperature as a factor.
Neither the dimensions of nodes of Ranvier nor the
specific membrane properties of the nodes were examined
in the present study, but either or both could be
involved in the CV changes observed. Rydmark (1982) has
demonstrated clear differences in his morphometric data
comparing nodal dimensions of cat ventral and dorsal
root fibres, and his techniques should be applied to the
present experimental model. Species differences of
conductance channel density between frog, rat, cat and
rabbit nerve have been demonstrated by direct electrical
measurements (Neumcke, 1983) and saxitoxin binding has
been used to calculate sodium channel density for rabbit
sciatic nerve (Ritchie & Rogart, 1977). It is not known
whether the area of exposed nodal axolemma and the
number or density of sodium conductance channels differ
for axons supplying different muscles.

A role for muscle afferent connexions?
Such axolemmal differences in excitability could
provide a mechanism by which the SOL axons increase
their CV when cross reinnervated to FDL muscle. The
quite different results for FDL axons either self or
cross reinnervating soleus suggest that the signal for
expression of nodal or Na^+ channel differences probably
lies in the muscle. Nerve growth factor seems to be
involved in retrograde signalling for regulation of gene
expression (Varon, 1975; Thoenen & Barde, 1980) and in
the survival or death of mammalian motor neurons
(Nurcombe & Bennett, 1982). It is not known whether
nerve growth factor production differs for mammalian
fast and slow muscle but the selective or predominant
uptake by sensory nerves has been suggested (Thoenen et
al., 1980). After division and reunion of peripheral
nerve afferent connexions are re-established early, but
function abnormally (Luff, Gregory & Proske, 1982).

Because their response pattern is bizarre and their numbers reduced, Lewis et al. (1977) suggested that this abnormal afferent input might contribute to the observed CV differences in SOL axons x FDL muscle.

In the present experiment after deafferentation the significant differences in the distribution of soleus conduction velocities (or their mean or modal values) between the self and cross-reinnervating populations are absent. This result, together with the apparent preferential involvement of sensory fibres in the effects of electric field stimulation on regenerating nerve fibres (Ziegenbein et al., 1983) suggests a regulatory role for sensory connexions in determining the expression of some motor axon characteristics.

The apparently inappropriate dimensional changes observed in cross and self reinnervating SOL and FDL axons may be better analysed in future in terms of the volume of myelin comprising each internode i.e. the surface area of the axolemma beneath the myelin sheath (Smith, Blakemore, Murray & Patterson, 1982).

REFERENCES

Aitken, J.T., Sharman, M. and Young, J.Z. J. Anat. 81, 1-22.

Bagust, J., Lewis, D.M. & Westerman, R.A. (1981). J. Physiol. 313, 223-235.

Boyd, I.A. and Davey, M.R. (1968). "Composition of Peripheral Nerves." Edinburgh, Livingstone.

Buller, A.J., Eccles, J.C. and Eccles, R.M. (1960). J. Physiol. 150, 399-439.

Close, R.F. (1972). Physiol. Rev. 52, 129-197.

Cragg, B.G. and Thomas, P.K. (1961). J. Physiol. 157, 315-327.

Czeh, G., Gallego, R., Kudo, N. and Kuno, M. (1978). J. Physiol. 281, 239-252.

Finkelstein, D.I. (1982). Unpublished M.Sc. Qualifying Thesis. Monash University, Department of Physiology.

Finkelstein, D.I., Sriratana, D. and Westerman, R.A. (1983) Proc. Aust. Physiol. Pharmacol. Soc. 14, 30P.

Grafstein, B. (1975). Exp. Neurol. 48, 32-51.

Gregory, J.E., Luff. A.R. & Proske, U. (1982). J. Physiol. 331, 367-383.

Jeffrey, P.L., Leung, W.N. and Rostas, J.A.P. (1981). In: "New approaches to nerve and muscle disorders. Basic and applied contributions". Edited by A.D. Kidman, J.K. Tomkins and R.A. Westerman. Excerpta Medica, Amsterdam, p. 66-79.

Koles, Z.J. & Rasminsky, M. (1972). J. Physiol. 227, 351-364.

Kuno, M., Miyata, Y. & Munoz-Martinez, E.J. (1974) J. Physiol. 242, 273-288.

Lascelles, R.G. and Thomas, P.D. (1966). J. Neurol. Neurosurg. Psychiatry, 29, 40-44.

Lewis, D.M., Bagust, J., Webb, S., Westerman, R.A. & Finol, H. (1977). Nature, 270, 745-746.

Neumcke, B. (1983) In: "Membrane permeability: experiments and models". Edited. by A.H. Bretag, Adelaide, Techsearch Inc.

Nurcombe, V. & Bennett, M.R. (1982) Neuroscience Letters Suppl. 8, S12.

Paintal, A.S. (1978). In: "Physiology and pathobiology of axons". Edited by S.G. Waxman. Raven Press, New York. p. 131-144.

Rasminsky, M. & Sears, T.A. (1973). In: "New developments in Electromyography and clinical Neurophysiology", Edited by J.E Desmedt. Vol. 2, 158-165.

Ring, G., Shugerman, H. and Rotshenker, S. (1983) Neuroscience Letters 35, 18-24.

Ritchie, J.M. & Rogard, R. (1977). Proc. Nat. Acad. Sci. 74, 211-215.

Rogart, R. & Ritchie, J.M. (1977). In: "Demyelinated nerve fibres". Edited by P. Morell. Plenum, New York. p. 353-383.

Rogart, R. (1981). Ann. Rev. Physiol. 43, 711-725.

Russell, N.J.W. (1980). J. Physiol. 298, 347-360.

Rydmark, M. (1982). An ultrastructural morphometric analysis of the node of Ranvier in peripheral myelinated nerve fibres in the adult cat. Ph.D. Thesis, Karolinska Institute, Stockholm.

Sanders, F.K. & Whitteridge, D. (1946). J. Physiol. Karger, Basel, 105, 152-174.

Smith, K.J., Blakemore, W.F., Murray, J.A. & Patterson, R.C. (1982). J. Neurol. Sci. 55, 231-246.

Smith, R.S. & Koles, Z.J. (1970). Am. J. Physiol. 214, 1256-1258.

Sunderland, S. (1978) "Nerves and Nerve Injuries". 2nd Edition. Churchill-Livingstone, Edinburgh.

Tal. M. & Rotshenker, S. (1983) Neuroscience Letters 35, 25-31.

Thoenen, H. and Barde, Y.A. (1980) Physiol. Rev. 60, 1284-1335.

Varon, S. (1975) Exp. Neurol. 48, 75-92.

Watson, W.E. (1970). J. Physiol. 210, 321-343.

Watson, W.E. (1974). Brit. Med. Bull., 30, 112-115.

Waxman, S.G. (1978). In: "Physiology and pathobiology of axons". Edited by S.G. Waxman. Raven Press, New York, p. 169-190.

Waxman, S.G. (1980). Muscle and Nerve, 3, 141-150.

Westerman, R.A., Finkelstein, D.I. & Sriratana, D. (1983). In: "Molecular aspects of Neurological Disorders". Edited by L. Austin & P.L. Jeffrey. Academic Press, Sydney. p. 95-102.

Ziegenbein, R.W., Westerman, R.A., Silberstein, R., Kranz, H., Cassell, J., Finkelstein, D.I. & Bettess, D. In: "Molecular pathology of nerve and muscle" Edited by A.K. Kidman & J. Tomkins.

Note added in proof:

   The recent finding of Ring, Sugerman & Rotshenker (1983) and Tal & Rotshenker (1983) suggest that contralateral motor axons sprouting may follow unilateral deafferentation. If this occurs in the cat, then reinterpretation of the results of dorsal root ablation will be required, and all bilateral comparisons should be viewed with even more caution.

MORPHOMETRIC ASSESSMENT OF PERIPHERAL NERVE

S.ALLPRESS, M.POLLOCK,H.NUKADA

Department of Medicine, University of Otago

Medical School, Dunedin, New Zealand.

ABSTRACT

In the past, peripheral nerve morphometric techniques have been infrequently fully utilized. This has reflected the laborious and time-consuming nature of traditional peripheral nerve morphometry. Now with the availability of computer programmes and direct projection techniques, peripheral nerves can be rapidly and more completely assessed. In this paper we describe inexpensive contemporary techniques of morphometrically assessing peripheral nerve. Single teased nerve fibre analysis gives rapid quantitation of demyelination, remyelination, axonal degeneration and regeneration. A computerised analysis of internodal length provides such statistics as number, mean and coefficient of variation of internodal length and frequency distribution of internodal length. Binomial distribution is used to determine whether demyelinated or remyelinated internodes are grouped or randomly distributed. By using a particle analyser, densities and diameter histograms can be determined and plotted for total, small and large nerve fibre populations. Electron microscopic negatives when directly projected provide such parameters as axonal area, axonal perimeter, whole nerve fibre area, myelin perimeter, number of myelin lamellae, densities of axonal or Schwann cell organelles and indices of axonal or myelin circularity. The use of such morphometric techniques has greatly improved the assessment of peripheral nerve in clinical and experimental settings.

151

INTRODUCTION

Morphometric evaluation of peripheral nerve has seldom been fully exploited. In part, this relates to a lack of rigorous processing techniques to provide optimally fixed tissue and in part to the expensive and time-consuming nature of traditional morphometric methods. With the development of back projection techniques and the use of 35 mm strip film, comprehensive morphometric data can be obtained quickly and inexpensively. Utilising simple computer programmes full use can be made of measured data.

METHODS

Human Nerve Biopsy

Of the various peripheral nerves available for biopsy, the sural nerve has been most frequently biopsied, usually just proximal to the lateral malleolus (Dyck and Lofgren 1966, 1968; Thomas 1970; Asbury and Johnson 1978). An additional segment of sural nerve may also be removed in the mid calf region to substantiate a dying-back pathology (Moss et al 1979). Whole nerve biopsy is preferred as it is simpler, faster and less painful than fascicular biopsy and it enables whole nerve morphometry and pathology to be determined. Clinical and electro-physiological follow-up of 16 control subjects, at least five years after sural nerve biopsy, has shown no significant difference in sensory loss or sensory symptoms between whole nerve and fascicular biopsy (Pollock et al 1983a). For less experienced operators, the whole nerve biopsy technique reduces the risk of peripheral nerve crush or traction artefact. Once a 2-3 cm length of sural nerve has been removed for morphological study, the dissection may be extended caudally to provide further nerve for *in vitro* conduction studies, biochemical analyses, tissue culture or histochemistry.

Nerve Processing

The procedure recommended (Table 1) enables evaluation of epoxy and paraffin embedded tissue and routine analysis of individual teased nerve fibres from a single nerve specimen. For *in vitro* fixation peripheral nerve is

NERVE PROCESSING

Teased Fibre	Epoxy Embedding
2% Glutaraldehyde in 0.1M Cacodylate Buffer 10-15 min ▼	2% Glutaraldehyde in 0.1M Cacodylate Buffer 90 min ▼
0.1M Cacodylate Buffer 3 x 35 min washes ▼	0.1M Cacodylate Buffer 3 x 10 min washes ▼
1% Osmium Tetroxide in 0.1M Cacodylate Buffer 90 min ▼	1% Osmium Tetroxide in 0.1M Cacodylate Buffer 90 min ▼
0.1M Cacodylate Buffer 3 x 10 min washes ▼	0.1M Cacodylate Buffer 3 x 10 min washes ▼
66% Glycerol Overnight at 60°C ▼	1% p-Phenylenediamine in 70% Ethanol 30 min ▼
100% Glycerol Tease or Store at 4°C	10 min wash in each of:- 80%, 90%, 100%, 100% Ethanol ▼
	100% Propylene Oxide 2 x 10 min washes ▼
	50% Epoxy Resin in Propy- lene Oxide Overnight ▼
	100% Epoxy Resin 60 min ▼
	Embed in 100% Epoxy Resin ▼
	Check orientation after 2h Cure at 65°C for 48h

All processing done at 20-25°C and at pH 7.4

Table 1.   *Processing schedule for concurrent*
preparation of teased fibres and
epoxy embedded nerve.

suspended using weighted hooks (200 mg) and fine silk
sutures (6-0) (Dyck and Lofgren 1966) to minimise collagen
shortening. The period of primary glutaraldehyde fixation
of the nerve segment reserved for teasing should not exceed
10-15 mins to avoid over-fixed "woody" nerve fibres which
are difficult to separate and prone to stretch artefact.
Thus each nerve specimen following the initial fixation
period is gently removed from glutaraldehyde and sectioned
on a moist soft wax block to provide a 1 cm segment for
teased nerve fibres and an 0.5 cm nerve segment for
embedding in paraffin. Nerve segments damaged by hooks
and sutures are discarded and distal nerve ends marked by
an oblique cut. Biopsy specimens of peripheral nerve
prepared for teased fibre analysis are suitable even after
prolonged storage, for quantitation of peripheral nerve
collagen (Myers et al 1977). The remainder of the nerve
specimen, following its more prolonged fixation in glutaraldehyde, is divided into fascicles, and cut into 1 mm
lengths to ensure optimum penetration of osmium. A 2 mm
segment of whole nerve is reserved for measurement of
whole nerve area. Routine enhancement of osmium staining
with p-phenylenediamine allows direct light microscopic
evaluation of epoxy embedded tissue.

Teased Nerve Fibres

On the day following the nerve biopsy, 2-3 hours is
required to tease 100 single nerve fibres in glycerol,
using a pair of fine curved watchmaker forceps. A more
representative distribution of teased fibres can be obtained when 100 single fibres are obtained equally from 50
strands of endoneurium (Dyck et al 1982). To retain proximal - distal orientation nerve fibres are transferred to
slides with minimum amounts of glycerol. Each internode is
measured in length, using an ocular micrometer and
graded descriptively (Dyck 1975). This information, together with each nerve fibre grade, is entered directly into
a computer. Statistics may be obtained for all 100
teased nerve fibres, or for specific categories of internodes or nerve fibres. Two examples of data that may be
generated are:

(a)   the number, mean, standard deviation and coefficient
       of variation of internodal length of normal inter-
       nodes

(b)   the frequency distribution of mean internodal lengths
       of remyelinated nerve fibres.

Using the number of abnormal internodes divided by
the total number of internodes as the probability of internodal abnormality, it is possible to determine whether
abnormally graded internodes are randomly distributed, or
clustered along particular nerve fibres.

Myelinated Nerve Fibre Diameters

Transverse sections of the epoxy embedded fascicles,
approximately 1 μm thick, are used to determine density
and size distribution of myelinated nerve fibres. A
minimum of 1000 myelinated nerve fibre diameters (axon plus
myelin) are measured on non-overlapping photographic enlargements (x 1200) using a particle size analyser with 48
intervals (Zeiss TGZ-3). A computer is used to plot
frequency or percentage histograms of myelinated nerve
fibre size distributions, and to calculate the density of
myelin fibres per mm^2 or per whole nerve. The programme
is able to use data from multiple cases and create composite histograms. The mean, standard deviation, cumulative
frequency and percentage of nerve fibre diameters is also
obtained. Diameter distribution histograms are compared
statistically, using the Kolmogorov-Smirnov two sample
test (Siegel 1956) based on the agreement between two
cumulative frequency distributions. This test is also used
to compare small diameter (less than or equal to 7 μm) and
large diameter (greater than 7 μm) nerve fibre distributions.

Ultrastructural Morphometry

A minimum of 100 myelinated nerve fibres (Bronson et
al 1978) are photographed as encountered serially in X and
Y traverses of at least 5 different electronmicroscopic
grid spaces. Using a motorised film strip projector, (Fig1)
35 mm electronmicrographic negatives are back projected and
axonal and nerve fibre perimeters measured with a computerised X-Y digitiser. The number of myelin lamellae and
axonal or Schwann cell organelles may also be determined
from back projected negatives. However, because of the
high number of neurofilaments in large myelinated nerve

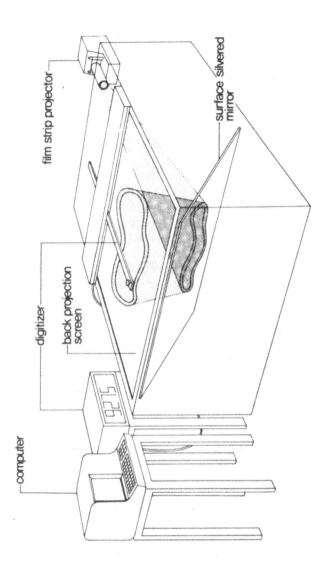

Figure 1.   *Diagram of digitizer and back projection sys-*
tem used to count organelles and myelin lamellae in peri-
pheral nerve and to measure nerve fibre area and circum-
ference.

fibres, these are counted only in a selected axonal area drawn across the largest diameter of each nerve fibre (Pollock and Dyck 1976). A computer calculates and compares means, standard deviations and distributions of measured parameters and determines myelin periodicity, indices of circularity, and regression analyses (relating number of myelin lamellae to axonal areas and perimeters).

A qualitative electronmicroscopic review of nerve sections is normally all that is required to assess unmyelinated nerve fibres. However, where there has been prominent loss of pain and temperature or autonomic dysfunction, quantitation of unmyelinated fibres may be required. Unmyelinated nerve fibres are sensitive to preparation artefact and reliable morphometry depends on good fixation and an absence of surgical trauma. 35-40 random non-overlapping 35 mm electronmicrographs are taken at low magnification (nerve area per micrograph equals 600 um^2). Each negative is then back projected and the number of unmyelinated nerve fibres counted. Numbers of Schwann cells, fibroblasts, macrophage nucleii, clusters of denervated Schwann cells and collagen pockets are also determined.

To obtain an unmyelinated nerve fibre diameter histogram a further 10-15 photographs are taken at higher magnification including as many unmyelinated nerve fibre clusters as possible. On the prints made at a final magnification of approximately 12,000, all unmyelinated nerve fibres are measured with a particle size analyser.

By this method 0.02-0.025 mm^2 of nerve (i.e. 2.5-3.0 % of the mean whole nerve area) is sampled to obtain a density of unmyelinated nerve fibres and 300-500 unmyelinated nerve fibres (i.e. 1-2% of the mean number of unmyelinated nerve fibres) measured to obtain an unmyelinated fibre size distribution histogram.

DISCUSSION

The present approach to peripheral nerve morphometry is aimed at reducing the cost and time of each evaluation while obtaining the maximum information from each biopsied nerve. An advantage of the present fixation technique is

that it allows concurrent processing of several nerve
specimens.

An analysis of single teased nerve fibres by descrip-
tive grading and measurement of individual internodes
provides data not obtainable by qualitative analysis alone.
Thus in cold injured nerve normally graded internodes were
shown to have significantly shorter mean internodal lengths
(Nukada et al 1981). Dyck and colleagues (1982) have shown
that less than one quarter of demyelinated nerve fibres
clearly identified by examination of teased fibres, were
recognised in transverse sections of peripheral nerve.
Teased nerve fibres with short, regular, thinly myelinated
internodes also provide strong evidence of peripheral nerve
regeneration. Analysis of the distribution of demyelinated
or remyelinated internodes determines whether these are
randomly distributed, suggesting an abnormality of Schwann
cells, or occur in groups along particular nerve fibres,
suggesting demyelination as a consequence of a primary
axonal atrophy (Dyck et al 1981a). Thus on the day following nerve biopsy a report on the frequency of teased nerve
fibres exhibiting axonal degeneration, demyelination,
remyelination, regeneration or tomaculae can be given and
on the following day a full internodal statistical report
can be provided.

Myelinated nerve fibre density and nerve fibre size
distribution histograms can be obtained on the fourth day
following nerve biopsy. It is preferable to measure myelinated nerve fibre size exponentially to accentuate the
small nerve fibre population. The plotting of percentage
diameter histograms allows visual comparison of nerve
fibre distributions from nerves with markedly different
nerve fibre densities. Impressions of abnormalities in
nerve fibre diameter distribution histograms can be
statistically compared using the Kolmogorov-Smirnov two
sample test. This detects in a quantifiable way subtle
shifts of nerve fibre populations.

Use of 35 mm microscopic roll film has the advantage
of low cost, speed (40 negatives per electron-microscopic
cassette) and suitability for rapid digitization. A
motorised roll film projector with remote control for fast
forward and reverse allows large areas of peripheral nerve
to be quickly surveyed. Reflecting the image with a high

quality mirror onto a horizontal back projection screen in
a darkened room preserves sufficient resolution to allow
the counting of myelin lamellae and cellular organelles.
Thus it is possible in 3 days to complete an electron-
microscopic morphometric analysis of 100 myelinated nerve
fibres. Regression analysis and indices of circularity
(Dyck et al 1980) provide valuable statistical evidence for
or against demyelination, remyelination, nerve fibre oedema
or axonal atrophy.

A problem continuing to face the morphologist is the
accurate evaluation of unmyelinated nerve fibre densities.
In part this is due to the large number and irregular
clustering of Remak cells. It is also a manifestation of
the difficulty of differentiating unmyelinated nerve fibres
from Schwann cell processes and regenerating myelinated
nerve fibres. Moreover, we have no ready means of distinguishing in peripheral nerve biopsies nociceptive
afferents from post ganglionic sympathetic fibres. The
present technique of measuring and counting only 1-3%
of unmyelinated nerve fibres and 10 % of myelinated nerve
fibres may prove to be an insufficient sample. The advent
of video and computer interfacing with the electron
microscope will improve nerve morphometry by allowing
direct rapid counting and digitization of nerve fibres.

Nerve biopsy is a painful procedure, at least at the
moment when the nerve is transected or interfascicular
branches are cut. Moreover sural nerve biopsy may result
in sensory loss in the lateral sole, leading rarely to
ulcer formation in the analgesic heel. While long term
pain or paraesthesias are uncommon following sural nerve
biopsy there is a high incidence of tactile-induced
dysesthesias (Pollock et al 1983). In view of these
complications is sural nerve biopsy clinically justified?
We believe it is provided patients are carefully selected
and there is local expertise in taking, processing and
morphometrically evaluating peripheral nerve. Quantitative
histological study of nerve is a more sensitive method of
detecting early or mild neuropathy than sophisticated
neurophysiological investigation (Behse and Buchthal 1978).
In syndromes where there are variable clinical manifestations and morphological specificity (e.g. Type I and II
hereditary sensory neuropathies) peripheral nerve biopsy
will settle the diagnosis (Nukada et al 1983). Nerve

biopsy will also establish the diagnosis of hereditary
neuropathy when it is the only abnormality in affected kin
(Dyck et al 1981b). Finally, nerve biopsy is required when
a suspected neuropathy has a distinctive histological
picture (Pollock et al 1983).

However, it is important that the specifity of each
peripheral nerve "work-up" be recognised to avoid number
"crunching" so easily obtained with computerisation. The
direction of each morphological attack will initially
depend on clinical and neurophysiological findings and
subsequently on the early results of morphometric assessment.

REFERENCES

Ashbury, A., and Johnson, P. (1978). In "Pathology of
    Peripheral Nerve" (J. Bennington, ed.) p. 268.
    W.B. Saunders, Philadelphia.
Behse, F., and Buchthal, F. (1978). Brain 101, 473.
Bronson, R., Bishop, Y., and Hedley-White, E. (1978).
    J. Comp. Neurol. 178, 177.
Dyck, P. (1975). In "Peripheral Neuropathy" (P. Dyck,
    P. Thomas and E. Lambert, eds.), p. 296. W.B. Saunders,
    Philadelphia.
Dyck, P., and Lofgren, E. (1966). Mayo Clin. Proc. 41, 778.
Dyck, P., and Lofgren, E. (1968). Med. Clin. North Amer.
    52, 885.
Dyck, P., Low, P., Sparks, M., Hexman, L., and Karnes, J.
    (1980). J. Neuropathol. Exp. Neurol. 39, 285.
Dyck, P., Lais, A., Karnes, J., Sparks, M., Hunder, H.,
    Low, P., and Windebank, A. (1981a). Ann. Neurol. 9, 575.
Dyck, P., Oviatt, K., and Lambert, H. (1981b). Ann. Neurol.
    10, 222.
Dyck, P., Lais, A., Hansen, S., Sparks, M., Low, P.,
    Parthasarathy, S., and Baumann, W. (1982). Exp. Neurol.
    77, 359.
Moss, J., Meckler, R., and Moss, W. (1979). Am. J. Surg.
    138, 736.
Myers, D., Pollock, M., and Calder, C. (1977). Acta Neuro-
    pathol. (Berl.) 37, 7.
Nukada, H., Pollock, M., and Allpress, S. (1981). Brain,
    104, 779.

Nukada, H., Pollock, M., and Haas, L. (1983). *Brain, 105,* 647.

Pollock, M., and Dyck, P. (1976). *Arch. Neurol. 33,* 33.

Pollock, M., Nukada, H., Taylor, P., Donaldson, I., and Carroll, G. (1983). *Ann. Neurol. 13,* 65.

Siegel, S. (1956). *In* "Non parametric statistics for the behavioural sciences", p. 127. McGraw Hill, Tokyo.

Thomas, P. (1970). *J. Neurol. Sci. 11,* 285.

II. Toxic Models of Disease

SELECTIVE DEFECTS IN AXONAL TRANSPORT

IN NEUROPATHOLOGICAL PROCESSES

John W. Griffin*, Juan C. Troncoso[+],
Irma M. Parhad[+], and Donald L. Price[+]

*Departments of Neurology and Neuroscience,
The Johns Hopkins University School of
Medicine, Baltimore, MD., U.S.A.
[+]Departments of Neurology and Pathology

INTRODUCTION

This presentation will review some of the roles of
axonal transport abnormalities in the pathogeneses of
axonal degenerations. Slowly evolving degeneration of
peripheral nervous system or central nervous system axons
occurs in a variety of human neurological diseases.
Examples include heritable processes such as Friedreich's
ataxia and Charcot-Marie-Tooth Disease, sporadic disorders
such as amyotrophic lateral sclerosis (motor neuron
disease), and diseases caused by neurotoxins. In these
disorders, the pathogenetic mechanisms responsible for the
axonal changes have been conjectural. Defects in the
maintenance of the axon have been hypothesized to result
from abnormalities of axonal transport systems. Early
studies of axonal transport in experimental models of
chronic axonal disease produced conflicting and generally
disappointing results, with only limited correlation
between axonal transport abnormalities and axonal
pathology. Rapid recent advances in understanding these
processes reflect the use of more focused strategies to
detect partial or selective transport defects. In
particular, recent studies have sought to identify
alterations in specific modes of transport or in transport
of specific axonal organelles. The major thesis of this

review will be that, at least in some models of axonal
disease, there are selective defects in axonal function;
in these models the specific type of axonal transport
defect correlates with -- and probably underlies -- the
early pathological changes. Before presenting evidence
supporting this generalization, the relationships between
axonal structures and modes of axonal transport in normal
nerve fibers will be summarized, and the major types of
ultrastructural changes in axonal degenerations will be
reviewed.

NORMAL TRANSPORT OF AXONAL ORGANELLES

Normal axonal transport is now generally accepted to
involve, at least in large part, the translocation of the
assembled axonal organelles rather than dissolved proteins
or subunits (Lasek and Hoffman, 1976; Black and Lasek,
1980; but also see Ochs, 1982). For example, particulate
organelles can be followed by microcinematography as they
are transported through axoplasm. Similarly, available
evidence indicates that the neurofilament proteins are
transported as assembled filaments (Morris and Lasek,
1982). Each organelle tends to move within a range of
rates characteristic of that type of organelle, ranging
from 400 mm/day to less than 1 mm/day. This conclusion
derives from isotopic studies, which have consistently
demonstrated multiple waves of transport leaving the cell
body and proceeding down the axon at distinct rates.
Electron microscopic (EM) autoradiography and
electrophoretic gel fluorography have been used to
identify the organelles carried in the two best defined
waves, fast and slow transport.

Fast anterograde transport carries small vesicles and
tubules which are approximately 15 nm in diameter and are
bounded by smooth membranes (Tsukita and Ishikawa, 1980).
These structures appear to insert into the racemose smooth
endoplasmic reticulum of the axon (Droz, Rambourg, and
Koenig, 1975) and into the axolemma (Bennett, et al.,
1973; Tessler, Autilio-Gambetti, and Gambetti, 1980;
Griffin, et al., 1981). Fast transport carries materials
at rates up to 400 mm/day. A closely related system,
retrograde transport, carries materials from the nerve
terminals toward the cell body at rates approaching those
of fast anterograde transport. Organelles carried by this

retrograde system include the prelysosomal vesicles and
dense bodies (Tsukita and Ishikawa, 1980).

Rapid bidirectional transport requires local
oxidative metabolism, but the mechanism of transport
remains unknown. The cytoskeletal elements implicated in
normal transport of particulate organelles include
microtubules; rapidly transported organelles are spatially
associated with microtubules (Papasozomenos, et al., 1982;
Griffin, et al., 1983), and depolymerization of
microtubules halts the process. However, it is possible
that microtubules provide only a "scaffolding" along which
transported organelles move; the force-generating
mechanism may involve an actin-based intracytoplasmic
motility system (Isenberg, Schubert, and Kreutzberg,
1980).

In contrast, the main slow transport peak moves at
rates of 0.3 to 3 mm per day; the specific rate varies
with the axons under study, the age of the animal, and the
temperature. This main slow transport peak (SC_a of
Lasek and Hoffman, 1976) carries the two major
cytoskeletal proteins of the axon: the neurofilament
proteins and tubulin, the subunit of microtubules. The
main slow component peak is preceded by a more rapidly
moving front, SC_b of Lasek and Hoffman, which contains
actin (Black and Lasek, 1979), clathrin, and a number of
glycolytic enzymes (Brady and Lasek, 1981).

THE SPECTRUM OF EARLY PATHOLOGIC CHANGES IN DISEASED AXONS

A wide spectrum of early structural changes have been
described in axonal degenerations. These abnormalities
have been most extensively studied in toxic axonopathies,
but occur in heritable, metabolic and nutritional
disorders as well. The polar extremes of this spectrum
occur in a pure form in relatively few model systems. At
one extreme is the intraaxonal accumulation of tubular and
vesicular elements bounded by smooth membranes. Model
systems producing these changes included thiamine
deficiency (Prineas, 1970) and intoxication with
tri-ortho-cresylphosphate (Prineas, 1969a), zinc
pyridinethione ZPT (Sahenk and Mendell, 1979), and
p-bromophenylacetylurea (BPAU) (Blakemore and Cavanagh,
1969; Ohnishi and Ikeda, 1980; Troncoso, et al., 1982).

The other extreme of the spectrum is characterized by the intraaxonal accumulation of neurofilaments. Examples include intoxication with β,β'-iminodipropionitrile (IDPN) (Chou and Hartmann, 1964, 1965; Griffin and Price, 1980), 2,5-hexanedione (HD) (Saida, Mendell, and Weiss, 1976; Spencer and Schaumburg, 1977; Cavanagh and Bennetts, 1981), carbon disulfide (Seppalainen and Haltia, 1980), and several inherited disorders of animals (Cork et al., 1982) and man (Asbury et al., 1972).

Not every disorder fits neatly into these categories. For example, perhaps the most extensively studied neurotoxic model, acrylamide neuropathy, produces a more complex pathology, including both multifocal accumulations of particulate organelles and also regions of modest neurofilament accumulations (Prineas 1969b; Schaumburg, et al., 1974; Chretien, et al., 1981). In addition, some rapidly evolving toxic disorders such as Vacor administration in the rat produce no distinctive changes before the onset of Wallerian-like degeneration.

It might be suspected that the early changes found in a given model could be a function of the time course of intoxication. For example, rapid high dose administration of a toxin might produce one type of change whereas continuous low dosage, with more slowly evolving pathology, might produce the other. On the contrary, the evidence to date suggests that the early changes are agent-specific and largely independent of the time course of exposure. This issue was addressed specifically by Troncoso et al. (1982) in the the BPAU model. Groups of rats were compared following intoxication with a single large dose or following repeated small doses. The time course of the disease varied markedly, with distal weakness and pathologic changes well developed by seven days in the first group and developing only over many months in the latter. Yet, in both groups, ultrastructural studies showed similar accumulations of tubulovesicular profiles in the distal axons. This agent specificity is also seen in neurofilamentous models. For example, IDPN produces neurofilamentous axonal swellings following either single large dose administration or continuous low dose exposure to the toxin (Clark, Griffin, and Price, 1980; Griffin, Hoffman, and Price, 1982); the time course is different, but the primary pathological changes are similar.

Table 1

EARLY ULTRASTRUCTURAL CHANGES IN AXONAL DISORDERS

Neurofibrillary Changes	Accumulations of Tubulo-vesicular Organelles
PROXIMAL AXON	**FOCAL**
o amyotrophic lateral sclerosis*	o nerve section or crush
o hereditary canine spinal muscular atrophy*	o focal cooling of nerve
o β,β'-iminodipropionitrile (IDPN) toxicity	o local application of spindle inhibitors (colchicine, vincristine) or inhibitors of oxidative metabolism
o 3,4-dimethyl-2,5-hexanedione (DMHD) toxicity	
o aluminum toxicity*	
DISTAL AXON	**DISTAL AXON**
o human giant axonal neuropathy	o thiamine deficiency
o canine giant axonal neuropathy	o zinc pyridinethione (ZPT) toxicity
o hexacarbon neurotoxicity (2,5-hexanedione (HD))	o p-bromophenylacetylurea (BPAU) toxicity
o carbon disulfide	o acrylamide
o acrylamide	
	AXOTERMINAL NEUROAXONAL DYSTROPHY (NAD)
	o aging (e.g., gracile tract)
	o human NAD
	o canine NAD
	o vitamin E deficiency

*These disorders also have neurofilament accumulations within the nerve cell bodies.

NEUROFIBRILLARY AXONAL CHANGES

Neurofilamentous accumulations may occur in either proximal or distal axons or both. The differences in distribution of the neurofilamentous axonal swellings among various models are listed in Table 1. The underlying transport abnormalities have been most extensively investigated in the proximal neurofibrillary neuropathies produced by IDPN and 3,4-dimethyl-2,5-hexanedione (DMHD); this latter model has recently been developed by Anthony, et al. (1983a,b,c). Both agents have the ability to impair neurofilament transport severely (Griffin, et al., 1978, 1982; Griffin, et al., submitted). The transport changes are both qualitatively and quantitatively similar in the two models. For example, administration of either agent in a short-term, high-dose schedule reduces the rate of neurofilament transport two- to ten-fold. Other slow component constituents, including tubulin and a variety of SC_b marker proteins, are retarded only by 10-50%, compared to controls (Griffin, et al., submitted).

This defect in neurofilament transport is present all along the course of nerve fibers, not only in the proximal regions. This has been shown in studies in which animals were labeled 1-35 days before IDPN administration, with the nerves removed 7-21 days after IDPN administration (Griffin, 1978). In these studies, the main slow component peak failed to move distally in the interval after IDPN administration; that is, it was retained at about the site expected at the time of administration of the toxin. These transport kinetics have suggested the following reconstruction of the development of the neurofilamentous swellings in the IDPN and DMHD models: the toxins impair neurofilament transport all along the course of the nerve fibers, but as new neurofilaments, which continue to be synthesized in the cell bodies, enter axons, they cannot be transported beyond the most proximal region. This region consequently becomes distended with accumulated neurofilaments.

Vulnerability to development of neurofilamentous axonal swellings following administration of IDPN or DMHD varies markedly in different fiber populations. Morphometric studies of these models have shown that

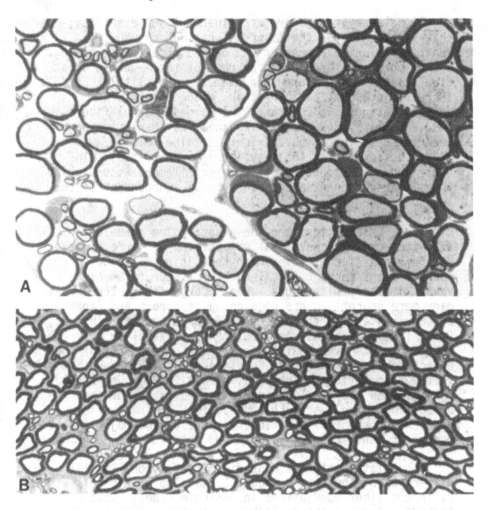

Fig. 1   Neurofilamentous axonal swellings produced by IDPN
         administration.
         A.   Proximal L5 ventral root of a young rat 6 days
              after intraperitoneal injection of IDPN
              (2g/kg).
         B.   Control Ventral Root.
              Note the marked increase in caliber of the
              large fibers in the IDPN-treated nerve; these
              swellings are filled with densely packed
              neurofilaments. In contrast, there is little
              change in the caliber of the small fibers.
Both magnifications x1,300.

axonal caliber is a major determinant of vulnerability;
that is, the larger the fiber before IDPN or DMHD
administration, the greater the degree of axonal swelling.
For example, in the L5 ventral root of the 7-week-old rat,
fibers less than 4 microns in diameter show little
increase in axonal caliber at any stage after IDPN
administration. In contrast, the largest normal fibers
(those normally 8-9 microns in axonal caliber) may reach a
peak increase in caliber of four- to nine-fold in
cross-sectional area (Stanley, et al., submitted). In
these models, susceptibility to neurofilament accumulation
is caliber-dependent and appears to be independent of the
length of the fiber.

These observations provide a satisfying correlation
with the normal cytoskeletal composition of large fibers.
Morphometric studies have shown that in normal fibers
neurofilament content (total number of neurofilaments)
varies linearly with axonal area. Large fibers thus have
many more neurofilaments undergoing transport and capable
of accumulating in the presence of toxic agents. In fact,
it is likely that a large complement of axonal
neurofilaments are required for the occurrence of the IDPN
effect on slow transport. Consistent with this hypothesis
is the observation of Yokoyama, et al. (1980), who showed
that, in the small-caliber unmyelinated fibers of the
dorsal motor nucleus of the vagus, IDPN administration
produced no abnormalities in transport of the major slow
component constituents, tubulin and actin.

The distribution of neurofilamentous axonal swellings
differs among the various models, and also within
different fiber populations in a single model. What
factors determine the distribution of the neurofilamentous
accumulations along the length of affected fibers? At
least three variables have been proposed to play roles.
First, Anthony, et al. (1983a) have suggested that the
relative potency of the neurotoxin determines the site of
initial formation of swellings. HD produces axonal
swellings in a predominantly distal distribution.
Anthony, et al. found that the dimethylated analogue,
DMHD, produced neurotoxicity at total doses of a 1/20th to
1/40th of those required for HD, with a time course of
neurotoxicity which was substantially compressed. The
swellings appeared in a predominantly proximal

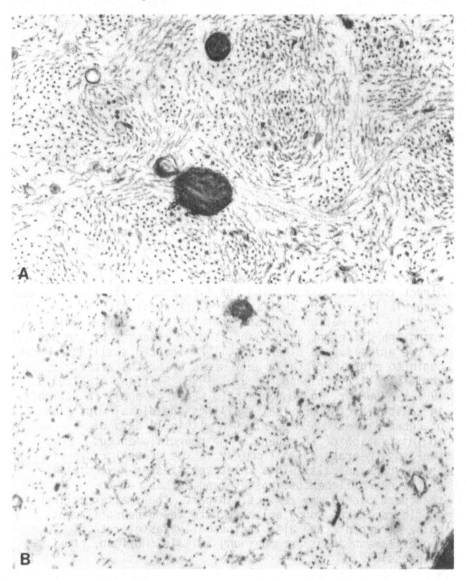

Fig. 2   Electron micrograph of an nerve fiber from an
         IDPN-treated (A) and a normal rat (B). Note the
         increase in number and density of neurofilaments
         in the IDPN-treated nerve. Both magnifications
         x34,500

distribution, very similar to the distribution produced by IDPN administration. It seems likely that if the neurofilament transport defect is established quickly and is relatively complete, the swellings will appear at the level of the proximal fiber. With less potent agents, such abrupt and profound effects on neurofilament transport may be precluded by nonspecific lethal effects of the very high doses which would be required. Cumulative exposure of axoplasm over many days or weeks as it moves down the nerve fiber might be required to produce neurofibrillary changes.

The second factor influencing the distribution of the swellings may be the extent of reversibility of the neurofilament accumulation. When the toxic agents, like IDPN and HD, are withdrawn, neurofilamentous masses break up and migrate distally (Chou and Hartmann, 1964; Shinomo, et al., 1978; Griffin and Price, 1981; Cavanagh, 1982). Direct comparisons regarding the time course of reversibility of the swellings are not available, but current information suggests that the time course varies among the different agents and is also affected by the age of the animals. In older rats, IDPN-induced swellings begin to migrate distally only weeks or months after administration (Shimono, et al., 1978; Griffin, et al., 1981). However, in young rats (3 weeks of age), reduction in caliber of the proximal swellings and distal migration of neurofilamentous masses begin within 14 days of administration of the agent. The neurofilamentous swellings migrate up to 1 mm/day in the ventral roots of these young animals. This relatively faster reversibility of the neurofilamentous masses (and perhaps of the transport block) may reflect, in part, the smaller caliber of fibers in the young animals, with fewer neurofilaments to be "trapped", and also the normally faster rate of neurofilament transport in young animals (Hoffman, et al., in press).

The third variable affecting distribution of neurofilamentous swellings appears to be local mechanical factors along the course of the nerve fiber. Spencer and Schaumburg (1977) pointed out the tendency for neurofilamentous axonal swellings in HD neuropathy to appear in the proximal paranodal regions. In large

myelinated nerve fibers, there is a normal constriction in
the region of the myelin sheath attachment sites and the
node of Ranvier. As neurofilament transport becomes
defective, these sites may be the regions of initial
accumulation of neurofilaments. In slowly developing
lesions, the caliber of the constricted segment is often
not altered. In more severe, rapidly evolving lesions,
however, the proximal myelin sheath attachment sites and
the node of Ranvier show substantial enlargements, and the
changes in calibre extend to the myelin sheath attachment
sites of the distal heminodes. This is most often seen in
the IDPN model, where the first few internodes on large
motor fibers may each enlarge to 50-150 microns in
diameter and become nearly spherical (Griffin, et al.,
1982).

   Mechanical factors may also play a role in
determining the localization of swellings within the optic
nerve. These neurons are unusual in that, in most
species, the nerve fibers have a long intraretinal
nonmyelinated segment; the myelin sheath is acquired only
distal to the lamina cribosa. Administration of IDPN
results in axonal swellings which form where the optic
nerve passes from its ocular portion into the lamina
cribosa. It is reasonable to presume the lamina cribosa
represents an area of mechanical constraint which is
unable to accommodate modest increases in axonal caliber
(Parhad, et al., 1982).

   The mechanisms by which IDPN, DMHD, and HD alter
neurofilament transport are beginning to be explored.
Morphologic studies by Papasozomenos, et al. (1981) first
demonstrated the reorganization of the cytoskeleton which
IDPN produces. Microtubules congregate in the center of
the axon with neurofilaments arrayed in a subaxolemmal
ring. These changes can be produced by local
administration of the agent directly into the endoneurial
space of the nerves (Griffin, et al., 1983), and HD
produces very similar changes (Griffin, et al., 1983).
This segregation of neurofilaments from the rest of the
cytoskeleton is likely to underlie the defect in
transport.

   The biochemical basis responsible for cytoskeletal
reorganization and defective neurofilament transport is

under intensive investigation. The possibility that the
responsible agents inhibit axonal enzymes involved in
energy metabolism has been examined. Both GAPDH (Sabri,
et al., 1979) and neuron-specific enolase (Howland, et
al., 1980) activities can be altered by HD, but the role
of these effects in pathogenesis of HD neurotoxicity are
unresolved. Anthony, et al. (1983b,c) have recently
presented evidence that HD and DMHD are capable of
covalently binding to ϵ-amino groups of proteins by
formation of pyrrole rings. Such pyrrole rings may well
be formed upon the neurofilaments themselves. These
findings thus provide an important basis for detailed
analysis of pathogenesis at a molecular level. Graham, et
al. (1982) suggested that the pyrrole groups may undergo
oxidation and nucleophilic attack resulting in covalent
crosslinking of neurofilaments. Alternatively,
intramolecular pyrrolization might prevent the
neurofilaments from interacting normally with the sidearms
of other neurofilaments and of microtubules, resulting in
their segregation of the rest of the cytoskeleton. IDPN
itself should not undergo similar reactions, but it is
possible that the neurotoxicity of IDPN depends upon
formation of a neurotoxic metabolite. The resolution of
this issue awaits further studies.

In summary, these neurofilamentous disorders appear
to represent examples of organelle-specific transport
defects. At least in the cases of IDPN and DMHD, the
underlying defect is in neurofilament transport; transport
of other slow component constituents, as well as fast
transport, are relatively little altered. The striking
caliber-dependence of vulnerability to these agents
probably reflects the direct relationship between numbers
of neurofilaments and fiber diameter. The greater the
neurofilament number in a given fiber, the greater the
vulnerability. The distribution of the resulting
neurofilamentous swellings depends upon the potency of the
toxin, the interval after administration, and on local
mechanical factors. The morphologic basis for the
transport impairment may well be the segregation of
neurofilaments from microtubules. The molecular
pathogenesis remains uncertain, but, at least in the cases
of HD and DMHD, formation of pyrrole rings involving
neurofilament peptides may well be involved.

ACCUMULATIONS OF TUBULOVESICULAR PROFILES

Table 1 lists a variety of disorders in which
accumulations of particulate organelles are found within
axons. In each of these disorders, the accumulations tend
to be most prominent in the distal regions of axons. The
simplest ultrastructural changes found in these disorders
are accumulations of vesicular and racemose smooth
membrane-bound profiles (Fig. 3). More complex changes
are seen in some disorders in which laminated sheets and
whorls of membranous structures are found (Fig. 4). When
extensive, these distal accumulations of vesicular and
lamellar membranes correspond to the changes often
referred to as axoterminal neuroaxonal dystrophy
(Seitelberger, 1971).

In normal nerve fibers, smooth membrane-bound
vesicles are carried by fast axonal transport, as
indicated previously. A simple model of focal
accumulation of these organelles has been produced by
axotomy (nerve crush or transection). A "pellet" of
particulate organelles begins to form at the interrupted
ends of the nerve fibers, and the size of these pellets
increases with time (Zelena, et al., 1968). EM
autoradiography has confirmed the association of rapidly
transported radioactivity with these organelles (Droz, et
al., 1973, Griffin, et al. 1977).

These "pellets" are the structural consequence of the
accumulation of rapidly transported organelles at the site
of axonal interruption. This conclusion is supported by
studies of focal cooling of nerve segments. Focal cooling
is known to halt fast transport within the cooled segment.
This system has been particularly instructive because of
the superior structural preservation and the ability to
reverse the accumulations by rewarming. Using this
procedure, Tsukita and Ishikawa (1980) have shown that
vesicular organelles accumulate proximal and distal to the
cooled segment.

In both the axotomy and focal cooling models, the
organelles which accumulate on the distal side of the
transport block are different from those on the proximal

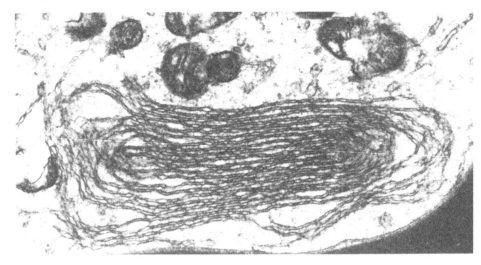

Fig. 3   Accumulation of tubular profiles and
         membranous masses in the distal region of a nerve
         fiber from a rat given BPAU intraperitoneally.
         Magnification x17,000

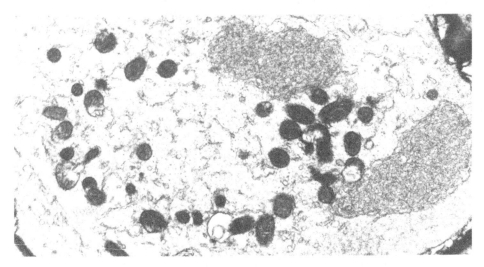

Fig. 4   Lamellar membranous material in an axon from a
         BPAU-treated rat.   Magnification x26,500

side. The distal side consists of dense bodies,
prelysosmal structures, and large vesicular organelles
(Tsukita and Ishikawa, 1980). These organelles accumulate
in this location because of the focal interruption of
retrograde transport from distal regions of the nerve and
nerve terminals.

Axonal transport studies have been reported in
several toxic models in which particulate organelles
accumulate in distal regions. Many of these studies have
found abnormalities of fast bidirectional transport which
appears to be most prominent in distal nerves. Applying
the method of Bisby (1976) to the ZPT model, Sahenk and
Mendell (1979) found delayed return of radiolabeled
materials which were carried into the distal nerve regions
by fast anterograde transport and returned by retrograde
transport. Jacobsen and Brimijoin (1981) reached similar
conclusions in studies of the BPAU model in rat sciatic
nerves. These approaches do not allow precise anatomical
localization of the site of the defect (fast anterograde
transport in preterminal regions, "turn-around" in the
nerve terminal, or retrograde transport in the distal
axon). However, at this time, it seems likely that these
accumulations of particular organelles represent the
structural consequence of defective transport in distal
nerve regions, involving one, two, or all three of these
steps.

Modest accumulations of particulate organelles are
also seen in the acrylamide model. In the ciliary nerves
of chicks intoxicated with acrylamide, abnormal aggregates
of rapidly transported organelles were prominent changes.
The derivation of these accumulations from focal regions
of impaired fast transport was shown by the EM
autoradiographic studies of Chretien, et al (1980).

In these disorders, the molecular basis for the
transport changes remains uncertain. A basic question is
whether the toxic agents interact directly with the
organelles undergoing transport, or instead affect the
transport mechanism. Some of the postulated defects, such
as interference with oxidative metabolism in distal nerve
regions, would clearly fall into the latter category.
These issues can be resolved with existing approaches.

DISCUSSION

The available data raise many issues. Three problems of both theoretical and pathogenetic importance are the following:

First, can multiple pathogenetic mechanisms produce similar structural changes? The mechanisms described to date reflect defective intracellular distribution of organelles (abnormal axonal transport). In theory, similar accumulations of neurofilaments, in particular, could result from reduced turnover. Normal neurofilament degradation appears to involve calcium-activated proteolysis in nerve terminals. Defective degradation could in theory produce distal neurofibrillary changes.

Second, are there modality-specific disorders of transport? At least in the case of neurofibrillary disorders, the defects in neurofilament tranport described so far appear to be organelle-specific. Whether the defects in fast bidirectional transport noted in the ZPT and BPAU models should be considered modality-specific awaits detailed models correlative studies of slow transport in.

Third, are there secondary effects of selective transport defects? It is axiomatic that the axon functions as an integrated unit with interactions among its organelles. Thus, disruption of the transport and distribution of one organelle is likely to affect other organelles at some stage. In the case of HD intoxication, the giant axonal swellings become sites of "trapping" of rapidly transported organelles. Such considerations may be important in understanding the basis for late breakdown and loss of nerve fibers.

ACKNOWLEDGEMENTS

Dr. Griffin is the recipient of an NIH Research Career Development Award (NS-00450). Studies from our laboratories were supported by NIH grants NS-14784 and NS-18687.

REFERENCES

Anthony, D.C., Giangaspero, F., and Graham, D.G., (1983a).
    J. Neuropathol. Exp. Neurol., in press.
Anthony, D.C., Boekelheide, K., and Graham, D.G., (1983b).
    Toxicol. Appl. Pharmacol., in press.
Anthony, D.C., Boekelheide, K., Anderson, C.W., and
    Graham, D.G., (1983c). Toxicol. Appl. Pharmacol., in
    press.
Asbury, A.K., Gale, M.K., Cox, S.C., Barnger, J.R. and
    Beg, B.O. (1972). Acta Neuropathol. (Berl.) 20, 237.
Bennett, G., Giamberardino, L.D., Koenig, H.L., and Droz,
    B. (1973). Brain Res. 60, 129.
Bisby, M.A. (1976). Exp. Neurol. 50, 628.
Black, M.M., and Lasek, R.J. (1980). J. Cell Biol. 86,
    616.
Black, M.M., and Lasek, R.J. (1979). Brain Res. 171, 401.
Blakemore, W.F., and Cavanagh, J.B. (1969). Brain 92, 789.
Brady, S.T., and Lasek, R.J. (1981). Cell 23, 515.
Cavanagh, J.B., and Bennetts, R.J. (1981). Brain 104,297.
Cavanagh, J.B. (1982). Neuropathol. Appl. Neurobiol. 8,19.
Chou, S-M, and Hartmann, H.A. (1964). Acta Neuropathol. 3,
    428.
Chou, S-M, and Hartmann, H.A. (1965). Acta Neuropathol. 4,
    590.
Chretien, M., Patey, G., Souyri, F., and Droz, B. (1981).
    Brain Res. 205, 15.
Cork, L.C., Griffin, J.W., Choy, C., Padula, C.A. and
    Price, D.L. (1982). Lab. Invest. 46, 89.
Droz, B., Koenig, H.L., and DiGiamberardino, L. (1973).
    Brain Res. 60, 93.
Droz, B., Rambourg, A., and Koenig, H.L. (1975). Brain
    Res. 93, 1.
Griffin, J.W., Anthony, D.C., Fahnestock, K., Hoffman,
    P.N. (1983). (Submitted for publication.)
Griffin, J.W., and Price, D.L. (1980). In "Experimental
    and Clinical Neurotoxicology" (P.S. Spencer and H.H.
    Schaumburg, eds.), p. 161. Williams and Wilkins,
    Baltimore.
Griffin, J.W., and Price, D.L. (1981). Lab. Invest. 45,
    130.
Griffin, J.W., Hoffman, P.N., and Price, D.L. (1982). In
    "Axoplasmic Transport in Physiology and Pathology"
    (D.G. Weiss and A. Gorio, eds.), p. 109.
    Springer-Verlag, Berlin.

Griffin, J.W., Fahnestock, K.E., Price, D.L., and Hoffman,
     P.N. (1983). J. Neurosci. 3, 557.
Griffin, J.W., Price, D.L., Drachman, D.B., and Morris, J.
     (1981). J. Cell Biol. 88,205.
Griffin, J.W., Price, D.L., Engel, W.K., and Drachman,
     D.B. (1977). J. Neuropathol. Exp. Neurol. 36, 214.
Griffin, J.W., Anthony, D.C., Fahnestock, K.E., Hoffman,
     P.N., and Graham, D.C. (Submitted for publication).
Griffin, J.W., Gold, B.G., Cork, L.C., Price, D.L., and
     Lowndes, H.E. (1982). Neuropathol. Appl. Neurobiol. 8,
     351.
Griffin, J.W., Hoffman, P.N., Clark, A.W., Carroll, P.T.,
     and Price, D.L. (1978). Science 202, 633.
Hoffman, P.N., Lasek, R., Griffin, J.W., and Price, D.L.
     (in press). J. Neuroscience.
Howland, R.D., Ivy, L.V., Lowndes, H.E., and Argentieri,
     T.M. (1980). Brain Res. 207, 131.
Isenberg, G., Schubert, P., and Kreutzberg, G.W. (1980).
     Brain Res. 194, 588.
Jakobsen, J., and Brimijoin, S. (1981). Brain Res. 229,
     103.
Lasek, R.J., and Hoffman, P.N. (1976). Cold Spring Harbor
     Conferences on Cell Proliferation 3, 1021.
Morris, J.R., and Lasek, R.J. (1982). J. Cell Biol. 92,
     192.
Ochs, S., (1982). "Axoplasmic Transport and its Relation
     to Other Nerve Functions" Wiley, New York.
Ohnishi, A., and Ikeda, M. (1980). Acta Neuropathol.
     (Berl.) 52, 111.
Parhad, I.M., Griffin, J.W., Price, D.L., Clark, A.W.,
     Cork, L.C., Miller, N.R., and Hoffman, P.N. (1982).
     Lab. Invest. 46, 186.
Papasozomenos, S.Ch., Autilio-Gambetti, L., and Gambetti,
     P. (1981). J. Cell Biol. 91, 866.
Papasozomenos, S.Ch., Autilio-Gambetti, L., and Gambetti,
     P. (1982). J. Neuropathol. Exp. Neurol. 41, 371.
Prineas, J. (1970). Arch. Neurol. 23, 541.
Prineas, J. (1969a). J. Neuropathol. Exp. Neurol. 28, 571.
Prineas, J. (1969b). J. Neuropathol. Exp. Neurol. 28, 598.
Sabri, M.I., Moore, C.L., and Spencer, P.S. (1979). J.
     Neurochem. 32, 683.
Sahenk, Z., and Mendell, J.R. (1979). Neurology 29, 590.
Sahenk, Z., and Mendell, J.R. (1979). J. Neuropathol. Exp.
     Neurol. 38, 532.

Schaumburg, H.H., Wisniewski, H.M., and Spencer, P.S.
    (1974). J. Neuropathol. Exp. Neurol. 33, 260.
Seitelberger, F. (1971). Acta Neuropathol. (Berl.)
    (Suppl.) V, 17.
Seppalainen, A.M., and Haltia, M. (1980). In "Experimental
    and Clinical Neurotoxicology" (P.S. Spencer and H.H.
    Schaumburg, eds.), p. 356. Williams and Wilkins,
    Baltimore.
Shimono, M., Izumi, K. and Kuroiwa, Y. (1978). J.
    Neuropathol. Exp. Neurol. 37, 375.
Spencer, P.S., and Schaumburg, H.H. (1977). J.
    Neuropathol. Exp. Neurol. 36, 276.
Stanley, E.F., Griffin, J.W., and Fahnestock, K.E.
    (Submitted for publication).
Tessler, A., Autillio-Gambetti, L., and Gambetti, P.
    (1980). J. Cell. Biol. 87, 197.
Troncoso, J.C., Griffin, J.W., Price, D.L. and
    Hess-Kozlow, K.M. (1982). Lab. Invest. 46, 215.
Tsukita, S., and H. Ishikawa (1980). J. Cell Biol., 84,
    513.
Tsukita, S., and Ishikawa, H. (1981). Biomedical Res. 2,
    424.
Yokoyama, K., Tsukita, S., Ishikawa, H. and Kurokawa, M.
    (1980). Biomed. Res. 1, 537.
Zelena, J., Lubinska, L., and Gutmann, E. (1968). Z.
    Zellforsch. Mikrosk. Anat. 91, 200.

AMYOTROPHIC LATERAL SCLEROSIS

TOXIC AND ANIMAL MODELS

A.D. Kidman, A. Gow, R.T. Johanson,
N.A. Cooper and C.A. Morris

Neurobiology Unit, NSW Institute of Technology

Westbourne St. GORE HILL NSW 2065 Australia

Amyotrophic Lateral Sclerosis (ALS) is a disease of motor nerve cells. It generally affects both the upper motor neurons, i.e. those nerves spreading from the brain to the medulla or spinal cord, and the lower motor neurons i.e. those neurons leading from the spinal cord to the muscles of the body. There is a progressive wasting and weakness of those muscles which have lost their nerve supply and also signs of spasticity and exaggerated reflexes (Varon, 1981).

In different individuals the emphasis of the disease may be as follows:

(a) Upon the lower motor neurons (LMNs) of the limbs when the syndrome is described as progressive muscular atrophy.

(b) Upon the upper motor neurons (UMNs) when it is known as primary lateral sclerosis. When the LMNs of the bulbar musculature are affected, it is also called progressive bulbar palsy. When the UMNs controlling bulbar function are affected, it is called progressive pseudo bulbar palsy.

Although these different syndromes can be recognised in the early stages of the disease, eventually most parts of the motor system are affected and thus two terms are used synonomously to describe this disorder: Amyotrophic

185

Lateral Sclerosis or Motor Neuron Disease.

There is still debate about the classification of the disease according to recent publications (Kurtzke, 1982; Rowland, 1982). Munsat and Bradley (1979) suggest that ALS is a disease confined solely to the voluntary motor system with progressive degeneration of the cortical spinal tract and alpha motor neurons characterised by UMN and LMN signs. Both must be present for a positive diagnosis. ALS is defined as much by the absence of other neurological involvement as it is by the degeneration of the voluntary motor nerves. Even in far advanced and terminal stages, ALS patients show a remarkable absence of sensory, intellectual, cerebellar and extra-pyramidal involvement. These exclusions further help define the disease. Other organs, such as the cardiovascular, renal, gastrointestinal and haemopoietic systems are normal. There is also sparing of certain voluntary motor functions such as extraocular movement and sphincter control.

EPIDEMIOLOGY

Average annual incidence rates for ALS are mostly about 1 to 1.5 per 100,000 population. Prevalence rates are about 5 per 100,000. Normally, the age of onset of ALS is between fifty and sixty years. However, cases as young as the late teens and older than eighty years have been reported. The male to female ratio or sporadic ALS is approximately 3:2.

There are a number of places in the world where the incidence rates are as much as twenty to fifty times higher than those normally observed. The two most inten- sively studied are on the Island of Guam and on the Kii Peninsula of South Eastern Honshu, Japan, (Kurtzke, 1982: Kurtzke and Beebe, 1980). Guamanian ALS appears clinic- ally and pathologically similar to sporadic ALS. Another high incidence focus is seen among the Auyu and Jaki people of West New Guinea. This was first described by Gajdusek and Salazar (1982). Parkinson-dementia complex and other Parkinsonian syndromes have been seen in a high incidence that parallels ALS in all three foci (Hudson, 1981).

Apart from these high incidence areas which are small in number, the disease appears to be uniformly distributed throughout the world.

CLINICAL ASPECTS

Amyotrophic Lateral Sclerosis was first described by the famous French neurologist, Charcot, in the late nineteenth century. The cause of the disease is still unknown and there is no effective treatment.

Five to ten percent of patients have a family history of ALS with an apparent autosomal dominant pattern of inheritance. Progress of the disease is constant and unfortunately rapid. The average duration from diagnosis to death is three to five years.

Approximately one third of patients with ALS notice the disease onset because hands become clumsy and there is difficulty in performing fine tasks. One third present with weakness of legs and they trip over things because of a mild foot drop. Another third present with difficulty of speech and maybe difficulty in swallowing as a result of bulbar symptoms. Distal muscle involvement is often more severe than proximal, but this may proceed to virtual complete paralysis except for the extraocular muscles of the eyes.

The frequent and often prominent occurrence of fasciculations in ALS is not understood (Layzer, 1982). These are rapid uncontrolled twitching of muscles in the arms and legs. They may be related to the great degree of collateral sprouting which occurs when motor neurons die. Healthy adjacent neurons send out sprouts from the tips of their axons to reinnervate the muscle fibres that have lost their innervation during the progression of the disease.

Munsat (1982) has reported that the rate of deterioration in a number of patients observed at his clinic has been constant at approximately three to six per cent per month. This is an important finding because the effects of therapeutic intervention may then be evaluated. One can also predict the future course of the disease after about four months.

CURRENT HYPOTHESES

1.   Viral: One hypothesis which has received a great

deal of support in the past is that ALS is caused by a
slow acting virus. Other neurological disorders such as
Kuru and Creutzfeldt-Jakob disease are now known to be
caused by such agents. Polio virus has been shown to destroy anterior horn cells, hence the suggestion that ALS
may be caused by a virus (Johnson and ter Mulen, 1978). Up
until now, however, no one virus has been consistently
isolated from ALS patient tissue.

2.   Disorder Specific Neurotrophic Hormone: Appel (1981)
has suggested a unifying hypothsis for the cause of ALS,
Parkinsonism and Alzheimer's Disease. He suggests that
each of these disorders is due to a lack of disorder
specific neurotrophic hormone. The hormone would be elab-
orated or stored in the target of the affected neurons. It
would be released by the post synaptic cell and then exert
its effect in a retrograde fashion after being taken up by
the presynaptic terminal. In the motor neurons of ALS
patients, failure of muscle cells to release the appropriate neurotrophic hormone would result in impaired
function of the anterior horn cells. The close association
between Parkinsonian and motor neuron symptoms in the high
incidence foci of ALS adds weight to this unifying
hypothesis.

3.   Environmental Agents: Yase (1972) and others have
carried out extensive studies on Guam and the Kii peninsula and have suggested that low levels of calcium and
magnesium, along with relatively high levels of aluminium
and manganese in the environment could play a role in the
aetiology of ALS. Calcium and magnesium levels in the well
water used by the ALS patients in West New Guinea were also
low according to Gajdusek and Salazar (1982). Yase (1980)
has suggested that the low intake of calcium and magnesium
may result in changes of calcium concentration in muscle
which may lead to muscle degeneration, followed by neural
degeneration. This hypothesis is consistent with the
neurotrophic hormone proposal. Such changes in mineral
concentrations may also disrupt the neuronal cytoskeleton
and axoplasmic flow, or even interfere with the DNA in the
cell body.

A history of exposure to lead, and less frequently
mercury and other heavy metals, has been obtained from a
number of patients with ALS.   Herrero (1972)

noted that welders, plumbers, farmers and oil and electrical equipment workers had a higher incidence of ALS than
the rest of the population. A causal relationship has not
been established and treatment based on increasing the
excretion of lead (D-penicilamine or EDTA chelation) has
mostly been ineffective (Conradi et al, 1982).

4.   DNA Hypothesis: Bradley and Krasin (1982) have proposed the DNA hypothesis of the aetiology of ALS. These
workers suggest that ALS is due to a deficiency in the
normal DNA repair mechanisms with resultant accumulation
of damaged DNA. This causes abnormal transcription of RNA
leading either to translation of abnormal proteins or
failure of synthesis of specific proteins. Studies by
Davidson and Hartman (1981 a; 1981 b) on the RNA of ALS
motor neurons and by Bradley and Kresin (1982) on RNA and
protein metabolism in motor neurons of the Wobbler mouse
may provide direct evidence for this hypothesis. It is
likely that the loss of thirty to forty per cent of neuronal RNA and the decrease of adenine in RNA reported in
both these studies reflect abhorrent transcription caused
by unrepaired damage in DNA. However, neuronal degeneration is relatively restricted to the motor system in ALS.
This hypothesis therefore presumes that the DNA repair
mechanisms differ from that in other neurons.

     If the deficiency in DNA repair mechanisms is the
primary cause of ALS, other factors such as toxins,
viruses, ageing and heavy metals could precipitate the
disease by a variety of mechanisms which cause an increase
in the number of translations and transcriptions. These
mechanisms could include an increase in DNA damage, a
decrease in DNA repair enzymes or an increase in metabolic
demand on the cell.

     The hypothesis is interesting and certainly requires
further testing.

5.   Other Significant Factors: Kurtzke and Beebe (1980)
studied the relationship between service personnel con-
tracting ALS and their illness history. They used control
groups of servicemen, matching for age, date of entry into
military service and branch of service. Military records
were extracted for information about preservice demographic
and other factors, the physical examination for entry into
the service and the history and factors characterising

their military careers during World War II. Admissions to hospital during service for trauma (especially fractured limbs) was the only factor in excess among patients with ALS. Kurtzke and Beebe (1980) therefore conclude that trauma, particularly major trauma of the limbs, is a risk factor for ALS. This could explain the relative preponderance of males with ALS, but the relationship to pathogenesis is unknown.

MODELS

Hereditary Canine Spinal Muscular Atrophy

Hereditary Canine Spinal Muscular Atrophy is a dominantly inherited lower motor neuron disease which was first recognised in Brittany spaniels (Cork et al, 1981). The disorder has clinical and pathological features in common with ALS. These include weakness, muscle atrophy, fibrillations, fasciculations and structural abnormalities in the ventral horn cells (Lorenz et al, 1979). Cork et al (1982) have shown that selected motor neurons are distinguished by chromatolysis and neurofibrillary abnormalities. These occur in the perikarya, dendrites and most strikingly in the proximal axons. Dendrites and axons were segmentally enlarged by accumulations of neurofilaments. The axonal swellings usually involved internodes and were constrained by the initial segment or nodes of Ranvier. The disorganised neurofilaments appeared to trap mitochondria and other organelles. Cork et al (1982) suggest that the neurofibrillary changes in this canine genetic disorder are associated with an abnormality of the cytoskeletal constituents of motor neurons.

The Wobbler Mouse

Genes of the Wobbler mouse (WR) arose by spontaneous mutation in an inbred strain of mice in Edinburgh. This resulted in a slowly progressive form of neural atrophy of autosomal recessive inheritance which affected primarily the motor neurons of the brain stem and the ventral horn of the cervical cord. This mutant may serve as an experimental model of motor neuron disease in man. The first sign of the disease is a head tremor which appears at about three weeks of age. There is progressive wasting and paralysis of the fore limbs. The mean age at death is

eight months compared with two to three years for the
normal mouse. Pathological studies by Bradley et al(1979)
show early vacuolation of the anterior horn cells with
progressive degeneration and loss of spinal motor neurons
leading to denervation atrophy of the muscles of the upper
limbs and to a lesser extent of the lower limbs. Axonal
transport studies were carried out more than ten years ago
by Bird et al (1971) and Bradley et al (1971). The techniques for axonal transport studies were such that the
results were somewhat inconclusive, however, on balance
it appeared that there was no alteration in either fast or
slow transport. However, it is important that axonal
transport in this model be re-examined in the light of
newer techniques and information that is available.

Toxic Agents

Lathyrogen intoxication initiated studies with the compound β,β'-iminodipropionitrile (IDPN). IDPN is a deriv-
ative of a compound extracted from the chick-pea (Lathyrus
odoratus) and was shown by Chou and Hartman (1964; 1965)
to produce dramatic enlargements of the proximal portion
of large axons in many regions of the nervous system.
Neurofilamentous swellings similar to those identified in
ALS are reproduced by IDPN and also aluminium intoxication
(Griffin et al, 1982). Within two days after a single
intraperitoneal injection of IDPN, axonal swellings occur.
These involve internodes, however, initial segments in
nodes of Ranvier are relatively spared. The first internode often enlarges into a massive spheroid measuring up
to one hundred and fifty millimicrons in diameter. The
axonal swellings are to a large extent reversible when
intoxication is stopped. They contain massive increases
of neurofilaments arranged in disorientated whorls and
spirals. Within this region, mitochrondria, membrane
bound vesicles, smooth endoplasmic reticulum and other
particulate organelles are retained to a variable extent.
Frequently, a channel of longitudinally orientated axonal
constituents including microtubules, vesicles and mitochondria is found in the centre of the fibre (Griffin et
al, 1982). Griffin et al (1978), using radioactive
labelling techniques, showed that rapidly transported
axonal proteins were not affected by IDPN intoxication,
whereas slowly transported axonal proteins which are presumed to make up the cytoskeleton were stopped. The transport of neurofilament proteins is most severely affected.

Evidence suggests that the primary defect may be in the
transport of the neurofilament proteins. Localised intraneural injections of IDPN in the rat sciatic nerve produced similar pathological changes to the systemic injection procedure. Many axons showed the central channel of
longitudinally oriented microtubules surrounded by subaxolemmal rings of chaotically oriented neurofilaments.
This abnormality appeared within two hours, reached a
maximum within six hours and became less prominent between
twenty-four and seventy-two hours. Griffin *et al* (1982)
argue that their results are consistent with a direct
effect on the axon which does not appear to require the
intervention of the cell body.

We have studied the effect of systemic IDPN intoxication on the transport of two enzymes, acetylcholinest-
erase (AChE) and choline acetyltransferase (CAT). AChe
is associated with the rapid phase, while CAT is associated with the slow phase of axonal transport. The rate of
movement of both these enzymes is not affected by the
disruption to the neurofilament elements (Kidman *et al*,
1982). These results do not contradict those of Griffin
et al (1978) since CAT travels with the slow component b
(SCb) fraction according to Lasek's transport classification scheme (Brady and Lasek, 1981). Both microtubules
and neurofilaments move at a slightly slower rate (SCa
fraction) in this scheme.

The question of cytoskeletal disruption and pathology
produced by IDPN is very important, although the relationship between these changes and those observed in ALS is
not clear. It would be desirable to be able to relate the
changes observed in the IDPN and aluminium models and
those observed in ALS to a common underlying mechanism.
Perhaps a defect in energy metabolism in the axon allows
intracellular concentrations of calcium to rise to levels
which are able to interfere with neurofilament interactions
and hence cause the observed cytoskeletal disruption
(Schlaepfer and Micko, 1979). Yase (1980) has postulated
that chronic nutritional deficiencies of calcium and magnesium such as found in West New Guinea, Guam and the Kii
Peninsula cause abnormal mineral metabolism suggestive of
secondary hyperparathyroidism. The presence of excessive
levels of divalent or trivalent cations such as manganese
and aluminium results in the mobilisation of bone calcium
which, along with aluminium, is deposited as hydroxyapa-

tites in nervous tissue (Kumamoto et al, 1975). Yase
(1980) has demonstrated elevated levels of calcium and
aluminium in ALS autopsy tissue using neutron activation
analysis.

Central to any hypothesis of ALS must be an explanation as to why nervous tissue is affected to a greater
extent than other tissues. As energy is required to maintain intracellular homeostasis in all tissues, energy
metabolism in nervous tissue must reflect an increased
vulnerability to mineral/toxin effects. The possible
targets are glycolytic or other energy related enzymes
which display different characteristics in nervous tissue
and hence may be more sensitive to the effects of aluminium or IDPN. We are currently testing this hypothesis.

REFERENCES

Appel, S. (1981). *Ann. of Neurol. 10,* 499.
Bird, M., Shuttleworth, E. Koiestner, A. and Reinglass, J.
    (1971). *Acta Neuro. Path., Berlin, 19,* 39
Bradley, W. and Krasin, F. (1982). *Arch. Neurol. 39,* 677.
Bradley, W., Munsat, T., Pelham, R., Rasool, C., Baruah,J.,
    Chatterjee, A., Silder, S. and Kugelman, K. (1979).
    In *"Muscle, Nerve and Brain Degeneration"* (A. Kidman
    & J. Tomkins, Eds.) p. 67. Excerpta Med. Int. Cong.
    Ser. 473, Amsterdam.
Bradley, W., Murchison, D. and Day, M. (1971). *Brain Res.
    35,* 185.
Munsat, T. (1982). *"Workshop on Pathogenesis of ALS".*
    Vth Int. Congress on Neuromuscular Disease, Marseille.
Munsat, T. and Bradley, W. (1979). In *"Current Neurology"
    Vol. 2.* (H. Tyler and D. Dawson, Eds.) p.79.
    Haughtonmifflin, Boston.
Brady, S. and Lasek, R. (1981). *Cell 23,* 515.
Chou, S. and Hartman, H. (1964). *Acta Neuropathol.(Berlin)
    3,* 428.
Chou, S. and Hartman, H. (1965). *Acta Neuropathol.(Berlin)
    4,* 590.
Conraid, S., Ronnevi, L., Nise, G. and Vesterberg, O.(1982)
    Acta Neurol. (Scandinav.) 65, 203.
Cork, L., Griffin, J., Choy, C., Padula, C. and Price, D.
    (1982). *Lab. Invest. 46,* 89.
Cork, L., Price, D., Griffin, J., Choy, C. and Padula, C.
    (1981). *J. Neuropathol. Exp. Neurol. 40,* 314.

Davidson, T. and Hartman, H. (1981a). *J. Neuropathol.*
    Exp. Neurol. 40, 187.
Davidson, T. and Hartman, H. (1981b). *J. Neuropathol.*
    Exp. Neurol. 40, 193.
Gajdusek, D. and Salazar, A. (1982). *Neurol. 32*, 107.
Griffin, J., Cork, L., Toncoso, J. and Price, D. (1982).
    Adv. Neurol. 36, 419.
Griffin, J., Hoffman, P., Clark, A., Carroll, P. and
    Price, D. (1978). *Science 202*, 633.
Herrero, F. (1972). *Lancet 2*, 1036.
Hudson, A. (1981). *Brain 104*, 217.
Johnson, R. and ter Mulen, V. (1978). *Adv. Int. Med. 23*,
    353.
Kidman, A., Cooper, N., Gow, A. and Morris, C. (1982).
    Vth Int. Cong. on Neuromuscular Diseases (Marseille)
    Abs. No. TH83.
Kumamoto, T., Nakagaura, S., Suematsu, C., Shimizu, E.,
    Yata, Y. and Hiroahata, T. (1975). *Acta Histochem.*
    Cytochem. 8, 294.
Kurtzke, J. (1982). *Brit. Med. J. 284*, 141.
Kurtzke, J. and Beebe, G. (198)). *Neurol. 30*, 453.
Layzer, B. (1982). *Adv. Neurol. 36*, 23.
Lorenz, M., Cork, L., Griffin, J., Adams, R. and Price, D.
    (1979). *J. Amer. Vet. Med. Assoc. 175*, 833.
Rowland, L. (1982). *Adv. Neurol. 36*, 1.
Schlaepfer, W. and Micko, S. (1979). *J. Neurochem. 32*,
    211.
Varon, M. (1981). In *"ALS - Current Research Status"*, p.1
    ALS Society of America, Cal. U.S.A.
Yase, Y. (1972). *Lancet 2*, 292.
Yase, Y. (1980). *Neurotoxicol. 1*, 101.

EXCITOTOXINS

Graham A.R. Johnston

Department of Pharmacology, University of Sydney,

NSW, 2006, Australia

The majority of neurones in the mammalian central nervous system are now known to use relatively simple amino acids as synaptic transmitters. The acidic amino acids L-glutamate and L-aspartate act as excitatory transmitters while the neutral amino acids 4-aminobutyric acid and glycine act as inhibitory transmitters. Many neurotoxins are structurally related to these amino acid transmitters and may act adversely of the synaptic receptors, transport carriers and metabolising enzymes associated with such transmitters (Johnston, 1974).

At the present time there is considerable interest centred around "excitotoxins" which may be able to "excite neurones to death". The neurotoxic action of L-glutamic acid has been linked to its excitatory on CNS neurones in Olney's concept of "excitotoxins" (Olney et al., 1971). A variety of acidic amino acids, structurally related to L-glutamic acid and able to depolarise neurones on local administration, can act as neurotoxins. Activation of one or more of a number of different classes of excitatory receptors leading to prolonged depolarisation of susceptible neurones appears to result in cell death. The detailed mechanisms contributing to cell death are not known but are likely to involve influx of sodium and calcium ions and depletion of ATP stores.

Excitotoxins, in particular kainic acid, are being used extensively in neurobiology to produce selective neuronal lesions (McGeer, Olney and McGeer, 1978; Coyle, 1978; McGeer and McGeer, 1982), and their actions appear to mimic many of the changes observed in human degenerative disorders (Sanberg and Johnston, 1981; Coyle, 1982). Studies of the possible involvement of excitotoxins, both exogenous and endogenous, in neuronal degenerative disorders are likely to lead to significant advances in our understanding of the etiology of such disorders and to their treatment by more rational therapies.

EXOGENOUS EXCITOTOXINS

There are a number of excitotoxins that have been isolated from plant, but not as yet animal sources. These toxins are thus classified as exogenous to the CNS. They may gain access to the CNS by injestion in the diet, as in the case of 3-N-oxalyl-L-2,3-diaminopropionic acid which is found in the chick pea Lathyrus sativus and has been linked to the disease neurolathyrism, or by administration as part of an experimental or therapeutic procedure, e.g. kainic acid, from the seaweed Digenea simplex, has been used in Taiwan to treat intestinal worms. Ibotenic acid, from the mushroom Amanita muscaria, has been used to produce highly localised neuronal lesions on direct injection into the brains of experimental animals. These substances have in common the ability to excite CNS neurones on local administration and to cause neuronal degeneration. On direct injection they destroy the somal and dendritic components of adjacent neurones but spare axons of passage and glial cells. Nerve terminals are spared providing the somal and dendritic components of the neurones are remote from the injection site. Thus intrinsic neurones in the injected brain region are destroyed and their terminals in that and other regions degenerate, while the axons and terminals of neurones projection from other regions and axons of passage are spared. When used in conjunction with other chemical and physiological evidence, such excitotoxin lesioning experiments can provide a great deal of information regarding neuronal pathways projecting to, within, and from particular brain regions (Coyle, 1978).

Glutamic acid is itself a major constituent of many foodstuffs and thus may represent an exogenous excitotoxin even though it occurs in mammalian brain in high concentration. This is because the neuronal excitant receptors activated by glutamic acid are extracellular and endogenous glutamic acid is stored intracellularly such that it excites neurones only after it is released from these stores. As its monosodium salt MSG, glutamic acid is widely used as an additive enhancing flavour and improving palatibility of many foods. Japanese workers have introduced the concept of "UMAMI", the 5th taste in addition to the 4 commonly accepted tastes of sweet, salty, sour and bitter (Yamaguchi and Kimizuka, 1979). UMAMI is considered to represent the fundamental taste properties of MSG and to play a major role in the flavour of foods. Tomatoes and parmesan cheese are particularly rich in glutamic acid which may explain their usefulness in enhancing the flavour of other foods. Glutamic acid has been used in Far Eastern cookery since ancient times as the active constituent of an indigenous seaweed and more recently as MSG, and is now used extensively in Western cooking, hundreds of thousands of tonnes of MSG being consumed yearly. This widespread use of glutamic acid may not present a problem to healthy adults when consumed in a balanced diet.

Popular interest in MSG arose from what became known as the "Chinese Restaurant Syndrome". This is an inappropriate name since an objective survey of unpleasant symptoms experienced after eating specific foods identified Mexican-Spanish, American and Italian cuisines as associated with the largest number of unpleasant symptoms with pizza, tacos, spaghetti and hot dogs as the "ethnic" foods receiving the most complaints (Kerr et al., 1979). This survey indicated that less than 2% of the population had ever experienced the characteristic symptoms of "Chinese Restaurant Syndrome" of "burning", "tightness" and/or "numbness" in the chest, neck or face. The likelihood of a small percentage of glutamic acid-sensitive individuals within a population of human or non-human primates seems high, but very difficult to objectively investigate. Dietary glutamic acid is unlikley to constitute a health risk to most healthy adults. It should be considered as a possible problem in conditions where the

blood brain barriers, which normally protect the CNS from
high levels of glutamic acid in the circulation, are likely
to be impaired e.g. in severe malnutrition.

MSG is listed by the US Food and Drug Administration
as "generally regarded as safe" (GRAS) and for many years
was added liberally to processed infant foods. In 1969,
when the neurotoxic effects of oral MSG in neonatal animals
were demonstrated (neonates being much more susceptible to
systemic glutamic acid than adults probably due to slow
development of blood brain barriers compared to the
development of neuronal glutamic acid receptors), baby food
manufacturers stopped adding MSG to baby foods. Protein
hydrolysates were substituted, rich is glutamic and
aspartic acids, to maintain the free glutamic acid content
in the baby foods at flavour levels to which the maternal
palate had been conditioned. In 1976, a scientific advisory
committee of the Federated American Societies for
Experimental Biology, reviewing the safety of GRAS food
additives, advised the US Food and Drug Administration that
neither glutamic acid nor protein hydrolysates could be
considered safe for use in baby or junior foods (See Olney,
1979). Glutamic acid occurs naturally in human milk, but
the glutamic acid content of some baby food was such that 1
jar (4.5 oz) would contain 20-25 times the glutamic acid in
one feeding of human milk and one quarter of the oral load
known to destroy hypothalamic neurones in infant mice
(Loney, 1979). The addition of glutamic acid to baby or
junior foods, either as MSG or as part of a protein
hydrolysate, appears to meet no health or nutritional need,
and may constitute an unnecessary risk without benefit.

Certain brain regions known collectively as
circumventricular organs (CVOs), which lie outside blood
brain barriers, appear to be selectively susceptible to
increased blood levels of glutamic acid. CVOs in both
infant and adult animals are vulnerable to glutamic acid,
although the effective dose in adults is higher perhaps due
to the greater capacity of the adult liver to metabolise
glutamic acid. The arcuate nucleus and median eminence have
been the CVOs most intensively investigated because of the
neuroendocrine disturbances associated with glutamic
acid-induced damage in these areas, but other CVOs
including the subfornical organ and area postrema appear
just as vulnerable to glutamic acid-induced damage.

Glutamic acid and related excitotoxins can be used as
neuroendocrine probes (Olney, 1979) since the arcuate
nucleus of the hypothalamus is a neuroendocrine regularory
centre. Glutamic acid can be used in either a provocative
or ablative approach to study neuroendocrine regulatory
function. At subtoxic doses glutamic acid may provoke
neuronal activity in the arcuate nucleus which could
influence pituitary hormonal output. At toxic doses
glutamic acid ablates arcuate neurones producing changes in
pituitary, thyroid and adrenal status, including decreased
prolactin levels in the pituitary of neonatal female mice
and obesity. Subtoxic doses of glutamic acid given
subcutaneously to adult rats result in appreciable
elevations of serum luteinizing hormone (Olney, 1979). Some
of these endocrine effects persist for many hours after
administration of glutamic acid (Blake et al., 1978), which
may be relevant to the clinical finding of two cases of
life-threatening attacks of asthma 11 to 14 hours after
injestion of glutamic acid as 2.5 g of MSG (Allen and
Baker, 1981).

ENDOGENOUS EXCITOTOXINS

Glutamic acid is the major excitatory neurotransmitter
in mammalian brain (Roberts, Storm-Mathisen and Johnston,
1981) and it is possible that synaptically release glutamic
acid in certain circumstances could be neurotoxic leading
to neuronal degeneration and neuroendocrine abnormalities.
Prompted by the similarities between the changes in the rat
striatum following intrastriatal injection of glutamic acid
and the changes in human striatum in Huntington's disease,
McGeer and McGeer (1976) proposed that overactive glutamic
acid pathways in the striatum may be responsible for the
striatal neuronal degeneration in Huntington's disease.
This was supported by Olney and de Gubareff (1978), who
further proposed that an adult-onset disturbance in
glutamic acid inactivation via intracellular uptake might
underlie this neurodegenerative syndrome. An inhibitor of
the high affinity uptake of glutamic acid, threo-3-hydroxy-
aspartic acid (Balcar et al., 1977), has been shown to be
toxic to striatal neurones (McBean and Roberts, 1982)
indicating that impaired inactivation of glutamic acid can
also lead to neuronal degeneration. The "glutamic acid
model" of Huntington's disease has considerable

experimental support (Sanberg and Johnston, 1981). Recently
Plaitakis et al. (1982) have provided evidence that for a
defect in glutamic acid metabolism in another hereditary
neurodegenerative disorder olivopontocerebellar atrophy
(OPCA). Patients with this disorder showed a 50% decrease
in leucocyte and fibroblast glutamic acid dehydrogenase
activity and increased serum levels of glutamic acid
following oral consumption of MSG.

There has been much speculation regarding the
occurence in mammalian brain of endogenous ligands for what
have become known as kainic acid receptors. Kainic acid,
one of the most potent excitants known, appears to act on a
relatively minor subpopulation of receptors for glutamic
acid and it is possible that the natural ligand for these
receptors is not in fact glutamic acid. Using radioligand
binding studies with tritiated kainic acid, a number of
substances have been found to compete with kainic acid for
binding sites; these include various derivatives of folic
acid (Ruck et al., 1980), and certain pyrethroids (Staatz
et al., 1982). In addition, electrophysiological studies
have provided evidence for the antagonist action of
paracetamol and related compounds on kainic acid receptors
(Headley and West, 1983). Endogenous inhibitors of kainic
acid binding have been reported in extracts of rat brain
(Skerritt and Johnston, 1981; Tsujimura et al., 1982) and
bovine brain has been reported to contain kainic acid-like
excitatory activity (Luini et al., 1982). A study of
Huntington's disease patients failed to detect kainic
acid-like molecules in urine, serum or CSF using a kainic
acid binding assay (Beutler et al., 1981). There is
considerable evidence for a multiplicity of receptors of
kainic acid and thus the possibility for more than one
endogenous ligand; in this context it appears that
derivatives of folic acid interact with kainic acid binding
sites in the cerebellum but not in the striatum, consistent
with folic acid being toxic to cerebellar but not striatal
neurones (Longoni et al., 1982).

CONCLUSIONS

Excitotoxins may well kill neurones by exciting them
to death but exactly how they do this is far from clear.
These substances can be very useful in experimental studies

of "how the brain is wired together" and of "animal models" for neurodegenerative diseases. Our understanding of the nature of possible endogenous excitotoxins, other than glutamic acid is poor, and much work remains to been done to develop more rational therapies for the treatment of nervous system disorders than may involve these substances.

ACKNOWLEDGEMENT

Our work on possible endogenous ligands in mammalian brain for excitotoxin receptors is supported by the National Health and Medical Research Council of Australia

REFERENCES

Allen, D.H., and Baker, G.J. (1981) Med. J. Aust. 2, 576.

Balcar, V.J., Johnston, G.A.R., and Twitchin, B. (1977). J. Neurochem., 28, 1145.

Beutler, B.A., Noronha, A.B.C., Poon, M.M., and Arnason, B.G.W. (1981) 51, 355.

Blake, J.L., Lawrence, N., Bennet, J., Robinson, S. and Bowers, C. (1978) Neuroendocrinology 26, 220.

Coyle, J.T. (1978). Trends Neurosci. 1, 132.

Coyle, J.T. (1982). Trends Neurosci. 5, 287.

Headley, P.M., and West, D.C. (1983) Brit. J. Pharmac. in press.

Johnston, G.A.R. (1974). In "Neuropoisons, Their Pathophysiological Actions" (L.L. Simpson and D.R. Curtis, ed.), p. 179, Plenum Press, New York.

Kerr, G.R., Wu-Lee, M., El-Lozt, M., McGandy, R., and Stare, F.J. (1979). In "Glutamic Acid: Advances in Biochemistry and Physiology" (L.J. Filer et al., ed.) p. 375, Raven Press, New York.

Longoni, R. Mulas, A., Spina, L., Loi, I., Di Chiara, G., and Spano, P.F. (1982) Neurosci. Letters, 10, S297.

Luini, A., Goldberg, O., Tal, N. and Teichberg, V.I. (1982) Abstracts 13th CINP, 454.

McBean, J., and Roberts, P.J. (1983). Brit. J. Pharmac., in press.

McGeer, P.L., and McGeer, E.G. (1982). CRC Crit. Rev. Toxicol. 10, 1.

McGeer, E.G., and McGeer, P.L. (1976). Nature 263, 517.

McGeer, E.G., Olney, J.W., and McGeer, P.L. (1978). "Kainic
    Acid as a Tool in Neurobiology", Raven Press, New York.
Olney, J.W. (1979). In "Glutamic Acid: Advances in
    Biochemistry and Physiology" (L.J. Filer et al., ed.)
    p. 287, Raven Press, New York.
Olney, J.W., and de Gubareff, T. (1978). Nature 271, 557.
Olney, J.W., Ho, O.L., and Rhee, V. (1971). Exp. Brain Res.
    14, 61.
Plaitakis, A., Berl, S., and Yahr, M. (1982) Science,
    216, 193.
Roberts, P.J., Storm-Mathisen, and Johnston, G.A.R. (1981).
    "Glutamate: Transmitter in the Nervous System" Wiley,
    New York.
Ruck, A., Kramer, S., Metz, J., and Brennan, M.J.W. (1980)
    Nature 287, 852.
Sanberg, P.R., and Johnston, G.A.R. (1982). Med. J. Aust.
    2, 460.
Skerritt, J.H., and Johnston, G.A.R. (1981). Proc. Aust.
    Neurosci. Soc., 1, 65C.
Staatz, C.G., Bloom, A.S., and Lech, J.J. (1982).
    Toxicol. Appl. Pharmac. 64, 566.
Tsujimura, R., Nomura, J., and Hatotani, N. (1982).
    Neurochem. Res. 7, 870.
Yamaguchi, S., and Kimizuka, A. (1979). In "Glutamic Acid:
    Advances in Biochemistry and Physiology" (L.J. Filer
    et al., ed.), p. 35, Raven Press, New York.

TOXIC EFFECTS OF GLUTAMIC ACID ANALOGUES

ON RETINAL NEURONS

Ian G. Morgan

Department of Behavioural Biology,

R.S.B.S. Australian National University

ABSTRACT

The toxic effects of kainic acid and N-methyl-D-aspartic acid on chicken retinal neurons are described. Kainic acid appears to directly kill horizontal cells and OFF-bipolar cells, and to indirectly kill amacrine cells. N-methyl-D-aspartic acid destroys amacrine cells alone. Evidence is presented suggesting that there are two types of kainic acid-preferring receptors in vertebrate retina, one linked to hyperpolarizing and one linked to depolarizing responses. The implications of the results for retinal transmitter circuitry and for the mode of action of kainic acid are discussed.

INTRODUCTION

The neurotoxic properties of the excitatory amino acids were first documented on retinal tissue (Lucas and Newhouse, 1957). Despite the obvious advantage of working on a tissue with the defined neuronal population and neuronal interactions which are reflected in the elegant lamination of the vertebrate retina, few papers followed up this phenomenon (see Olney, 1974 for review). Even after, and in fact as a result of the renewed burst of interest in excitatory amino acid neurotoxicity, and its relationship in the striatum to Huntington's disease, and in the brain as a whole to epileptogenic cell death and other degenerative phenomena (for reviews see McGeer et al. 1978a; Coyle et al. 1981; Coyle, 1982), little attention was paid to the retina as a system for studying the general nature of excitatory amino acid neurotoxicity, as well as for analysing neuronal interactions in the retina at bio-chemical and physiological levels. The latter topic has been reviewed in detail recently (Morgan, 1983) and only selected elements will be dealt with here.

In 1974, Olney pointed out the strong correlation between the physiological excitatory properties of the excitatory amino acids and their neurotoxic properties, and coined the term "excitotoxic amino acids". He formulated the exitotoxic hypothesis in which neurotoxicity depended upon an interaction of the excitotoxic amino acids with receptors for glutamic acid on a cell, which produced a profound and often sustained depolarization, which ultimately led to cell death. The framework of this theory remains unchallenged, although complicating factors have been introduced. Toxicity appears, at least in some cases, to require intact inputs (Biziere and Coyle, 1978a; McGeer et al. 1978b; Streit et al. 1980) which might imply synergism between on-going input and the neurotoxic compound, or possibly an effect of the neurotoxic compound on pre-synaptic, as well as post-synaptic activity (Ferkany et al. 1982). The recognition of cell death far removed from the injection site, particularly with kainic acid, has led to the suggestion that not all cell death need result from direct effects of kainic acid. Instead it has been suggested that the hyperexcitation induced by kainic acid and other excitatory amino acid analogues might kill other cells which receive input from the excited cells (Schwob et al. 1980; Ben-Ari et al. 1979; Nadler and Cuthbertson, 1980).

Further complexity has been introduced by the recognition of several types of excitatory amino acid receptors. Watkins and Evans (1981) have proposed that there are three distinguishable receptors with preferential affinities for N-methyl-aspartic acid (NMDA), quisqualic acid or kainic acid. 2-Amino-5-phosphonovaleric acid (2APV) is a selective antagonist at NMDA-preferring receptors, while D-γ-glutamyl glycine (DGG) tends to block kainic acid - and NMDA-preferring receptors. Glutamic acid diethylester (GDEE) in some situations blocks quisqualic acid-preferring receptors specifically. Piperidine-2,3-

dicarboxylic acid (PDA) is a potent antagonist at all three receptors.

EFFECTS OF KAINIC ACID ON CHICKEN RETINA

Schwarcz and Coyle (1977) showed that kainic acid injected intravitreally caused extensive cellular destruction in the chicken retina. The amacrine cells were particularly affected, although they cautioned that other cell types were also destroyed. The relative potencies of a series of glutamic acid and aspartic acid analogues in causing destruction of retinal neurons correlated well with the neurotoxic potencies determined in the striatum (Schwarcz et al. 1978). More precise data on the pattern of cell sensitivities to intravitreal kainic acid were obtained in a series of studies (Ehrlich and Morgan, 1980; Morgan and Ingham 1981; Ingham and Morgan, 1983). Most amacrine cells (including the displaced amacrine cells) and over half the bipolar cells were extremely sensitive to intravitreal kainic acid. Horizontal cells were destroyed by higher amounts. Glial cells, photoreceptors, ganglion cells and the remaining bipolar and amacrine cells appeared to be totally resistant to exposure to kainic acid.

Two forms of kainic acid induced cell death seem to be involved in generating this pattern of sensitivity. The effects on bipolar and horizontal cells seem to be direct, since intravitreal injections of Co^{++} ions did not prevent the neurotoxic effects of kainic acid on these cells. By contrast, the effects of kainic acid on amacrine cells were significantly reduced in the presence of Co^{++} ions, suggesting that the effects of kainic acid are mediated by, or at least require on-going synaptic activity. Amacrine cell destruction was also selectively prevented by pretreatment with barbiturates and benzodiazepines (Imperato et al. 1981; cf. Ben-Ari et al. 1979), presumably as a result of potentiation of inhibitory influences at the level of the inner plexiform layer.

While the effects of kainic acid on both amacrine and bipolar cells were extremely rapid, at very short times after the injection bipolar cells were more significantly affected than amacrine cells, suggesting a primary effect on the bipolar cells. The pattern of sensitivity of amacrine cell sub-classes to intravitreal kainic acid provided evidence

of a correlation between probable bipolar cell input and
sensitivity to kainic acid. Most strikingly, the dopa-
minergic amacrine cells known not to receive bipolar cell
input in many species (Dowling and Ehinger, 1978; Dowling
et al. 1980, Adolph, 1980; Holmgren-Taylor, 1982) appear
to be totally resistant to kainic acid. Thus direct
effects of kainic acid on receptors located on bipolar
cell and horizontal cell dendrites seem to account for the
destruction of these cells, while the amacrine cells are
destroyed by kainic acid-induced hyperactivity in bipolar
cells.

     This view of the mode of action of kainic acid enables
two features of the pattern of sensitivity to kainic acid
to be explained. The greater sensitivity of the bipolar
cells compared to the horizontal cells may be related to
the higher gain at photoreceptor-bipolar cell synapses as
compared to the gain at photoreceptor-horizontal cell
synapses (Ashmore and Falk, 1979). To explain the partial
survival of the bipolar cells, we postulated that kainic
acid might mimic the effects of the photoreceptor transmitter, depolarizing, and according to the excitotoxic
hypothesis destroying the OFF-bipolar cells (and the
horizontal cells), while hyperpolarizing the ON-bipolar
cells which might survive. This postulate has been confirmed by the demonstration that kainic acid permanently
eliminates OFF components from the light responses mediated
by a lesioned retina, while ON components continue to be
transmitted (Dvorak and Morgan, 1983). Electrophysiological studies in other vertebrates have demonstrated that
kainic acid hyperpolarizes ON bipolar cells (Shiells, Falk
and Naghshineh, 1981). OFF-bipolar cells have not been
studied, but the horizontal cells, which have a similar
response to light, are depolarized by kainic acid (Shiells,
Falk and Naghshineh 1981; Lasater and Dowling, 1982;
Rowe and Ruddock, 1982a).

     The nature of the receptors mediating the kainic acid
neurotoxicity has been investigated in two ways. Kainic
acid is more than 50 times more effective than quisqualic
acid and N-methyl D-aspartic acid in causing morphological
destruction of bipolar cells. The toxic effects of kainic
acid on the bipolar cells could be blocked by PDA and DGG
but were not reduced by 2APV and GDEE. Thus the effective
receptor on the OFF-bipolar cells appears to correspond to
the kainic acid-preferring receptor defined by

physiological studies in the spinal cord (for review see
Watkins and Evans, 1981; McLennan, 1981). In more quantitative measures of the indirect destruction of amacrine
cells, kainic acid was also more effective than quisqualic
acid or N-methyl D-aspartic acid (Morgan and El-Lakany, 1982)
although the latter compounds appeared to be more
effective than expected from the less precise morphological
assessments, and from their ability to compete in kainic
acid binding assays (London and Coyle, 1979).

EFFECTS OF N-METHYL D-ASPARTIC ACID
ON CHICKEN RETINA.

Intravitreal N-methyl D-aspartic acid causes extensive
lesions of the chicken retina. In contrast to kainic
acid, these lesions do not involve the bipolar cells, but
seem to be restricted to the amacrine cells. The effects
of NMDA were effectively antagonised by DGG, 2APV and PDA
but not by GDEE, suggesting that the neurotoxic effects
were mediated by an NMDA-preferring receptor.

While the studies carried out so far on NMDA are not
as complete as those on kainic acid, the same transmitter-
specific classes of amacrine cells seem to be destroyed by
the two agents. It is not known whether the effects of
NMDA are direct, since Co^{++} interferes with direct interaction of NMDA with NMDA receptors, as well as blocking
indirect effects (Watkins and Evans, 1981).

Since excitatory amino acids are good candidates as
transmitters of the bipolar cells, and since it has been
specifically proposed that aspartic acid might be a bipolar
cell transmitter (Ikeda and Sheardown, 1982), one possibility
was the presence of NMDA receptors on amacrine cells might
be related to a bipolar cell input which used an aspartic
acid-like transmitter. The effects of kainic acid could
be explained by direct interaction of kainic acid with
kainic acid-preferring receptors on bipolar cell and
horizontal cell dendrites in the outer plexiform layer.
The stimulated release of the aspartic acid-like transmitter from OFF-bipolar cell terminals in the inner plexiform layer would then cause the indirect destruction of
amacrine cells. One prediction of this scheme is that 2APV
should block the effects of kainic acid on the amacrine
cells, just as it blocks the effects of NMDA on the
amacrine cells. However while the effects of kainic acid

on amacrine cells were reduced, the reduction was only
partial, and appeared to show some specificity for different
amacrine cell classes. As yet, it is not clear whether
this means that the organization of transmitters in the
inner plexiform layer is quite different. The results
might be explained within the framework of our postulated
scheme, by invoking different thresholds for neurotoxicity
in different types of amacrine cells, perhaps based on
different patterns of excitatory and inhibitory input to
the cells.

IMPLICATIONS FOR RETINAL TRANSMITTER CIRCUITRY

From the results reported above, it would appear that
OFF-bipolar cells possess kainic acid-preferring receptors
at which DGG and PDA act as antagonists. The effects of
kainic acid and its antagonists on OFF-bipolar cells have
not been examined in any species using the intracellular
recordings necessary to obtain definitive physiological
results. Kainic acid depolarizes fish and amphibian
horizontal cells, whose response to the photoreceptor
transmitter is similar to that of the OFF-bipolar cells
(Shiells et al. 1981; Lasater and Dowling, 1982; Rowe and
Ruddock, 1982a). However DGG did not appear to be an
effective antagonist (Rowe and Ruddock, 1982b).

Kainic acid does not appear to destroy the ON-bipolar
cells, probably because it hyperpolarises them. This
unusual hyperpolarizing effect of the analogue of a so-
called excitatory amino acid on the ON-bipolar cells has
been directly demonstrated by intracellular recording in
fish (Shiells et al. 1981), and glutamic acid, while much
less potent, has a similar effect (Murakami et al. 1975).
Unfortunately the selective antagonists have not been
tested on the ON-bipolar cells, but the receptor involved
appears to be different. 2-Amino-4-phosphonobutyric acid
acts as a powerful hyperpolarizing agent on the ON-bipolar
cells, just like kainic acid and the photoreceptor transmitter, while it is without effect on the OFF-bipolar cells
(Slaughter and Miller, 1981).

These results suggest that there may be in fact two
sorts of kainic acid-preferring receptors in the chicken
retina, whose properties are outlined in Table 1. No
binding studies are yet available to test for the existence
of these two types of receptor, although kainic acid-

preferring receptors in the retina have been demonstrated (Biziere and Coyle, 1979). The use of the selective agonists and antagonists should enable their identity to be confirmed or disconfirmed. One important point is that, while the evidence on a given species is incomplete, the partial data available on fish (Shiells et al. 1981; Lasater and Dowling, 1982; Rowe and Ruddock, 1982a, b), amphibia (Slaughter and Miller, 1981), birds (Dvorak and Morgan, 1983) and mammals (Neal et al. 1981; Schiller, 1982) suggest that the features of the receptors outlined in Table 1 are common to all vertebrate species.

TABLE 1

Kainic acid-preferring receptors in chicken retina.

response	depolarizing	hyperpolarizing
cellular localization	horizontal cells and OFF-centre bipolar cells	ON-centre bipolar cells
agonists	kainic acid photoreceptor transmitter?	kainic acid 2-amino-4-phosphonobutyric acid photoreceptor transmitter?
antagonists	piperidine 2,3-dicarboxylic acid D-γ-glutamylglycine	?

These observations clearly have some implications for the nature of the photoreceptor transmitter. Kainic acid mimics the effect of the photoreceptor transmitter by depolarizing horizontal and OFF-bipolar cells and by hyperpolarizing the ON-bipolar cells. It is much more effective than glutamic and aspartic acids, and appears to interact with a kainic acid-preferring receptor. It therefore seems reasonable to suggest that the photoreceptor transmitter or transmitters is likely to be a molecule structurally related to glutamic and/or aspartic acid, with a preferential affinity of the kainic acid-preferring receptor. Studies on the ability of the selective agonists and antagonists to interfere with light responses in bipolar cells will be necessary to further establish this possibility.

At the level of the inner plexiform layer, amacrine cells
clearly possess NMDA receptors. Whether they are related
to bipolar cell input, or are related to other inputs to
the amacrine cells, remains to be established. The further
implication would be that the likely transmitter is a
compound structurally related to aspartic acid, or aspartic
acid itself. There does appear to be a correlation between
bipolar cell input and the sensitivity of the amacrine cells
to kainic acid. Thus in the case of an amacrine cell whose
synaptic inputs have not yet been defined, if it is
sensitive to kainic acid, it may be tentatively assumed
that it receives bipolar cell input.

IMPLICATIONS FOR THE MODE OF ACTION
OF KAINIC ACID

As outlined above, in the retina there may in fact
be two pharmacologically distinct kainic acid-preferring
receptors, one linked to depolarizing and the other to
hyperpolarizing responses. Whether these two types of
receptor exist in other parts of the nervous system is not
known. The pattern of toxicity of bipolar cells in the
retina suggests that only the OFF-bipolar cells, which are
depolarized by kainic acid, are destroyed following an
interaction with one receptor type which corresponds to
that defined in spinal cord and hippocampus. The ON-bipolar
cells, which are known to be hyperpolarized by kainic acid,
survive. This is consistent with the initial excitotoxic
hypothesis of Olney (1974), by suggesting that depolarizing
responses are obligatory for neurotoxicity.

Active pre-synaptic terminals do not seem to be
necessary for the kainic acid-induced destruction of bipolar
cells. Intravitreal injections of doses of Co^{++} which
completely block light-evoked responses have no effect on
the destruction of the bipolar cells by kainic acid.
Similarly varying photoreceptor activity by varying ambient
lighting conditions does not shift the kainic acid-neuro-
toxicity dose-response curve. By contrast, pre-synaptic
activity, probably induced in bipolar cells by kainic acid,
appears to be essential for the destruction of amacrine
cells. This activity on its own may be sufficient to
destroy those cells, although further work needs to be
carried out to establish this point. The indirect cell
death seems to be prevented by barbiturates and benzodiazepines, presumably as a result of activation of GABA-

ergic inhibitory phenomena in the inner plexiform layer.
In many species, the synapses of GABAergic amacrine cells
are widely distributed in the inner plexiform layer (Lam
et al. 1979; Brandon et al. 1979; Famiglietti and Vaughn,
1981; Yazulla and Brecha, 1981). One obvious morphological
substrate for these protective effects is the GABAergic
amacrine cell feed-back synapse onto bipolar cell terminals
which exists in many species. Although these indirect
effects of kainic acid are similar in some ways to the
distant cell death induced by kainic acid in the brain, it
is not clear how closely related the two phenomena are.

   One interesting point is that while the ganglion cells
show rapid responses to both kainic acid and N-methyl-D-
aspartic acid, neither compound destroys them (Morgan and
Ingham, 1981; Ingham and Morgan, 1983; unpublished results).
It is not clear why the ganglion cells survive, particularly
since the resistance of ganglion cells is not observed in
all species (Goto et al. 1981; Hampton et al. 1981; Hughes
and Wienawa-Narkiewicz, 1980; Lessell et al. 1980; Yazulla
and Kleinschmidt, 1980). The survival of ganglion cells
in birds may be related to the exceptional complexity of
the avian inner plexiform layer (Dubin, 1970). It is
possible that ganglion cells are protected because they
receive relatively little direct bipolar cell input.
Alternatively the relative balance of excitatory and
inhibitory inputs to a cell may be important, and avian
ganglion cells may be protected by a high level of inhibitory amacrine cell input.

   These results do not directly clarify the intracellular
events which follow the interaction of kainic acid with
membrane-bound receptors and ultimately lead to cell
destruction. However anatomical studies have demonstrated
pronounced swelling of cell processes in the retina as one
of the earliest detectable effects of kainic acid (Ingham
and Morgan 1983; Morgan and Ingham, in preparation). Biochemical studies have shown rapid losses of ATP and phos-
phocreatine after exposure to kainic acid (Biziere and
Coyle, 1978b). Both these responses to kainic acid have
been reported in other parts of the nervous system
(Nicklas et al. 1980; Retz and Coyle, 1980). In the case
of the retina, other compounds appear to have related neurotoxic properties. In frog retina, veratrine, which
chronically activates voltage-sensitive sodium channels,
eliminates spike-generating neurons (Schwartz, 1982).

In chicken retina, ouabain, which blocks the operation of (Na^+, K^+)-ATPase leads to pronounced swelling of retinal neurons, and eventually to neuronal destruction. Since at least in the short term, ouabain would be expected to increase rather than decrease ATP levels as a result of its ability to block (Na^+, K^+)-ATPase, this may not be the crucial element in neurotoxicity of the kind mediated by all these compounds. Rather the crucial element may be the cellular oedema induced in the case of kainic acid by receptor-mediated opening of sodium channels, in the case of veratrine by the chronic activation of voltage-sensitive sodium channels, and in the case of ouabain by failure of the sodium pump. In this perspective, the excitotoxic compounds would be only one specific trigger for a chain of intracellular events, including cell swelling, which leads eventually to neuronal destruction.

CONCLUSIONS

The use of the vertebrate retina, with its defined neuronal population and neuronal interactions, and the systematic use of the presently available range of relatively selective and potent excitatory amino acid agonists and antagonists, has enabled combined biochemical, morphological and physiological studies of the role of the excitatory amino acids as transmitters in this tissue. Progress has been particularly facilitated by the ease with which physiologically relevant inputs to the retina (light stimuli) can be controlled, and by the ease with which the retinal output (ganglion cell activity) can be monitored. In lower vertebrates, the large size of the retinal neurons facilitates intracellular recording of the effects of the selective agonists and antagonists. These studies have led to some novel conclusions:

1. In the retina, the so-called excitatory amino acids can provoke hyperpolarizing responses, as well as the more commonly observed depolarizations.
2. In the retina these hyperpolarizing responses appear to be associated with a form of kainic acid-preferring receptor pharmalogically distinct from that associated with the depolarizing responses.
3. In the retina, kainic acid-preferring receptors and NMDA-preferring receptors have distinct cellular localizations, the former on the bipolar and horizontal cells, the latter on amacrine cells and probably

ganglion cells.

Many of these conclusions may have implications for the role of kainic acid-preferring receptors, and for the role of the "excitatory" amino acids as transmitters in many other parts of the nervous system.

REFERENCES

Adolph, A., Dowling, J.E., and Ehinger, B. (1980). *Cell Tissue Res.* <u>210</u>, 269.

Ashmore, J.F., and Falk, G. (1979). *Vision Res.* <u>19</u>, 419.

Ben-Ari, Y., Tremblay, E., Ottersen, O.P., and Naquet, R. (1979). *Brain Res.* <u>165</u>, 362.

Biziere, K., and Coyle, J.T. (1978a). *Neurosci. Lett.* <u>8</u>, 303.

Biziere, K., and Coyle, J.T. (1978b). *J. Neurochem.* <u>31</u>, 513.

Biziere, K., and Coyle, J.T. (1979). *Neuropharmacol.* <u>18</u>, 409.

Brandon, C., Lam, D.M., and Wu, J.Y. (1979). *Proc. Natl. Acad. Sci. USA* <u>76</u>, 3557.

Coyle, J.T. (1982). *Trends in Neuroscience* <u>5</u>, 287.

Coyle, J.T., Bird, S.J., Evans, R.H., Gulley, R.L., Nadler, J.V., Nicklas, W.J., and Olney, J.W. (1981). *Neurosci. Res. Prog. Bull.* <u>19</u>, 331.

Dowling, J.E., and Ehinger, B. (1978). *J. comp. Neurol.* <u>180</u>, 203.

Dowling, J.E., Ehinger, B., and Floren, J. (1980). *J. comp. Neurol.* <u>192</u>, 665.

Dubin, M.W. (1970). *J. comp. Neurol.* <u>140</u>, 479.

Dvorak, D.R., and Morgan, I.G. (1983). *Neurosci. Lett.* in press.

Ehrlich, D., and Morgan, I.G. (1980). *Neurosci. Lett.* <u>17</u>, 43.

Famiglietti, E.V., and Vaughn, J.E. (1981). *J. comp. Neurol.* <u>197</u>, 129.

Ferkany, J.W., Zaczek, R., and Coyle, J.T. (1982). *Nature* (Lond.) <u>298</u>, 757.

Goto, M., Inomata, N., Oho, H., Saito, K.I., and Fukuda, H. (1981). *Brain Res.* <u>211</u>, 305.

Hampton, C.K., Garcia, C. and Redburn, D.A. (1981). *J. Neurosci. Res.* <u>6</u>, 99.

Holmgren-Taylor, I. (1982). *Invest. Ophthalmol. vis. Sci.* <u>22</u>, 8.

Hughes, A., and Wienawa-Narkiewicz, E. (1980). *Nature* (Lond.) 284, 468.

Ikeda, H., and Sheardown, M.J. (1982) *Neuroscience* 7, 25.

Imperato, A., Porceddu, M.L., Morelli, M., Fossarello, M., and Di Chiara, G. (1981). *Brain Res.* 213, 205.

Ingham, C.A., and Morgan, I.G. (1983). *Neuroscience*, in press.

Lam, D.M.K., Su, Y.Y.T., Swain, L., Marc, R.E., Brandon, C., and Wu, J.Y. (1979). *Nature* (Lond.) 278, 565.

Lasater, E.M., and Dowling, J.E. (1982). *Proc. Natl. Acad. Sci. USA.* 79, 936.

Lessell, S., Craft, J.L., and Albert, D.M. (1980). *Exp. Eye Res.* 30, 731.

London, E.D. and Coyle, J.T. (1979). *Mol.Pharmacol.* 15, 492.

Lucas, D.R., and Newhouse, J.P. (1957). *Arch. Ophthalmol.* 58, 193.

McGeer, E.G., Olney, J.W., and McGeer, P.L. (1978a). *Kainic Acid as a Tool in Neurobiology,* (Eds.). Raven Press, New York.

McGeer, E.G., McGeer, P.L., and Singh, K. (1978b). *Brain Res.* 139 381.

McLennan, H. (1981). in *Glutamate as a Neurotransmitter*. Di Chiara, G., and Gessa, G.L. (Eds.). Raven Press, New York, p.253.

Morgan, I.G. (1983). in *Progress in Retinal Research*. Chader, G.L. and Osborne, N. (Eds.). Pergamon, Oxford, in press.

Morgan, I.G., and El-Lakany (1982). *Neurosci. Lett.* 34, 69.

Morgan, I.G., and Ingham, C.A. (1981). *Neurosci. Lett.* 21, 275.

Murakami, O., Ohtsu, K., and Shimazaki, H. (1975). *Vision Res.* 15, 456.

Nadler, J.V., and Cuthbertson, G.J. (1980). *Brain Res.* 195, 47.

Neal, M., Cunningham, J.R., James, T.A., Joseph, M., and Collins, J.F. (1981). *Neurosci. Lett.* 26, 301.

Nicklas, W.J., Krespan, B., and Berl, S., (1980). *Eur. J. Pharmacol.* 62, 209.

Olney, J.W., (1974). in *Heritable Disorders of Amino Acid Metabolism*. Nyham, W.H. (Ed.). John Wiley, New York, p. 501.

Retz, J.C., and Coyle, J.T., (1980). *Life Sci.* 27, 2495.

Rowe, J.S., and Ruddock, K.H. (1982a). *Neurosci. Lett.* 30, 257.

Rowe, J.S., and Ruddock, K.H., (1982b). *Neurosci. Lett.*
    30, 251.

Schiller, P. (1982). *Nature* (Lond.). 297, 580.

Schwarcz, R., and Coyle, J.T. (1977). *Invest. Ophthalmol.*
    vis. Sci. 16, 141.

Schwarcz, R., Scholz, D., and Coyle, J.T. (1978). *Neuro-*
    pharmacol. 17, 145.

Schwarcz, E.A., (1982). *J. Physiol.* 323, 211.

Schwob, J.E., Fuller, T., Price, J.L. and Olney, J.W.,
    (1980). *Neuroscience* 5, 991.

Shiells, R.A., Falk, G. and Naghshineh, S. (1981). *Nature*
    (Lond.). 294, 592.

Slaughter, M.M., and Miller, R.F. (1981). *Science* 211, 182.

Streit, P., Stella, M., and Cuenod, M., (1980). *Brain Res.*
    187, 47.

Watkins, J.C., and Evans, R.H., (1981). *Ann. Rev. Pharma-*
    col. Toxicol. 21, 165.

Yazulla, S., and Brecha, N. (1981). *Proc. Natl. Acad. Sci.*
    USA. 78, 643.

Yazulla, S., and Kleinschmidt, J. (1980). *Brain Res.* 182
    287.

III. Behavioral Neurology

STRESS HORMONES AND HEALTH

*G. Singer and W. Fibiger

*Department of Psychology & Brain-Behaviour Research Institute
CSIRO, Division of Chemical & Wood Technology

La Trobe University, Melbourne, Australia
Melbourne, Australia

ABSTRACT

In this paper a rationale will be provided for the use of urine hormone tests in the assessment of stress in industry and as a measure of outcome of stress management programs.

Recent research on differential patterns of hormone responses to physical and psychological stress, examples of the effect of automation and piece work payments on hormone levels and changes in hormone levels as a result of stress management programs will be presented.

It is argued that these biochemical measures will play an ever increasing role in stress assessment since they are more objective and have the additional advantage of providing a direct link with stress related illness.

I do not intend to enter into an argument on how to define stress. Biologists regard a number of environmental conditions such as extreme heat or cold or lack of oxygen in the atmosphere as "physical stress". Exercise can also produce physical stress whereas threatening environmental situations produce psychological stress. It has been suggested (Selye, 1976) that these various stresses give rise to a non-specific arousal the general adaptation syndrome. Later research (Levi et al., 1982) has shown that in addition to the general mobilisation of the body for activity (fight and flight) there are specific physiological responses attached to specific emotional states.

In this paper I will be concerned with the relationship of physiological factors (in particular neuroendocrine responses) and stressful situations. Dr Spillane in his paper will be more specific about the genesis of stressful factors in industrial settings. My specific topics for tonight which will be based mainly on findings from our own research will be:

1. Rationale for the use of hormone responses and examples from laboratory studies;

2. Patterns of hormone responses during physical and psychological stress;

3. Stress and health;

4. Examples of field studies in industry;

5. Hormone responses in stress management programs.

1. RATIONALE FOR USE OF HORMONES

Figures 1 and 2 show the simplified flow charts of the release of cortisol and catecholamines following the perception of threatening arousing or distressing stimuli. Two points need to be made here:

(a) The hormonal responses are preparing the organisms for activity (see Fig. 3). However, high levels of the fight-flight response are inappropriate in a modern society when these neuroendocrine responses are produced while sitting at a desk or working at a machine.

(b) These hormone responses will occur again at any time of the day or night when a person thinks or imagines the stressful situation which gave rise to the earlier hormone responses. If no activity is involved these hormone responses are inappropriate since they are neither conducive to problem solving nor to sleep.

First, I would like to give you an example of a laboratory study which shows the relationship between hormone responses and stressful situations. In an experiment

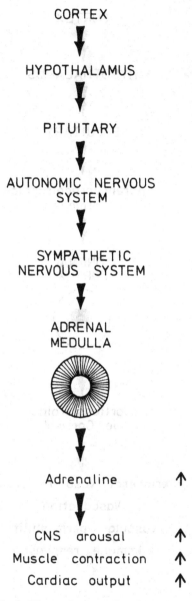

Figure 1. Simplified flow chart of adrenaline release
following a threatening stimulus.

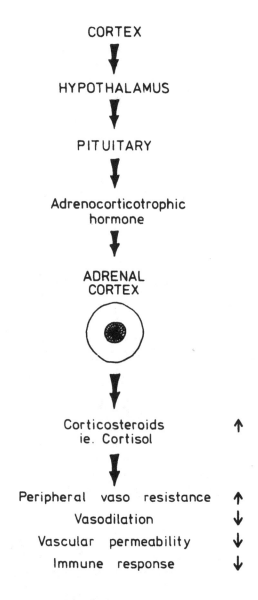

Figure 2. Simplified flow chart of cortisol release
following a distressing stimulus.

FIGHT-FLIGHT RESPONSE

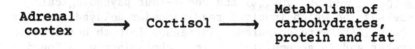

Adrenal cortex ⟶ Cortisol ⟶ Metabolism of carbohydrates, protein and fat

Adrenal medulla ⟶ Catecholamines: Adrenaline Noradrenaline ⟶ Circulatory system (H.R. B.P.) glucose release

Figure 3. Preparation for activity, fight-flight responses.

conducted by Frankenhauser and colleagues at the University of Stockholm a group of subjects were given a baseline test of the speed and accuracy of performance when the background noise was 76 db. During this session a baseline for physiological cost, heart rate, blood pressure, urine adrenaline, noradrenaline and cortisol were also established. In a second session on the following day the same subjects performed similar mental tests with an 86 db background noise which made this task by far more difficult to perform. Results showed that during the second session performance was maintained at the same level as baseline but that all parameters of physiological cost increased. In a second experiment baseline conditions were established in exactly the same way as in the first experiment. In a second session with 86 db background noise levels of aspiration of these subjects was lowered by warning them that nobody is expected to work at the same rate when conditions are so much more unpleasant and difficult. For this group performance levels dropped and all parameters of physiological cost remained at baseline level. These experiments show the effects of psychological factors on hormonal responses. There is a considerable body of data showing a similar relationship between psychological stress and hormone responses. Now I will turn to one of our more recent studies on the relationship between catecholamines in urine and hormonal responses to physical and psychological stress.

2. PHYSICAL AND PSYCHOLOGICAL STRESS

Changes in urine catecholamines, blood pressure and
heart rate during one hour physical exercise sessions
(35% VO_{2max} and 50% VO_{2max}) and one 1-hour psychological
stress session which involved reading under delayed auditory
feedback (DAF) were compared. Increases in both hemodynamic
parameter and in accumulation of catecholamines were found
in response to all three tests. The changes in adrenaline
did not differentiate between the tests. Noradrenaline
levels were significantly larger for physical exercise

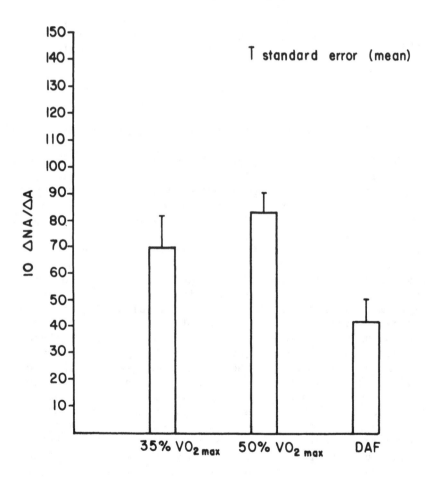

Figure 4. Mean ratio of pretest-post test difference scores
of Noradrenaline-Adrenaline for physical exercise and DAF
conditions.

conditions and graded according to the relative workload.
A ratio $\Delta NA/\Delta A$ was similar in both physical exercises but
statistically different for DAF (Fig. 4). Negative correlations for physical tests with hemodynamics parameters and
catecholamine accumulation were found, whereas correlations
between DAF and hemodynamic factors and catecholamines were
positive (Fibiger et al, 1983). These correlations suggest
a reasonable balance between secretion and reuptake in
sympathetic nerve endings and metabolism in tissues of both
hormones during physical effort contrasted with a surplus in
secretion and a less complete withdrawal of parasympathetic
tone during psychological stress.

3.   STRESS AND HEALTH

The most important question is how does stress and hormone secretion relate to health? A number of sociological
studies are available. Some examples are: studies of the
English public service show that the lower echelon of
the public service has a much greater incidence of both
morbidity and mortality, and there have been various other
studies relating coronary heart disease to occupational
groups and to various types of jobs (Henry and Stephens, 1978).
All of these provide correlational data and correlational
data are very interesting but do not imply causation. Let me
give you at least one example: in 1969 the Surgeon General
of the United States provided a report showing correlations
between cigarette smoking and lung cancer. The first
interpretation of this report, not only by the tobacco lobby
and by heavy smokers, was "well, there could be a selection
factor here; it does not imply a causal relationship". It
is totally possible to interpret this correlation by saying
that people who are prone to lung cancer have a craving for
cigarettes. This is an alternate scientifically respectable
interpretation of these results. Now we do not believe it
any more, and not because we have become less sceptical and
more suspicious of vested interests of people who are more
addicted to cigarette smoking, but simply because there is
now a whole body of experimental data which is derived from
animal and human experiments and very clearly shows that you
can only interpret this correlation as cigarette smoking
causing lung cancer and not vice versa. Dr Bassett will
report a series of elegant laboratory studies which show a
causal link between stress, catecholamines, steroids and

various forms of heart disease, thus providing a causal link for many of the correlational studies, like the study of English public servants cited earlier.

4.   EXAMPLES OF FIELD STUDIES IN INDUSTRY

In a study in the clothing industry we compared female operators on manual electric sewing machines with operators on automated machines. Questionnaire responses of job satisfaction and perception of health showed no difference between the two groups. Urine samples taken at 11, 14 and 16.30 hours showed significantly higher adrenaline and noradrenaline levels but not cortisol for the operators of automated machines at the two afternoon test sessions (see Figs. 5,6,7).

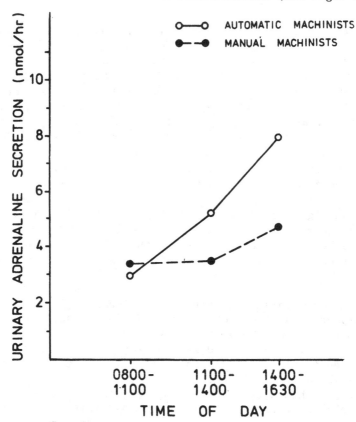

Figure 5. Mean Urinary Adrenaline levels for automated and manual operators in a clothing factory during a working day.

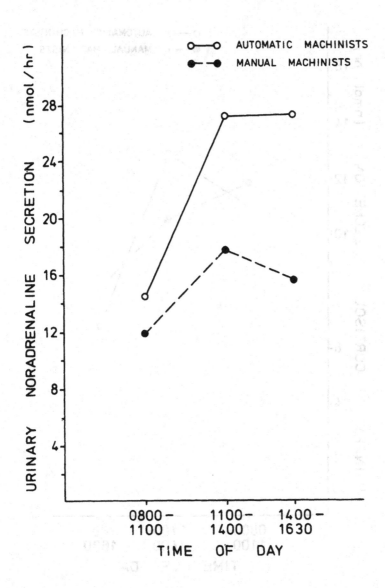

Figure 6. Mean Urinary Noradrenaline levels for automated and manual operators in a clothing factory during a working day.

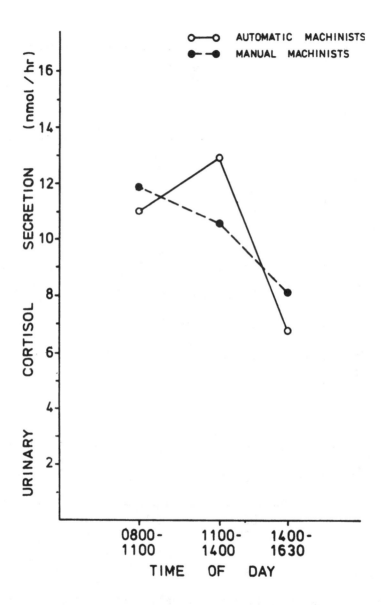

Figure 7. Mean Urinary Cortisol levels for automated and manual operators in a clothing factory during a working day.

There was also an increase in adrenaline for both groups of
operators at the last period of the day, at a time when
circadian rhythm research shows a decline in this hormone in
readiness for relaxation and sleep. For noradrenaline this
pattern was only present for operators of automatic machines.
These data aré consistent with reports by both groups of
workers of an inability to unwind when returning home after
work. Since both groups in this factory worked on a piece
rate incentive system it is possible that this arousal is
the   result   of   "psychological pacing".   In order to test
this hypothesis we compared these clothing workers with
manual and automated female operators in a munitions factory
where no incentive system was operating. The results (Fig. 8,9)

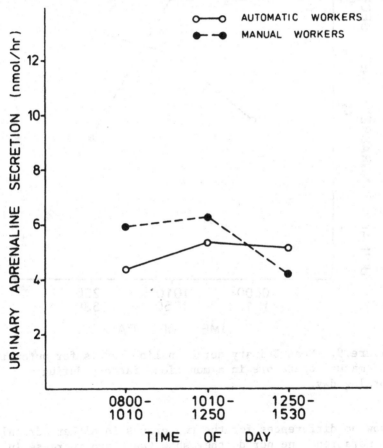

Figure 8. Mean Urinary Adrenaline levels for automated and
manual operators in a munitions factory during a working day.

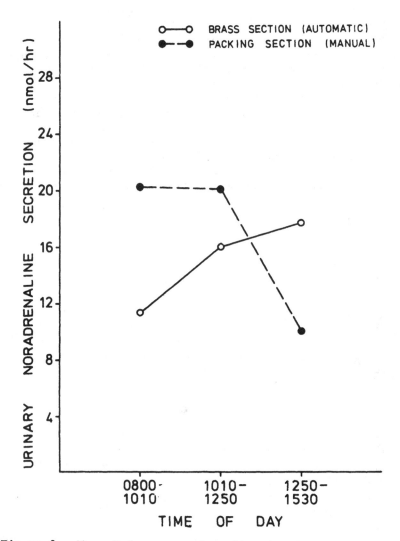

Figure 9. Mean Urinary noradrenaline levels for automated and manual operators in a munitions factory during a working day.

show no differences for the two groups in either adrenaline or noradrenaline nor do they show the sharp increase in hormones at the end of the day (Romas et al, 1983)

These studies are representative of our industrial

studies and suggest that hormonal responses may be more
sensitive in a number of stressful situations than questionnaire data.

5. HORMONE RESPONSES IN STRESS MANAGEMENT PROGRAMS

Kirk, Coleman and Singer (1981) conducted two experiments designed to evaluate the effect of the relaxation
response on the adrenal hormones cortisol, noradrenaline and
adrenaline. Both acute and chronic practice of the relaxation response were evaluated, and the results showed that
while cortisol and adrenaline decreased below basal levels
during the relaxation response noradrenaline did not change
(see Figs. 10,11,12).

We concluded that the results indicate the potential
for implementing relaxation techniques in the treatment of
stress-related disorders, especially those with disorders
relating specifically to the hormones cortisol and adrenaline
and that changes in hormone levels provide an independent
outcome measure for the success of these stress management
programs.

In an attempt to assess the effect of a 10-week stress
management program on the hormonal responses of police
recruits at a residential training centre a "stress management group" was compared with a control group. The recruits
spent 20 weeks living in at the police training academy but
were permitted to return to their homes at the weekends.
The stress management classes commenced for the experimental
group 10 weeks after they were admitted into the academy,
and were held every Tuesday from 8.50 am through to 10.20 am
for the remaining ten weeks of training. The control group
received no classes. The urine collection days were during
the first, tenth and twentieth week being the final week of
the recruits' training. Samples were collected at 6.00 am,
10.00 am and 2.00 pm. The group receiving the training
showed significantly lower levels of adrenaline and noradrenaline.

In both groups the levels of both adrenaline and
noradrenaline rose during the training course in the academy -
similar stress related changes have been reported for other
intensive training courses. The increase was significant

for the control groups but not for the stress management group.

These results indicate that those who received the stress management program showed smaller increases in hormonal response possibly because the programe enabled them to cope better with the pressure of the training course. These examples show that hormonal tests can be useful in stress assessment in industrial settings and in the assessment of the outcome of stress management programs. These neuroendocrine responses also provide a direct link between stress and illness.

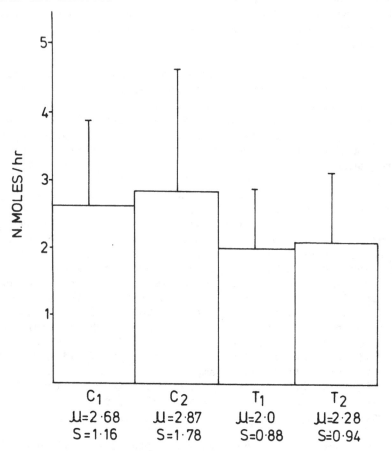

Fig. 10   ADRENALINE MEAN N.MOLES/hr FOR CONTROL
AND TREATMENT SESSIONS.   (P<0·05)

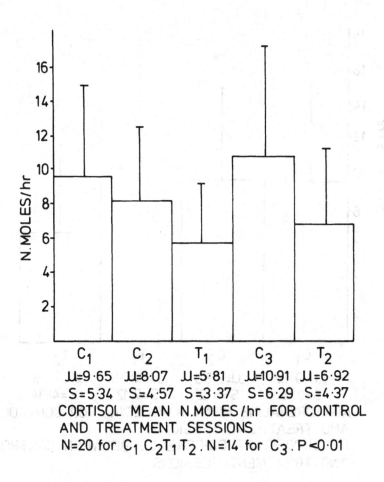

Figure 11.

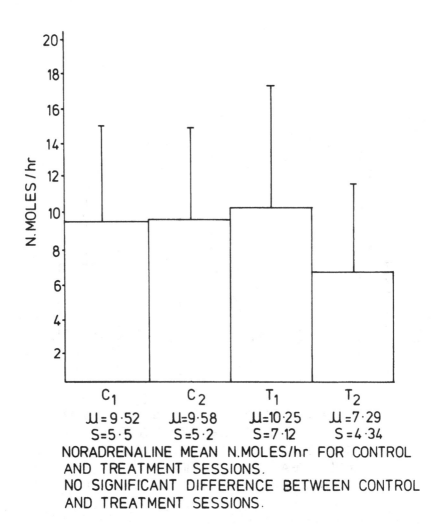

NORADRENALINE MEAN N.MOLES/hr FOR CONTROL
AND TREATMENT SESSIONS.
NO SIGNIFICANT DIFFERENCE BETWEEN CONTROL
AND TREATMENT SESSIONS.

Figure 12.

REFERENCES

Fibiger, W. and Singer, G. (1983), Physiological changes during physical and psychological stress (submitted International Journal of Psychophysiology.)

Henry, C.P. and Stephens, P.M. (1977), Stress Health and the Social Environment. Springer Verlag, NY Inc.

Kirk, A, Coleman, G and Singer, G. (in preparation 1983). Changes in neuroendocrine responses following the relaxation response in trained and untrained subjects.

Levi, L. Frankenhauser, M. and Gardell, B. (1982), Work stress related to Social Structures and Processes in G.R. Elliott and C. Eisdorfer, eds. Research on Stress and Human Health Springer Publishing Co. New York.

Romas, N., Beeby, M, Coleman, G., Spillane, R. and Singer, G. (in preparation 1983) The effects of automation and piece work on urinary catocholomine responses.

Seyle, H. (1976). Stress in health and disease, Butterworths, Boston.

Singer, G. (1980). Work environment stress, neuroendocrine changes and health in ed. J.W.G. Tiller and P.R. Martin Behavioural Medicine, Geigy Psychiatric Symposium, Melbourne. p. 49 - 59.

STRESS AND WORK BEHAVIOUR

Dr. Robert Spillane

Management Studies Centre
Macquarie University
North Ryde   NSW   2113
AUSTRALIA

ABSTRACT

     The aim of this paper is to overview research into
relationships between job satisfaction, work environment,
job content, occupational stress and health. Factors
which interfere with work effectiveness and are believed
to contribute to occupational stress are discussed. The
main theme of the research program is the application of
psychoneuroendocrine studies of occupational stress and
coping responses in Australian work environments. Interest
is focussed on the relationships between work environments
characterised by understimulation, overstimulation, lack
of personal control and psychobiological indices of stress
(adrenaline, noradrenaline, cortisol). The modulating
influence of controllability is considered in relation to
work settings, e.g. in highly mechanised and highly automated work processes. Implications of stress research for
the design of jobs and organisations in Australia are
discussed.

INTRODUCTION

     In the search for improvements in productivity, work
effectiveness, employee health and well-being are inextric-
ably linked. Thus it is not surprising that the study of
occupational stress has become a major topic in work
research. It has become commonplace to speak of stress-
related disorders threatening the health and well-being of
industrial man. This view is well supported by the dramatically high proportion of people who suffer from some form
of stress-related illness, such as hypertension or cardiac
disease. Moreover, people who are dissatisfied with their
work are more likely to suffer from a range of physical and
psychological disorders than are those whose work is interesting and challenging (Gardell & Johansson, 1981).
Researchers have found that the incidence of nervous diseases, problems of sleep, psychosomatic symptoms and use
of medication are highest among people with narrow, monotonous jobs which do not allow the individual to learn and
develop basic skills (Gardell, 1971; 1976; Kornhauser, 1965).
Furthermore, people with narrow and constrained jobs are
less likely to take part in social and cultural activities
outside the job (Karasek, 1981).

     Stress research, is not only a social, psychological
and medical topic. It is also a political topic which has

significant economic implications which extend beyond the
work organisation. When research moves from the laboratory
to the work organisation it becomes enmeshed in the politics
of industrial relations. Stress research has the potential
to influence industrial courts in matters of workers'
compensation, work-value judgements, job design and managerial
prerogatives. It may well become a major factor in work
reform in Australia in the next decade.

STRESS RESEARCH

If the 1960's was the decade of social democracy in
Western Europe, the 1970's was the decade of industrial
democracy. Experiments were conducted which took up the
challenge of changing work environments to promote increased effectiveness, job satisfaction, less work stress and
more involvement in the work process. Studies showed that
the social and human costs of improving productivity were
greater than had previously been acknowledged (Gardell,
1976; 1981). The following factors were associated with
psychosocial difficulties, ill-health, absenteeism and
poor work performance:
- Structural change.
- Physical and chemical factors in the work environment
  (e.g. inadequate lighting, excessive noise vibration,
  extremes of temperature, dust, fumes, physical and
  chemical hazards).
- Machine pacing of work rhythm and machine control of
  work methods.
- Monotonous and repetitive work.
- Authoritarian and detailed control of the individual
  (e.g. by foremen, supervisors, computer system etc).
- Piece-rate and related payment systems.
- Shift work and the effects of mechanisation.
- Lack of possibilities for contact with people at work.

Gardell (1981) believes that studies dealing with the
relationship between job content and work effectiveness
have shown that two dimensions are crucial:
- "the degree of discretion given to the individual
  to determine work layout, working methods, pace and
  social interaction; to perform a task in various
  ways, improve his performance and further develop
  any aptitudes he may have;

- the level of skill that the task requires of the
  individual; his know-how, initiative, and ability
  to initiate contacts - in short, all the creative
  talents needed to do a satisfactory job" (p. 7).

Where workers are obliged to work in low discretion
jobs with little opportunity to use creative talents feelings
of monotony, coercion and mental strain are reported.
These are more widespread and intense among workers whose
jobs are severely circumscribed as to autonomy, variety,
skill and social interaction. These results are valid
after allowances are made for age, sex, education, income,
quality of supervision and pay satisfaction. Studies of
white-collar workers confirm trends established for blue-
collar workers.

A breakdown of the results by age reveals that monotony
in relation to machine-paced and low-skilled jobs is more
pronounced among young and better educated workers. A
breakdown by income shows that income differences cannot
explain differences in monotony, powerlessness, mental
strain and social isolation (Blauner, 1964; Gardell, 1971;
1981).

HEALTH CONSEQUENCES OF JOB DESIGN

Evidence linking work environment, job content, stress
responses and ill-health is not as clearcut as that regarding
job dissatisfaction.   This is largely due to the probable
influence of confounding variables. For example, social
class and personality factors, company selection procedures,
health reasons for job mobility or terminations, may all
influence these relationships (Kasl, 1978). Further,
problems in determining and measuring exposure to stressors,
stress responses and longer-term problems are considerable.

However, there is sufficient evidence to demonstrate that
the following aspects of job design are important from a
health viewpoint (Frankenhaeuser & Gardell, 1976).

- 1. Quantitative overload (too much to do, time pressure,
  repetitious work flow).

- 2. Qualitative underload (too narrow job, little content,
  lack of variety, no demands on creativity).

-   3. <u>Lack of control</u> (over planning, work pace, work
       methods).

-   4. <u>Lack of social support</u> from significant others.

PHYSIOLOGICAL COST OF WORK

One technique used by Swedish researchers employs
urinary hormonal analysis to index the physiological cost
of work. This research strategy involves the following
assumptions:

(1)   there is a physiological cost attached to all work
       situations - in some cases the cost is large, in
       other cases it is small;

(2)   this cost varies with the type of situation and with
       the personality of the individual; and

(3)   this cost can be assessed independently of survey type
       job satisfaction questionnaires by analysis of the
       "stress hormones" (Singer, 1980).

One of the notions underlying the use of physiological
techniques in stress research is that one can determine the
emotional impact of specific factors in the environment by
measuring the activity of the body's organ systems. With the
development of biochemical techniques that permit the
determination of exceedingly small amounts of hormones in
blood and urine, stress research has been placed on a more
rigorous foundation.

Many jobs require workers to maintain performance
under difficult conditions. Those who achieve this goal
often do so at a cost. Adrenaline, noradrenaline, cortisol
levels, heart rate and blood pressure have been seen to
increase as a result of attempting to maintain job performance under conditions of job overload and job underload.
In short, performance is maintained but physiological cost
increases (Johansson <u>et al</u>, 1978).

An important issue in such research is whether hormonal
excretion patterns are causally linked to disease. Although
there is no direct evidence for such a causal relationship
data from several sources suggest that if secretion is
prolonged, damage to various organs may occur (Henry &

Stephens, 1977).

It is important to note that individuals differ with
regard to secretion patterns during and after exposure to
stressors. Field studies pursued the hypothesis that the
time for 'unwinding' varies predictably with the person's
state of well-being. In a group of industrial workers the
proportion of 'rapid decreasers' was significantly higher
after than before a vacation period which had improved
workers' physical condition and psychological state
(Johansson, 1976). In a study of overtime at work, Rissler
(1977) demonstrated that adrenaline excretion was significantly increased throughout an overtime period. An interesting finding, however, was the pronounced elevation of
adrenaline output in the evenings which were spent relaxing
at home. This was accompanied by an elevated heart rate
and feelings of fatigue and irritability. The results
showed that the effects of work overload may spread to
leisure hours and may accumulate gradually.

Swedish researchers (Frankenhaeuser, 1981; Frankenhaeuser
& Gardell, 1976) have found that the following factors
produce elevated levels of adrenaline and noradrenaline:

- machine-paced work
- short work cycles
- repetitive work with little task variation
- shift-work
- overtime
- long periods at video-display units
- piece-rated payment systems
- open-plan offices
- time-pressures (e.g. in bus driving)
- lack of control over work process.

In Australia Singer, Spillane and Romas (1982) studied
female operators in a clothing factory and found that women
operating semi-automated sewing machines had higher levels
of adrenaline and noradrenaline than did women operating
manual machines which allowed more control over the work
process. The results showed an increase in arousal for
both manual and automated workers at the end of the working
day. This is contrary to the normal 24 hour change patterns
of the hormones in which arousal levels should decline
towards the end of the afternoon in preparation for rest
and sleep during the evening. The hormonal patterns were

reflected in the operators' questionnaire reports which
revealed that "inability to unwind" after work was the best
predictor of job satisfaction and health. Singer and his
colleagues argue that the feeling of continued arousal may
have long term effects on health. The end of day arousal
was much greater for the automated workers than for manual
workers, although this difference could only be detected by
hormonal analysis. None of the questionnaire responses
revealed this difference which suggests that workers cannot
explain to themselves or to others the origin of these
feelings. In fact, a feature of this study was the high
levels of job satisfaction reported. Overseas studies have
reported an increase in hormonal levels at the end of the
day for workers who work on machine-paced operations
(Johansson et al, 1978). This suggests that arousal is
the result of work pace. Singer, Spillane and Romas (1982)
attribute the high end of day hormonal levels to the fast
pace originating in the incentive payment system (piece-
rates). They believe their results may constitute an early
warning signal of the effects of automation and payment by
results systems on health. In contrast to the usual
questionnaire type studies, hormonal analysis provides a
methodology for monitoring and detecting the risks which
may arise from new technologies, particularly where these
are paired with psychological pacing, as with incentive
schemes.

       This use of hormonal analysis in stress research
overcomes the difficulties associated with the use of job
satisfaction questionnaires.

       Spillane (1981) has argued that the use of job
satisfaction questionnaires may have had a conservative
influence on stress research due to the tendency of their
designers to ask questions about people's capacity to cope
with the present rather than their desire to anticipate and
plan for change. When general questions of satisfaction with
life are raised, responses are largely conservative - a
mixture of resignation and accommodation. But when questions
are raised about the future of work and what is needed to
understand and anticipate it responses are generally
more radical.

       Spillane (1981) argues that where people adopt the
policy of calling on their powers of adaptation they become
unreliable instruments for measuring the fitness of the

work environment, particularly for others who are not so
inured. The use of job satisfaction questionnaires as the
sole index of occupational stress carries with it the risk
of pointing us towards work environments which approach the
limits of human tolerance rather than toward better
conditions. Many researchers have come to the view that
what is needed in research are studies which tell us less
about how people can adapt to their work environments and
more about how these environments can be improved.

Many researchers and practitioners have accepted survey
results at face value and have not concerned themselves with
the psychological processes which underpin questionnaire
responses. A serious consequence of this research has been
the tendency to consider a small percentage of employees
as chronically dissatisfied and to attribute their dissatisfaction to maladjusted personalities rather than working
conditions. According to Vroom (1964), most of the empirical
work in the field of job satisfaction represents an effort
to show that those who are job dissatisfied are likely to
be neurotic or maladjusted and their dissatisfaction is
related to personality pathology.

CONTROLLABILITY

Many stress researchers believe that a key to effective
coping is controllability - the control an individual has
over job-related decisions. The control people have over
their situation is related to the effects of stress on body
and mind. The individual who is in a position to regulate
work load is able to maintain physiological and psychological activation at an optimum level (Frankenhaeuser & Gardell,
1976).

Karasek (1981) has pointed to the many contradictory
findings in stress research which can be traced to incomplete
models derived from two mutually exclusive research traditions.
One tradition focuses on job control and another considers
job demands. Job demands research rarely includes a discussion
of job control. Karasek believes that both job demands and
job control have to be analysed to avoid inconsistencies
such as the finding that both executives and assembly line
workers have stressful jobs, but the latter report lower
levels of job satisfaction. Consideration of differences
in job control might account for the differences in stress
symptoms and job satisfaction.

Karasek predicted that people working in high demand and low control jobs will report the highest frequency of stress symptoms (exhaustion, depression). His studies of Swedish and American workers confirm this view. Reductions in levels of job demand, however, lead to passivity among workers. Karasek argues that people working in low demand and low control jobs (i.e. passive jobs) may over time lose their ability to make judgements, solve problems and accept challenges. He found that people in passive jobs reported the highest degree of non-participation in 'active leisure' thus providing evidence for 'carry over' from work to leisure. The content of work experience has a significant association with rates of participation for socially active leisure activities. There is little evidence that deficiencies in the work environment are compensated for by choice of leisure activity.

The lowest levels of stress symptoms and the highest levels of participation in social activity are found in jobs which offer high levels of control. These findings have been confirmed by Gardell and his colleagues in studies of urban bus drivers, white-collar workers and hospital employees (Gardell, 1982).

Otto (1980) found that car plant workers in an Australian plant were under greater pressure and had less job control than workers from a government factory. Furthermore, the car plant workers experienced more stress and reported higher frequencies of psychological and physiological symptoms. Her study demonstrated clear links between (a) the quality of work environments, (b) stress and tension experiences, and (c) symptoms of impaired well-being. The study also revealed a relationship between stress and job dissatisfaction. The major stressors were:

- work pressure and work speeds over which workers have no control;

- supervisory and managerial practices which treat workers as objects rather than people;

- close supervision;

- tasks offering little scope for skill-utilisation;

- role conflict, particularly contradictory and unreasonable requests:

- adverse physical conditions.

In a study of occupational stress among high school teachers, Otto (1981) found the most prominent stressors were concerned with the alienating relationship between teachers and the Education Department. Ninety-six per cent of those questioned said they lacked influence over decisions which affected them while 79% said the Department showed them little or no appreciation, respect and consideration. Alienating circumstances within the school also affected the majority of those sampled. Lack of influence on organisational or policy decisions, lack of consultation and of appreciation by superiors were particular problems. Stress symptom levels were related to experiences of marked stress which teachers derive from various aspects of their jobs.

IMPLICATIONS FOR THE DESIGN OF JOBS AND WORK ORGANISATIONS

The following psycho-social guidelines for work organisation and job design based partly on the results of work stress research, served as the basis for Swedish legislation:

- Work should be arranged in a way which allows the individual worker to influence his own work situation, working methods and pace;

- Work should be arranged in a way which allows for overview and understanding of the work processes as a whole;

- Work should be arranged in a way which gives the individual worker possibilities to use and develop all his human resources;

- Work should be arranged in a way which allows for human contacts and co-operation in the course of work;

- Work should be arranged in a way which makes it possible for the individual worker to satisfy time claims from roles and obligations outside work, e.g. family, social and political commitments etc.

It is encouraging to note that more than 750 business organisations in Sweden alone have made various attempts to redesign work along these lines (Agure & Edgren, 1980; Swedish Employers Confederation, 1975). However, in Australia progress is very slow.

THE FUTURE

The 1980's will be a decade in which occupational stress research in Australia will mature. New, sophisticated techniques of data collection and analysis are already being used in research designs which have benefitted from the work of the Stockholm group. Research is underway in the sawmilling industry, clothing industry and the public sector where factors such as job content, piece-rates, shift-work, are the focus of attention (Bartley 1980, 1982).

Access to industrial settings will remain a problem. However, as the results of stress research become available to the general public, sponsorship of research can be expected to become more significant and diverse. Work stress research will become a major factor in Australian industrial relations as we become more aware of the psychosocial needs of all our citizens.

REFERENCES

Argue, S. & Edgren,J. (1980). "New Factories, Job Design
    through Factory Planning in Sweden". Swedish Employers
    Confederation, Stockholm.
Bartley, H. (ed) (1980). "Stress at Work". Brain Behaviour
    Research Institute, La Trobe Univ. Melbourne.
Bartley, H. (ed.) (1982). "Work Effectiveness". Brain
    Behaviour Research Institute, La Trobe Univ. Melbourne.
Blauner, R. (1964). "Alienation & Freedom". Chicago Univ.
    Press, Chicago.
Frankenhaeuser, M. & Gardell B. (1976). J. Human Stress,
    2, 3, 35-46.
Frankenhaeuser, M. (1981). In "Working Life: A Social
    Science Contribution to Work Reform". (B. Gardell &
    G. Johansson eds.) pp.213-234, John Wiley, Chichester.
Gardell, B. (1971). "Technology, Alienation & Mental Health".
    English summary in Acta Sociologica, 19, 83-93.
Gardell, B. (1976). "Job Content & Quality of LIfe", Prisma,
    Stockholm.
Gardell, B. (1981). In "Working Life:A Social Science
    Contribution to Work Reform" (B. Gardell & G. Johansson,
    eds.) pp.3-16, John Wiley, Chichester.
Gardell, B. (1982). In "Work Effectiveness" (H. Bartley ed.)
    pp.13-49. Brain Behaviour Research Institute, La Trobe
    Univ. Melbourne.
Henry, J. & Stephens, P. (1977). "Stress, Health & the
    Social Environment". Springer-Verlag, New York.
Johansson, G. (1976). Bio Psychology, 4, 157-172.
Johansson, G. Aronsson, G. & Lindstrom, B. (1978).
    Ergonomics, 21, 583-599.
Karasek, R. (1981). In "Working Life: A Social Science
    Contribution to Work Reform". (B. Gardell & G.
    Johansson, eds.) pp. 75-94. John Wiley, Chichester.
Kasl, S. (1978). In "Stress at Work". (C. Cooper & R. Payne
    eds.) John Wiley, Chichester.
Kornhauser, A. (1965). "The Mental Health of the Industrial
    Worker". John Wiley, New York.
Otto, R. (1980). "Occupational Stress among Factory Workers".
    La Trobe Univ. Melbourne.
Otto, R. (1981). "Occupational Stress among High School
    Teachers". La Trobe Univ. Melbourne.
Rissler, A. (1977). Ergonomics, 20, 13-16.

Singer, G. (1980). In "Stress at Work". (H. Bartley ed.)
    Brain Behaviour Research Institute, La Trobe Univ.
    Melbourne.
Singer, G., Spillane, R. & Romas, N. (1982) (unpublished).
    "Report on Automated Work in a Clothing Factory".
    La Trobe Univ, Melbourne.
Spillane, R. (1981). In "Work Effectiveness". (H. Bartley
    ed.) pp. 1-12. Brain Behaviour Research Institute,
    La Trobe Univ. Melbourne.
Swedish Employers Confederation (1975). "Job Reform in
    Sweden". Stockholm.
Vroom, V. (1964). "Work & Motivation" John Wiley, New York.

STRESS, CATECHOLAMINES AND ISCHAEMIC HEART DISEASE

J.R. BASSETT

Macquarie University

North Ryde, N.S.W. 2113, Australia

ABSTRACT

While emotional stress has been implicated in the pathogenesis of cardiovascular disease, controversy still exists as to how exposure to stressful situations can induce such pathological changes. Emotional, environmental and sensory stress are all associated with the activation of both the sympathetic-adrenal medullary system (resulting in the release of the catecholamines, adrenaline and noradrenaline) and the pituitary-adrenal cortical system (with the release of the glucocorticoids, cortisol and/or corticosterone). There is considerable evidence linking the emotionally induced release of catecholamines with ischaemic heart disease. But it is not the catecholamines alone; the glucocorticoids also play an important role. There is a marked intensification of the cardiotoxic effects of the catecholamines by a glucocorticoid-catecholamine interaction. The interaction between the glucocorticoids and the catecholamines appears to have two phases. The first phase occurs when the circulating level of steroid is high and results in a potentiation of the cardiac stimulating action of the catecholamines. Without an adequate compensatory dilation of the coronary vessels myocardial hypoxia and necrosis will occur. The enhanced myocardial sensitivity to the catecholamines appears to be mediated by a delay in the inactivation of the catecholamines following their release, probably via an inhibition of both neuronal and extraneuronal uptake. The second phase of the interaction occurs when the circulating

251

..evels of the glucocorticoids have adapted to a lower level.
Without the anti-inflammatory action of the steroids, the
catecholamines initiate the release of endogenous
inflammatory substances, the opening up of junctional gaps
in the endothelial lining of the coronary vessels, and the
aggregation of platelets. The resulting thrombosis and
deposition of lipids in the coronary artery wall leads to
myocardial infarction associated with coronary occlusion.

INTRODUCTION

For many years now exposure to emotional, environmental and sensory stress has been linked with the incidence
of degenerative disease states, especially those associated
with the cardiovascular system (Raab, 1966; Shimamoto, 1968;
Ratcliffe, Luginbuhl, Schnarr and Chacko, 1969; Landabura,
1971; Haft and Fani, 1973; Corley, Shiel, Mauck and
Greenhoot, 1973; Eliot, Clayton, Pieper and Todd, 1977).
However, while a link between psychological stress and the
disease state may have been accepted, controversy still
exists as to how exposure to stressful situations can induce
pathological changes. Exposure to stress results in the
disturbance of many endocrine systems (Mason, 1974; Pollard,
Bassett and Cairncross, 1976), but the main systems
associated with psychological stress are the sympathetic-
adrenal medullary system and the pituitary-adrenal cortical
system. It would appear that stress induced changes in these
two systems constitutes a primary factor in the etiology of
ischaemic heart disease.

SYMPATHETIC-ADRENAL MEDULLARY SYSTEM

The liberation of the sympathetic-adrenal medullary
catecholamines, adrenaline and noradrenaline, is well
established as a sequel to prolonged psychological and
sensory stress (see review by Mason, 1968b). Exposure to
stressful situations increases the activity of the
sympathetic nervous system, resulting in an increase
noradrenaline turnover (Rubenson, 1969), at the same time as
it stimulates the release of catecholamines from the adrenal
medulla. The catecholamine released from the adrenal medulla
appears to depend on the type of stimuli (Feuerstein and
Gutman, 1971). Adrenaline discharge is characteristic of
situations involving passive anxiety and apprehension, of

situations of uncertainty or unpredictable nature. In contrast noradrenaline is mobilized during attitudes of
aggression, anger, or where the psychological stress is
familiar. This association between the nature of catecholamine released from the medulla and the type of stressor
appears to be mediated via the hypothalamus since selective
release of the catecholamines can be demonstrated by the
stimulation of various hypothalamic areas (Redgate and
Gellhorn, 1953; Folkow and Von Euler, 1954).

The involvement of these stress induced elevated
catecholamine levels in myocardial pathology has been well
established. Hypoxic changes in ECG patterns and the
occurrence of necrotic foci can be produced by continued
elevation of circulating catecholamine levels, either
exogenously administered or following nerve stimulation
(Raab and Gigee, 1955; Johansson and Vendsalu, 1957;
Barger, Herd and Liebowitz, 1961; Moss and Schenk, 1970).
Similar changes can be observed in animals under experimental
conditions in which psychological or sensory stress is a
prominent feature (Raab, 1966; Corley et al. 1973; Schiffer,
Hartley, Schulman and Abelmann, 1976). The use of centrally
depressing, ganglion blocking, adrenergic blocking and
adrenergic depleting drugs have been reported to inhibit the
occurrence of such stress induced myocardial necroses with
differing degrees of effectiveness (Raab, 1966; Prabhu,
Sharma and Singh, 1972). Urinary excretion of both noradrenaline and adrenaline is found also to be greatly
elevated in cases of myocardial infarction (Staszewska-
Barczak and Ceremuzynski, 1968; Jewitt, Mercer, Reid, Valori,
Thomas and Shillingford, 1969), and there is a striking
correlation between the secretion of medullary adrenaline
and cardiac arrhythmias after infarction.

There appears, therefore, to be considerable evidence
linking an emotionally induced neurohormonal mechanism,
involving catecholamine discharge, with myocardial hypoxia
and necrosis. The foci of necrosis, whether produced by
emotional stress or by catecholamine administration, appears
to be regularly located in the subendocardium. This has led
to the suggestion that there is a stress-induced reduction
in coronary blood flow to the endocardial surface (Boerth,
Covell, Seagren and Pool, 1969), an hypothesis supported
by the observation of lowered creatine phosphate levels in
this region of the myocardium. Raab (1966), in his review of
emotional and sensory stress factors involved in myocardial

ɪathology, put forward the hypothesis that the hypoxic
changes seen in situations of psychological stress are due
to an inadequate compensatory dilatability of the coronary
arteries, particularly those supplying the left ventricle.
Discharge of catecholamines from the adrenal medulla and
from the cardiac sympathetic nerve terminals during
emotional stress produces an increased work load on the
heart, and thus an increased oxygen consumption by the
myocardium. If the dilation of the coronary arteries by the
catecholamines is insufficient to provide the oxygen
requirements of the excited heart, ventricular anoxia will
be produced and areas of myocardial necrosis will develop.

Activation of the sympathetic-adrenal medullary system,
however, cannot be the sole factor involved in stress
induced myocardial necrosis. Activation of this system
occurs in response to other situations apart from exposure
to emotional stress. Physical exercise also results in the
release of catecholamines from the sympathetic nerve endings
and the adrenal medulla but, under normal circumstances, is
not associated with myocardial pathology.

PITUITARY-ADRENAL CORTICAL SYSTEM

Activation of the pituitary-adrenal cortical system is
a characteristic feature of emotional stress. The release
of adrenocorticotropic hormone (ACTH) from the anterior
pituitary, and the subsequent release of the glucocorticoid
hormones, cortisol or corticosterone, from the zona
fasciculata of the adrenal cortex, have been accepted as an
index of stress (Mason, 1968a). The level of plasma
corticosteroid has been used as a measure of the intensity
of the stressor (Bassett, Cairncross and King, 1973). While
the pituitary-adrenal cortical axis is activated by a wide
range of psychological stressors, situations of uncertainty
or unpredictability produce by far the greatest elevation
in circulating corticosteroid level (Mason, 1968a; Bassett
et al. 1973).

The presence of elevated plasma levels of glucocorticoids has been linked with degenerative disease states of
the heart. Daily injections of the glucocorticoids to mice
or rats will produce myocardial necrosis together with
leucocyte invasion in the absence of other controlled stress
factors (Clarke, Ashburn and Lane Williams, 1968; Gorny,

1968). Troxler et al. (1977) found a significant correlation between plasma cortisol levels and other major risk factors normally associated with coronary artery disease.

Psychological stress then is associated with both an elevated level of catecholamines and an elevated level of glucocorticoids. However the important factor in stress induced ischaemic heart disease appears not to be the toxic effects of the two systems independently, but rather the interaction between the two systems. In acute stress there is a marked intensification of the cardiotoxic overproduction of catecholamines by a glucocorticoid–catecholamine inter-action.

CATECHOLAMINE–GLUCOCORTICOID INTERACTION

Selyé was the first to note that the glucocorticoids greatly aggravated the necrotic cardiotoxicity of both injected and stress induced catecholamines. Since then his findings have been confirmed by numerous other workers. There is a marked increase in the extent of myocardial destruction induced by psychological stressors or exogenously administered catecholamines when these factors are combined with exogenously administered glucocorticoids (Nahas et al. 1958; Raab and Bajusz, 1965; Raab, 1966). From clinical studies Liakhov et al. (1979) concluded that an increase in the level of 17-hydroxycorticosteroids in association with an increase in catecholamines was one of the main mechanisms in the development of post-operative myocardial infarction. Originally it was suggested that the cardiotoxic interaction between catecholamines and glucocorticoids may involve a disturbance in ionic balance. Prolonged isolation stress in rats produces a significant diminution of myocardial potassium (K^+) with a marked increase in myocardial sodium (Na^+) (Raab et al. 1968). Histochemical examination of the hearts of these rats showed a marked aggravation of adrenaline induced myocardial focal K^+ displacement and necroses. A single injection of adrenaline was shown to increase the intracellular Na^+ concentration of cardiac muscle while decreasing the K^+ concentration (Robertson and Peyser, 1951). This finding is consistent with the observation that adrenaline blocked the re-entry of K^+ into muscle cells (Hajdu, 1953), probably by an action on the specific transport system. Prolonged elevation of the glucocorticoids is also known to bring about the depletion

of myocardial K[+] levels (Nickerson, Karr and Dresel, 1961;
Prioreschi, 1962). It was proposed that the combination of
intramyocardial electrolyte shifts due to catecholamine-
induced local hypoxia, superimposed on a corticoid induced
depletion of myocardial K[+] may constitute the mechanism
involved in stress induced myocardial destruction. However
the interaction appears to be more complicated than just
superimposing electrolyte shifts.

POTENTIATION OF THE ACTION OF CATECHOLAMINES

The glucocorticoids themselves do not appear to exert
a positive inotropic or chronotropic effect on the myocardium
(Almirall Collazo and Miyares Cao, 1971), however they do
potentiate many of the effects of the catecholamines,
especially those on the cardiovascular system. Potentiation
by corticosteroids of the pressor effects of catecholamines,
and catecholamine induced vasoconstriction in certain
vascular beds, has been observed by many investigators (see
review by Ramey and Goldstein, 1957). The vasoconstrictor
response to adrenaline is enhanced by hydrocortisone in the
perfused hindquarters of the cat, and in the perfused
cephalic saphenous venous systems of the dog. However,
hydrocortisone is reported not to increase the constrictor
response to noradrenaline or sympathetic nerve stimulation
in these preparations, or in the perfused vascular beds of
the cat intestine or kidney (Kadowitz and Yard, 1970, 1971;
Yard and Kadowitz, 1972). The dilator response to
isoprenaline in these vascular beds also remains unaltered
by hydrocortisone (Yard and Kadowitz, 1972). Similarly, Hess
and Shanfeld (1963), using the open chest rat preparation,
were unable to demonstrate any potentiation of the effects
of adrenaline on blood pressure, or cardiac inotropic and
chronotropic responses following cortisol or corticosterone
administration. Conversely, in vitro studies using the
isolated aortic strip have reported that cortisol potent-
iates the response to both adrenaline and noradrenaline
(Besse and Bass, 1966; Kalsner, 1969b). Similar findings were
reported by Bettini et al. (1978 a,b) for the isolated
coronary artery.

With regard to psychological stress and myocardial
sensitivity to catecholamines, Bassett and Cairncross (1976a)
found that exposure to a stress procedure associated with a
large plasma corticosteroid elevation resulted in an enhanced

myocardial sensitivity to both noradrenaline and adrenaline.
The enhanced myocardial sensitivity appeared to relate to
the level of circulating glucocorticoids since it was not
apparent in animals exposed to a stressor associated with
only a moderate steroid elevation. This hypothesis is
supported by the finding that both cortisol and corticosterone will potentiate the inotropic action of noradrenaline
in a dose-dependent manner (Bassett, Strand and Cairncross,
1978). ACTH will also potentiate the inotropic action of
noradrenaline, the degree of potentiation being greater than
either of the glucocorticoids.

The enhanced sensitivity of the myocardium to the
catecholamines following exposure to the stressor persists
for at least 24 hours, even though the plasma glucocorticoid
levels have returned to normal values within 3 hours. While
high levels of circulating glucocorticoids may be necessary
to initiate the enhanced sensitivity of the myocardium to
catecholamines, continued steroid elevation (by continued
exposure to the stressor) is not required to maintain the
sensitivity change over a 24 hour period.

DELAY IN CATECHOLAMINE INACTIVATION

The potentiation of the cardiovascular response to the
catecholamines by the glucocorticoids may relate to a delay
in their inactivation following release. Such a delay would
make more catecholamine available to the receptor site and
would explain the observed enhanced sensitivity. Bassett and
Cairncross (1976b) reported a depletion of endogenous
noradrenaline and an absence of adrenaline in the myocardium
following exposure to stress. Their results are consistent
with an inhibition of catecholamine uptake into storage
sites. Depletion of cardiac noradrenaline and adrenaline has
been also reported following the systemic administration of
corticosteroids (Gorny, 1968).

Iversen (1967) demonstrated the existence of two
separate mechanisms for the uptake of catecholamines in the
heart, $Uptake_1$ and $Uptake_2$. $Uptake_1$ is associated with the
re-uptake into sympathetic nerve endings, occurs at low
concentrations of the catecholamines, and is much more
sensitive to noradrenaline than adrenaline (Iversen, 1967).
$Uptake_2$ is associated with extra-neuronal uptake and becomes
apparent only at high concentrations of the catecholamines

(Ehinger and Sporring, 1968; Kalsner, 1969a,b). Iversen
and Salt (1970) demonstrated a dose-dependent inhibition of
Uptake$_2$ by corticosterone, and Bassett and Cairncross (1976c)
found that the uptake of noradrenaline by Uptake$_1$ was
inhibited following exposure to stress.

The inhibition of catecholamine uptake, both neuronal
and extraneuronal, by the glucocorticoids would explain the
observed enhanced sensitivity. However, the possibility that
the steroids may exert their effect by a direct action on
the effector cell itself cannot be overlooked. Activation
of the β-adrenoreceptor involves the formation of cyclic
3-5 adenosine monophosphate (3-5 AMP) in the effector cell;
a substrate essential for the conversion of phosphorylase to
its active form. It is postulated that the formation of
cyclic 3-5 AMP following β-receptor activation is a common
step both in muscle glycolysis and in the enhanced mechanical
response of the effector cell (Lefkowitz, Limbird, Mukherjee
and Caron, 1976; Atlas, Volsky and Levitzki, 1980).
Glucocorticoids are known to increase cardiac but not skeletal muscle phosphorylase activity (Hess, Aronson,
Hottenstein and Karp, 1969) and to potentiate the adrenaline
induced rise in cardiac phosphorylase activity (Haugaard and
Hess, 1965; Hess et al. 1969). Exposure to chronic stress
is known to enhance mitochondrial oxidative and phosphory-
lative capacity in the heart (Stoner, Ressallat and Sirak,
1968), and defect in oxidative phosphorylation in cardiac
interfibrillar mitochondria has been shown to accompany
cardiomyopathy (Hoppel, Tandler, Parkland, Turkaly and
Albers, 1982).

Exposure to stress situations resulting in elevated
levels of circulating glucocorticoids will produce an
enhanced myocardial sensitivity to catecholamines and an
increased work load on the heart. If such a response is not
adequately compensated for by a similar enhanced coronary
blood flow, then myocardial ischaemia leading to necrosis
will occur. Such stress induced myocardial damage may be
produced without any apparent pathological changes in the
coronary vascular system. There are numerous reports to
suggest that myocardial ischaemia and necrosis can occur
with or without a major contribution from coronary
obstruction. Eliot et al. (1977) in a study of aerospace
workers at Cape Kennedy, a work situation with excessive
occupational stress, showed that the population exhibited a
higher than normal incidence of sudden cardiac death and

acute myocardial infarction. In this study acute myocardial
necrosis was much more frequently demonstrated than was
acute coronary obstruction of any type. Regan et al. (1975)
in their study reported a high incidence of toxic
cardiomyopathy in acute myocardial infarction without any
significant coronary obstruction, a finding supported by
Topolianski et al.(1978) who found normal coronary vessels
in patients with ischaemic heart disease. Similar findings
have been reported by Baroldi et al. (1974) and Bruschke
et al. (1973).

However, myocardial ischaemia, resulting from an
inadequate compensatory dilation of the coronary arteries,
would be greatly exacerbated if major obstructive disease
of the coronary vessels was present.

CHANGES IN THE CORONARY VASCULAR SYSTEM

(a) Role of the Catecholamines

The passage of large molecules across the endothelial
lining of the coronary system is generally confined to
vesicular transport rather than passage between endothelial
cells. The intact endothelium provides a barrier against
free exchange between the plasma and interstitial fluid of
large lipid molecules such as fatty acids, lipoproteins, and
cholesterol. It is only when the endothelium is damaged that
the levels of such molecules equilibrate rapidly between the
arterial wall and the plasma (Zilversmit, 1975). Exposure to
prolonged psychological stress opens up endothelial gaps and
allows the accumulation of lipid molecules in the compact
tissue of the media and adventitia of the vascular wall
(Bassett and Cairncross, 1975, 1977). It was proposed that
the stress induced release of the endogenous inflammatory
substances, histamine, bradykinin and serotonin, were
responsible for such an increase in coronary vascular permeability. The source of the inflammatory substances being
either the increase in mast cells reported to occur following
prolonged exposure to stress (Bassett and Cairncross, 1977)
or an intrinsic store of histamine within the endothelial
cells themselves (Schayer, 1963).

Venoconstriction also plays a part in such a histamine-
type leakage of lipid materials. The endogenous inflammatory
substances not only open endothelial gaps but also cause

venoconstriction in a number of veins including the coronary
veins (Rowley, 1964). In the stress situation catecholamine
induced arteriolar dilation, together with venoconstriction,
would raise the internal pressure within the coronary
vessels, thus enhancing the leakage of lipids through the
endothelial gaps. Congestion and dilation of coronary
vessels following prolonged exposure to stress have been
reported by Bassett and Cairncross (1975) and Prabhu et al.
(1972).

Elevated catecholamine levels play a vital role in the
changes in coronary blood flow induced by stress. The
accumulation of lipid materials in the arterial wall will
decrease its lumen size as well as greatly impede its ability
to dilate. While endogenous inflammatory substances are
involved in the opening up of junctional gaps and an
increased vascular permeability, the release of such
substances from their stores is triggered by increased
catecholamine levels (Heitz and Brody, 1975; Shimamoto, 1968).
Lipid accumulation in the arterial wall will be aggravated
by an elevation in the level of circulating lipids. High
plasma adrenaline levels are associated with high serum
levels of cholesterol (Sobel et al., 1962) and free fatty
acids (Ferguson and Shultz, 1975). Following prolonged
psychological stress the lipid content of the myocardium is
raised (Mascitelli-Coriandoli et al. 1958), similar effects
being seen after large doses of catecholamines (Maling,
Highman and Thompson, 1960). Noradrenaline infusion has been
shown to result in the accumulation of lipid droplets in
areas of cardiac myolysis (Moss and Schenk, 1970) and an
enhanced triglyceride uptake by the myocardium (Regan,
Moschos, Oldeuristfi, Weisse and Asokan, 1967; Hoak, Warner
and Connor, 1969).

As well as their effects on lipid accumulation the
catecholamines can induce haematological changes associated
with thrombosis. Noradrenaline infusion results in the
aggregation of platelets and occlusive platelet thrombi
(Haft, Kranz, Albert and Fani, 1972). Intravascular
aggregation of platelets, similar to that found after
noradrenaline infusion, has been observed in animals
subjected to stress (Haft and Fani, 1973; Bassett and
Cairncross, 1977). Nordoy, Gjesdal, Jaeger and Berntsen
(1975) observed both platelet aggregation, and increased
numbers of circulating platelets following the infusion of
either noradrenaline or adrenaline. It appears that the

levels of catecholamines released endogenously during stress period are sufficient to produce the observed platelet aggregation (Haft and Fani, 1973). Surface activation and aggregation of platelets are two of the earliest changes in the formation of most kinds of thrombosis.

(b) Role of the Glucocorticoids

High circulating levels of the glucocorticoids protect against most of the effects of the endogenous inflammatory substances and should prevent the leakage of lipid molecules and thrombotic complications. The glucocorticoids depress the vascular permeability response induced by histamine or serotonin (Garcia Leme & Wilhelm, 1975; Davies and Thompson, 1975) as well as stabilize the mast-cell membrane, preventing the release of the inflammatory agents (Jaques, 1975). Cortisol exerts a protective effect on the myocardium by reducing the extent of ischaemic injury and subsequent necrosis following coronary artery occlusion (Braunwald and Maroko, 1976; Maroko and Braunwald, 1976) and adrenaline administration (Kraikitpanitch et al, 1976). The glucocorticoids also prevent cell proliferation in the atherosclerotic plaque (Cavallero et al. 1976).

Inflammatory responses leading to coronary occlusion, therefore, will be inhibited by high circulating levels of the glucocorticoids and should not be manifest until adaptation of the steroid response to stress has occurred. A close correlation between the adaptation of the steroid response to stress and the onset of a progressive degeneration of the coronary vascular system leading to coronary occlusion has been observed (Bassett and Cairncross 1977).

CONCLUSION

Prolonged exposure to stress, in which the psychological parameters of anxiety or fear are prominent, is implicated in the etiology of ischaemic heart disease. Such an association between psychological stress and the disease state involves the overactivity of the sympathetic-adrenal medullary system (resulting in a increase in circulating catecholamines) together with an interaction with the glucocorticoids. There appears to be two phases in the involvement of the catecholamines and the glucocorticoids in ischaemic heart disease.

The first phase occurs when the circulating levels
of the catecholamines and glucocorticoids are both high.
This phase is associated with an enhanced myocardial
sensitivity to the catecholamines due to a catecholamine-
glucocorticoid interaction. There is an inadequate
compensatory dilation of the coronary arteries to match
the increased work load on the heart.

The second phase involves an inflammatory and
thrombotic response resulting in coronary occlusion. This
phase involves high circulating levels of catecholamines,
but only develops when the glucocorticoids released in
response to stress have adapted to a lower level. The
release of inflammatory substances, platelet aggregation,
thrombosis, and the induction of coronary arteriosclerosis
are prominent in this phase.

REFERENCES

Almirall Collazo, A., and Miyares Cao, C.M. (1971). Rev.
    Cuba Med. 10, 629.
Atlas, D., Volsky, D.J., and Levitzki, A. (1980). Biochim.
    Biophys. Acta. 597, 64.
Barger, A.C., Herd, J.A., and Liebowitz, M.R. (1961).
    Proc.Soc.exp.Biol.Med. 107, 474.
Baroldi, G., Radice, F., Schmid, G., and Leone, A. (1974).
    Am. Heart J. 87, 65.
Bassett, J.R., and Cairncross, K.D. (1975). Pharmac.Biochem.
    Behav. 3, 411.
Bassett, J.R., and Cairncross, K.D. (1976a). Pharmac.Biochem.
    Behav. 4, 27.
Bassett, J.R., and Cairncross, K.D. (1976b). Pharmac.Biochem.
    Behav. 4, 35.
Bassett, J.R. and Cairncross, K.D. (1976c).Pharmac.Biochem.
    Behav. 4, 39.
Bassett, J.R., and Cairncross, K.D. (1977). Pharmac.Biochem.
    Behav. 6, 311.
Bassett, J.R., Cairncross, K.D., and King, M.G. (1973).
    Physiol. Behav. 10, 901.
Bassett, J.R., Strand, F.L., and Cairncross, K.D. (1978).
    Eur. J. Pharmac. 49, 243.
Besse, J.C., and Bass, A.D. (1966). J.Pharmac.exp.Ther. 154,
    224.

Bettini, V., Aragno, R., Legrenzi, E., and Bizzotto, D.
    (1978a). Boll.Soc.Ital.Biol.Sper. 54, 2182.
Bettini, V., Legrenzi, E., Mayellaro, F., and Boscolo, S.
    (1978b). Boll.Soc.Ital.Biol.Sper. 54, 2297.
Boerth, R.C., Covell, J.W., Seagren, S.G., and Pool, P.E.
    (1969). Am.J.Physiol. 216, 1103.
Braunwald, E., and Maroko, P.R. (1976). Am.J.Physiol. 37,
    550.
Bruschke, A.V.G., Proudfit, W.L., and Sones, F.M. (1973),
    Circulation 47, 936.
Cavallero, C., Di Tondo, U., Mingazzini, P.L., Nicosia, R.,
    Pericoli, M.N., Sarti, P., Spagnoli, L.G., and
    Villaschi, S. (1976). Atherosclerosis 25, 145.
Clarke, T.D., Ashburn, A.D., and Lane Williams, W. (1968)
    Am. J. Anat. 123, 429.
Corley, K.C., Shiel, F. O'M., Mauck, H.P., and Greenhoot, J.
    (1973). Psychosom.Med. 35, 361.
Davies, G.E., and Thompson, A. (1975). J. Pathol. 115, 17.
Ehinger, B., and Sporrong, B. (1968). Experientia 24, 265.
Eliot, R.S., Clayton, F.C., Pieper, G.M., and Todd, G.L.
    (1977). Fed.Proc. 36, 1719.
Ferguson, J.H., and Shultz, T.D. (1975). Int.J.Biochem. 6,69.
Feuerstein, G., and Gutman, Y. (1971). Br.J.Pharmac. 43, 764.
Folkow, B., and von Euler, U.S. (1954). Circ.Res. 2, 191.
Garcia Leme, J., and Wilhelm, D.L. (1975). Br.J.exp.Path. 56,
    402.
Gorny, D. (1968). Acta Physiol. Polonica 19, 835.
Haft, J.I., and Fani, K. (1973). Circulation 48, 164.
Haft, J.I., Kranz, P.D., Albert, F.J., and Fani, K. (1972).
    Circulation 41, 698.
Haugaard, N., and Hess, M.E. (1965). Pharmac.Rev. 17, 27.
Hajdu, S. (1953). Am.J.Physiol. 174, 371.
Heitz, D.C., and Brody, M.J. (1975). Am.J.Physiol. 228, 1351.
Hess, M.E., Aronson, C.E., Hottenstein, D.W., and Karp, J.S.
    (1969). Endocrinology 84, 1107.
Hess, M.E., and Shanfeld, J. (1963). Biochem. Pharmac. 12,
    119.
Hoak, J.C., Warner, E.D., and Connor, W.E. (1969).
    Arch. Path. 87. 332.
Hoppel, C.L., Tandler, B., Parkland, W., Turkaly, J.S., and
    Albers, L.D. (1982). J.Biol.Chem. 257, 1540.
Iversen, L.L. (1967). "The uptake and storage of
    noradrenaline in sympathetic nerves". Cambridge University
    Press, Cambridge.
Iversen, L.L. and Salt, P.J. (1970). Br.J.Pharmac. 40, 528.

Jaques, L.B. (1975). Gen.Pharmac. 6, 235.
Jewitt, D.E., Mercer, C.J., Reid, D., Valori, C., Thomas,
    M., and Shillingford, J.P. (1969). Lancet 3, 635.
Johansson, B., and Vendsalu, A. (1957). Acta Physiol.Scand.
    39, 356.
Kadowitz, P.J., and Yard, A.C. (1970). Eur.J.Pharmac. 9, 311.
Kadowitz, P.J., and Yard, A.C. (1971). Eur.J.Pharmac. 13,281.
Kalsner, S. (1969a) Br.J.Pharmac. 36, 582.
Kalsner, S. (1969b) Circ.Res. 24, 383.
Kraititpanitch, S., Haygood, C.C., Baxter, D.J., Yunice, A.
    A., and Lindeman, R.D. (1976). Am.Heart J. 92, 615.
Landabura, R.H., Castellanos, D.E., Giavedoni, E., and
    Lo Presti, C.A. (1971). Acta Physiol. Latinoam. 21, 64.
Lefkowitz, R.J., Limbird, L.E., Mukherjee, C., and Caron,
    M.G. (1976). Biochim.Biophys.Acta 457, 1.
Liakhov, N.T., Zhivoderov, V.M., Milov, V.G., and Chernikov,
    S.A. (1979). Kardiologiia 19, 24.
Maling, H.M., Highman, B., and Thompson, E.C. (1960).
    Am.J.Cardiol. 8, 628.
Maroko, P.R., and Braunwald, E. (1976). Circulation 53, 162.
Mascitelli-Coriandoli, E., Boldrini, R., and Citterio, C.
    (1958). Nature 181, 1215.
Mason, J.W. (1968a). Psychosom.Med. 30, 576.
Mason, J.W. (1968b). Psychosom.Med. 30, 631.
Mason, J.W. (1974). In "Frontiers in Neurology and
    Neuroscience Research" (Seeman and Brown, eds.), p.68.
    Univ. Toronto Press, Toronto.
Moss, A.J., and Schenk, E.A. (1970). Circ.Res. 27, 1013.
Nahas, G.G., Brunson, J.G., King, W.M., and Cavert, H.M.
    (1958). Am.J.Path. 34, 717.
Nickerson, M., Karr, G.W., and Dresel, P.E. (1961).
    Circ.Res. 9, 209.
Nordoy, A., Gjesdal, K., Jaeger, S., and Berntsen, H.
    (1975). Thrombos.Diathes.Haemorrh. 33, 328.
Prabhu, S., Sharma, V.N., and Singh, V. (1972). Br.J.Pharmac.
    44, 814.
Prioreschi, P. (1962). Circ.Res. 10, 782.
Pollard, I., Bassett, J.R., and Cairncross, K.D. (1976).
    Neuroendocrinol. 21, 312.
Raab, W. (1966). Am.Heart J. 72, 538.
Raab, W., and Bajusz, E. (1965). Circulation 32, 174.
Raab, W., and Gigee, W. (1955). Circulation 3, 553.
Raab, W., Bajusz, E., Kimura, H., and Herrlich, H.C. (1968).
    Proc.Soc.Exp.Biol.Med. 127, 142.
Ramey, E.R., and Goldstein, M.S. (1957). Physiol.Rev. 37,155.

Ratcliffe, H.L., Luginbuhl, H., Schnarr, W.R., and Chacko, K. (1969). J.Comp.Physiol.Psych. 68, 385.

Redgate, E.S., and Gellhorn, E. (1953). Am.J.Physiol. 174, 475.

Regan, T.J., Moschos, C.B., Oldeuristfi, B.A., Weisse, A.B., and Asokan, S. (1967). J.Lab.Clin.Med. 70, 221.

Regan, T.J., Wu, C.F., Weisse, A.B., Moschos, C.B., Ahmed, S.S., Lyons, M.M., and Haider, B. (1975). Circulation 51, 453.

Robertson, W.V., and Peyser, P. (1951). AmJ.Physiol. 166,277.

Rowley, D.A. (1964). Br.J.Exp.Path. 45, 56.

Rubenson, A. (1969). J.Pharm.Pharmac. 21, 878.

Schiffer, F., Hartley, L.H., Schulman, C.L., and Abelmann, W.H. (1976). Am.J.Cardiol. 37, 41.

Schayer, R.W. (1963). Ann.N.Y.Acad.Sci. 103, 164.

Shimamoto, T. (1968). Am.Heart J. 76,105.

Sobel, H., Mondon, C.E., and Straus, R. (1962). Circ.Res. 11, 971.

Staszewska-Barczak, J., and Ceremuzynski, L. (1968) Clin. Sci. 34, 531.

Stoner, C.D., Ressallat, M.M., and Sirak, H.D. (1968). Circ.Res. 23, 87.

Topolianski, V.D., Alperovich, B.R., and Strukovskaia, M.V. (1978). Kardiologiia 18, 140.

Troxler, R.G., Sprague, E.A., Albanese, R.A., Fuchs, R., and Thompson, A.J. (1977). Atherosclerosis 26, 151.

Yard, A.C., and Kadowitz, P.J. (1972). Eur.J.Pharmac. 20, 1.

Zilversmit, D.B. (1975). Am.J.Cardiol. 35, 559.

HERBICIDES AND THE DEVELOPMENT OF BRAIN AND BEHAVIOUR

A STUDY IN BEHAVIOURAL TOXICOLOGY

Dr. L. Rogers,

Department of Pharmacology,

Monash University,

Clayton, Vic. 3168.

My aim is to demonstrate the importance of including behavioural tests as an essential part of all toxicological screening procedures. Studies conducted in my laboratory which have found behavioural abnormalities in animals exposed to the phenoxyacetic acid herbicides, 2,4,5 - trichlorophenoxyacetic acid (2,4,5-T) and 2,4 - dichlorophenoxyacetic acid (2,4-D) will be reported as one example of how to approach testing for toxicity on behaviour.

Toxic effects of chemicals on behaviour have been traditionally under-rated in preference to a focus on deformations in morphology, both macro-and microscopic, or biochemistry. I suspect this has a historical basis, since study of animal behaviour is a relatively recent area of science and people are just beginning to recognise its medical importance. I am certainly not suggesting that findings made in behavioural testing of animals should be directly extrapolated to humans. Rather, the presence of behavioural abnormalities can be used as sensitive indicators of toxic effects which must correlate with biochemical and/or structural abnormalities as yet undetected. Behavioural tests are frequently more sensitive in detecting neural disturbances than are presently available methods for brain biochemistry and anatomy (Norton, 1980, Mello, 1975). Screening for behavioural abnormalities should therefore be part of the regular programme of toxicity testing, and not simply

267

something possibly tacked on at the end of the screening
tests if the experimenter has been observant enough to
detect behavioural changes while conducting the other
standard toxicity tests (Loomis, 1978), or only if the
chemical being tested is assumed to be neurotoxic.
Behaviour can be altered acutely and chronically by direct
effects on neural tissue or by indirect effects on
extra-neural function or structure. As most chemicals
escape screening on behavioural tests, I suspect
that many more chemicals than presently believed will be
found to be behaviourally toxic and neurotoxic.

The common-place use of the concept of the "no-effect"
concentration used in assessing the safety of a compound
has   led   toxicologists to a situation in which they must
seek the most sensitive measures available for assessing
toxicity. It is useless to claim that a "no-effect" dose
has been determined if, as is commonly the case, only gross
morpholigcal deformities have been measured. Given the
sensitivity of brain function to disruption by chemicals,
toxins are often found to cause behavioural effects at
doses much lower than the doses which cause detectable
deformations in biochemistry or morphology (Sanderson &
Rogers, 1981; Spyker et.al. 1975). Thus the claimed
"no-effect" doses of many chemicals would be set many
magnitudes lower if comprehensive testing of behaviour
had been an essential part of the original toxicity
screening. Actually, application of the "no-effect"
concept in assessing safety to humans is of questionable
validity, since it is often found that some individuals
are highly susceptible to the toxic effects of a chemical,
as we found to be the case for 2,4,5-T (Sanderson & Rogers
1981). In such cases use of the "no-effect" dose in
extrapolating animal studies to assess safety for the
human species can generate misleading over-estimates of
safety particularly when the studies have not used
extremely large sample sizes (Loomis, 1978).

I will now cover some of the most important
considerations to be made in a programme of study testing
for behavioural toxicity.

1.   Choice of the animal species to be used in screening
     tests.

If the ultimate aim is to assess the safety of a

chemical to humans, it is essential to have conducted
tests on as closely a related species as possible.
However, it is not necessarily beneficial to commence a
toxicological study on the usual limited range of
laboratory mammals. Indeed, a lot more important
base-line information can often be obtained by a choice
of a species with special biological and/or behavioural
characteristics which might be expected to highlight the
effects being measured (Lagerspetz, 1981). By beginning
studies on species with specific and simplified
behavioural systems or by using species for which a good
range of easily applied tests is available, the
experimenter is better able to detect effects where they
exist and formulate behavioural models which can assist
the next step of testing for similar effects in mammalian
species.

We commenced searching for effects of 2,4,5-T on
behaviour using chickens, a choice determined by the
range of sensitive and easily applied behavioural tests
which we had on-going in our laboratory, the fact that
chickens develop rapidly and pass through relatively
discrete phases of neural and behavioural development,
and that the chicken foetus can be exposed to chemicals
in the egg without interaction between the maternal
animal and foetus causing complications.

2. Choice of the age of the animal when exposed

The developing brain is extremely sensitive to both
physiological and environmental influences on its pattern
of development. Disruption of the normal differentiation
can lead to permanent (teratogenic) deficits in its
function (Rogers, Drennen & Mark, 1974). Thus one of the
best approaches to begin testing a suspected neurotoxin
is to administer it at different times during brain
development.

Sanderson and I chose to administer 2,4,5-T (0.03 ppm
dioxin) to chicken eggs on days 8 and 15 of incubation
by injection into the egg avoiding the embryo itself, and
day 2 post-hatch by subcutaneous injection (Sanderson and
Rogers, 1981; Rogers and Sanderson, 1982). Day 8 of
incubation is the time at which neuronal cell division
is at its peak. By day 15 of incubation this cell division
is largely completed and synaptic proliferation is

occuring (Freeman & Vince, 1974). Synaptic proliferation
appears to be largely completed by day 2 post-hatch
(Rogers, Drennan & Mark, 1974). Chickens found to have
any morphological deformities were eliminated, as we
were interested in looking for behavioural deformities in
animals which were normal in gross morphology.

3. Choice of the best age to apply the tests

Since behaviour of animals can be influenced by many
variables apart from the biological ones resulting from
exposure to the chemical, one is always working against
a dynamic background of behaviour change determined by
past experience and other factors pertaining to a given
individual's environment. This tends to become a larger
variable the more experiences an animal has, or the
longer it lives. Interaction with environmental variables
can either enhance or diminish the magnitude of a toxin's
effect on behaviour. Being precocious, chickens can be
tested soon after hatching which circumvents some of
these problems. We tested the chickens in the first or
second weeks of post-hatch life.

4. Choice of the behavioural tests

It is important to begin with broad screening tests,
i.e. tests which depend on many behavioural variables,
and will therefore show changes if any one of these
variables is affected. Tests for activity fall into
such a category. Activity, scored either as a cumulated
measure of all movements (e.g. electronically) or
divided into ambulation, grooming, rearing, etc., can be
scored in an open field apparatus or in the home cage.
Many factors can contribute to an increase in ambulation
in the open field. Rats will ambulate more if they are
more exploratory or if they are more fearful (Candland &
Nagy, 1969; Whimbley & Denenberg, 1967). They may also
ambulate more if a chemical has directly facilitated
their somato-motor system (Iverson and Iversen, 1981).
We found increased open-field activity in chickens
exposed to 2,4,5-T on day 15 of incubation and day 2
post-hatch (see Sanderson and Rogers, 1981). Treatment
on day 8 of incubation produced no significant effects.
Escape jumps at the walls of the field proved to a
sensitive measure; a significant increase in jumping
was detected at a dose as low as 13 mg 2,4,5-T/kg of egg

weight given on day 15 of incubation.

Detection of activity changes should be taken as the impetus for further behavioural testing; yet toxicological researchers usually stop at this point. If they do take up the behavioural challenge they usually pursue it further through the standard tests made available by experimental psychology (e.g. operant conditioning tasks; Loomis, 1978). Almost certainly, it is the difficulties and time involved in training animals on these paradigms which deter most toxicological investigators. What we need are simple tasks which can be rapidly applied. This is where I believe the field of ethology can make an important contribution to toxicological studies on behaviour. By knowledge of the behaviour of a species in the field environment, an experimental ethologist designs behavioural tests for use in the laboratory. The operant conditioning apparatus of the experimental psychologist is far removed from any situation an animal may meet in the natural, or even semi-natural, environment. This contributes to the difficulties of training animals to perform in it and at the same time diminishes the probability of detecting any but gross behavioural deformations. To detect more subtle, and possibly more important, behavioural effects one must either apply very complex operant paradigms or turn towards behavioural tasks tailored along ethological lines. These latter will, I believe, become the tasks most useful to toxicologists, since they will be quicker and easier to apply which is an important criterion for toxicological screening. However, once behavioural abnormalities can be detected on a range of well designed ethologically based tests, operant procedures will only be applied at the later stages of a detailed behavioural study, when they can be useful in determining the exact nature of the behavioural lesion, not as part of the toxicological screening program itself.

One ethologically designed task on which we tested our chicks is a visual task requiring hungry chicks deprived of food for 3 hours to search for grains of chicken mash scattered on a back-ground of small pebbles which have been adhered to the floor (Rogers, Drennen & Mark, 1974). Within 60 pecks and less than 10 minutes one can obtain performance scores, which would take days to obtain in a standard operant apparatus. This is another broad screening test, since learning performance on the task can be disrupted by a range of variables (reduced motivation to feed, impaired memory formation, visual defects, etc.). Chickens which had received as little as 7 mg 2,4,5-T/kg of egg on day 15 of incubation were found to have impaired performance on this task (Sanderson and Rogers, 1981).

Next we considered it important to see whether we could find similar effects in a mammalian species, particularly given that, for the foetal state of a mammal to be exposed, the phenyoxacetic acid would need to cross the placenta. It is known that 2,4,5-T passes readily through the placental membrane (Fang et al, 1973).

Effects of phenoxyacetic acids on behaviour of rats

Sjodén and Söderberg (1972, 1975) have reported teratogenic effects on behaviour in rats given a single exposure of 2,4,5-T around day 8 of gestation (100 mg/kg given orally to the pregnant mother). When the pups were tested in the open field at 35 and 60 days of age ambulation and rearing scores were elevated above control levels, especially on the first day of testing. None of these rats showed any obvious morphological deformations; Khera & McKinley (1972) have reported an increased incidence of skeletal anomalies in pups born of mothers administered 100 - 150 mg 2,4,5-T/kg administered daily from day 6 to 15 of gestation (i.e. after receiving a total dose 10 times larger than that which Sjödén and Söderberg found to be behaviourally teratogenic). By cross fostering exposed pups to control mothers and vice versa, Sjodén and Söderberg (1975) demonstrated that these long-lasting changes in behaviour in rats exposed to 2,4,5-T and raised by their own mothers are due both to direct effects of the herbicide on the foetus and indirectly to effects on the mother rat. Exposed pups raised by control mothers showed increased ambulation and rearing, but less than those seen in exposed pups raised by treated mothers.

Crampton, Booth and I administered a single dose of 0.25 ml maize oil suspension of 2,4,5-T (Sigma; 95% pure; 0.03 ppm dioxin) to pregnant, female, hooded rats on day 8 of gestation. The doses of 2,4,5-T administered were 6,12,25 and 100 mg 2,4,5-T/kg. Controls received 0.25 ml of the vehicle alone.

Effects on maternal behaviour

As Sjödén and Archer (1976) and Sjödén et al (1979)
have reported that 2,4,5-T can induce taste aversion in
rats, we monitored the food and water intake of the
pegnant females to check the possibility that factors such
as these may be indirectly effecting the development of
the foetuses.   The consumption of each rat was measured
on a daily basis from day 8 until parturition. No
significant effects of treatment with 2,4,5-T were found.
However, there was an acute and significant reduction in
nesting behaviour after 2,4,5-T treatment. The pregnant
females were supplied with fixed quantities of cotton
wool and grass hay on day 8 of gestation. Each day until
parturition the volume of each nest was estimated by
measuring maximum length, width and height, and the
quality of nest was estimated by a ranking system similar
to that developed by Wolfe and Barnett (1977). Nest volume
and quality was reduced in females which had been treated
with 100 mg 2,4,5,-T/kg (nest volume mean and standard
error, was 4.2 (±0.3)1 for controls and 3.0 (±0.2)1 for
100 mg/kg treated females, $0.01 < p < 0.05$; nest quality
ranked as 11 ± 0.5 for controls and 4 ± 1 for 100 mg/kg
treated females, $p < 0.001$). The lower doses of 2,4,5-T
had no effect on nesting behaviour. By parturition these
acute effects of the 100 mg/kg treatment on nesting
behaviour had disappeared. It is therefore unlikely that
changed nesting behaviour in the mothers affects behaviour
of the exposed pups, as suggested by Sjödén and Sjöderberg
(1975).

Effects on litters, morphology etc.

All litters were culled to 8 pups on day 2 after birth,
and weaning occurred at 23 days. No significant effects
of 2,4,5-T were found on litter sizes, sex ratios,
gestation time, pup weights or gross morphology (Crampton
and Rogers, paper submitted). Brain weight after
perfusion on day 2 of life was found to be significantly
elevated in a small sample of the culled pups which had
been exposed to 100 mg/kg of 2,4,5-T (mean brain weight
and standard error was 0.55 ± 0.01 g for 9 treated
pups, and 0.49 ± 0.01g for 7 controls $p < 0.05$,
t-test). This could result from 2,4,5-T's
ability to cause transient hyperthyroidism

(Sjödén and Söderberg, 1978). However, no qualititative
or quantitative structural differences were detected in
the sizes of the cerebral cortex, hippocampus, cerebellum
or corpus callosum (measured by S. Singh, Monash
University). Also, this effect on brain weight may be
transient since no significant differences in perfused
brain weight were detected in a sample of adult brains
measured after completion of the behavioural testing
(6 controls and 6 rats exposed to 100 mg/kg on day 8 of
gestation).

Open field testing

Open field testing of the pups was conducted between
65 and 75 days after birth, according to the procedure
described by Sjödén and Söderberg (1975). Latency,
ambulation, rearing, grooming and defaecation were
scored in a 4 min period. Analysis of variance (sex x dose)
revealed significant main effects of sex and dose and
interaction between sex and dose for ambulation
($p < 0.05$ for each). T-tests between the control group
and treatment groups showed that the significant dose
effects were due to an elevation of ambulation in both
sexes of offspring of mothers which had been treated with
25 mg/kg 2,4,5-T ($0.01 < p < 0.025$), and in the male
offspring of mothers treated with 100 mg/kg 2,4,5-T
($0.025 < p < 0.05$): see Fig 1. Lower doses had no
significant effects. The main effects of sex were in the
expected direction (higher ambulation and rearing and lower
latency and grooming scores in females). This confirms
the previous reports by Sjödén and Söderberg (1972, 1975),
who reported effects in males but not in females. They
administrered only the 100 mg/kg dose of 2,4,5-T. Indeed,
in females the 25 mg/kg dose produced a marked elevation
in ambulation; whereas the 100 mg/kg dose had no effect.
It is possible that non-specific effects of 2,4,5-T on
open field behaviour may partially or completely mask
effects of higher doses.

Sjödén and Söderberg (1978) reported that the elevated
ambulation observed in male pups of females exposed to
100 mg/kg 2,4,5-T was confined to novel environments, and
interpreted it as increased exploration. As mentioned
earlier, increased fear may be the most important factor
contributing to this response the first time that rats are
tested in the open field, and a simple facilitation of

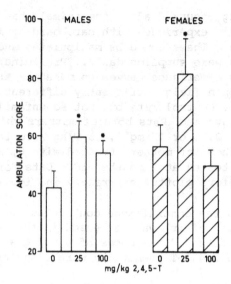

Fig. 1.

*Ambulation scores together with standard errors for male
and female pups tested in the open field. Asterisks
indicate significance of t-test comparison to controls
(p.01 < p < 0.025). The dose given to their mothers on
day 8 of gestation is presented on the x-axis. Lower
doses had no significant effects.*

somatomotor responses could also be the cause.   If
2,4,5-T is simply facilitating somatomotor responses this
should occur in all environments, even in the home cage,
but we measured activity in the home-cage by electronic
recording, and found that it was not effected.

Exploration

To test the possibility that exploration may be
increased we secured a small, plastic cylinder (6 cm in
diameter, 12 cm in length, grey with black circular 1 cm
stripes) in the centre of the open field arena
(76 x 76 cm with 10 cm high walls painted grey).   Over a
2 minute test period we scored latency to move from the
starting square, number of entries with 2 front paws into
a 24 cm zone containing the cylinder, number of times the
head was inserted into the cylinder up to the rats' eyes,
and defaecation.   Only males were tested (12 to 20 per

group). Testing occurred after the animals had been given
at least 3 week's experience with cardboard cylinders in
their home cage. These could be manipulated and chewed.
Fresh cylinders were supplied daily. Preliminary tests
found that this experience serves to make the stimulus
placed in the open field sufficiently different to deserve
investigation by control rats but not so unfamiliar as to
be fearful and avoided. Rats born of mothers which had been
treated with 0, 3, 6 or 12 mg 2,4,5-T/kg were tested at
65 days old. Those of mothers treated with 0, 25 or
100 mg/kg were tested at 5 months old. Data for these
groups is therefore plotted separately in Fig. 2.

Entry into the central zone containing the cylinder,
(i.e. exploration of it) was decreased in the rats which
had been exposed to 2,4,5-T doses of 6 mg/kg and above.
Pups exposed to 2,4,5-T prenatally were also less likely to

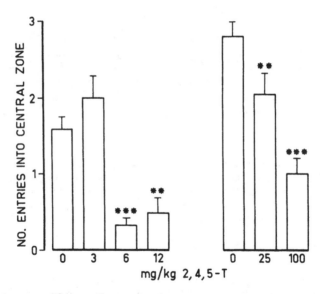

Fig. 2   *The number of times an individual enters a
zone in the centre of an open field containing a cylinder
is plotted against dose of 2,4,5-T exposure. The U-tests
were applied after significant heterogeneity was
calculated by Kruskal-Wallis Analysis of variance
(0.001 < p < 0.01). Asterisks indicate significant
difference from controls 2-tailed tests. *, p < .05;
** p < .01; *** p < .001.*

explore the novel object by placing their heads inside it;
43% of the controls inserted their heads in the pipe
compared to only 13% of the 25 mg/kg and 11% of the
100 mg/kg treatment groups (p = 0.019, Chi-squared test).
There were no significant effects on latency to move or
defaecation in this test.

Thus 4,5,6-T appears to decrease exploration rather
than increase it. Perhaps increased ambulation in the
open field is therefore due to increased fear.

Fear responsiveness

Welker (1957) suggested that increased activity in a
novel situation may represent attempts to escape. He
found that provision of a small dark box opening off one
corner of a well-illuminated open field resulted in rats
retreating into this enclosure. A fearful animal would
be expected to say in the dark box for longer. At 12
months of age we retested the groups exposed to 0, 12 and
100 mg 2,4,5-T/kg in the open field provided with a small,
dark box. In the week prior to testing all animals
received several minutes experience daily in an identical
small dark box. Over a 4 min. period, we scored the total
amount of time spent in the dark box and the number of
times the rat sniffed the entrance of the box but did not
enter (Fig. 3).

There was significant heterogeneity between groups for
each measure (Kruskal-Wallis, 0.02 < p < 0.05). The

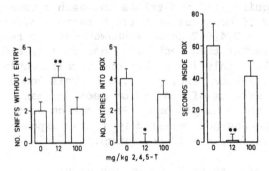

Fig. 3.
*Testing for levels of fear. See text for details.
Asterisks as in Fig. 2.*

100 mg/kg exposed group showed no significant difference
from controls, but the 12 mg/kg exposed group scored
increased sniffing and decreased entry and time spent
inside the box. This implies increased exploration of
the dark box but decreased fear responsiveness, a result
which does little to clarify the exact nature of the
behavioural lesion produced by 2,4,5-T. Are 2,4,5-T
exposed rats more thigmotaxic and more likely to explore
stimuli around the walls? Further testing is required.
Thus far we can eliminate any simple facilitation of the
somatomotor system by 2,4,5-T. Our findings indicate
a role for effects on higher brain mechanism related to
integration of decision making.

Effects on learning

     Sjödén & Söderberg (1978) suggest that 2,4,5-T exposed
rats have difficulty in changing their behaviour in response
to changing demands in the environment, a deduction based
on finding that treated rats have difficulties in reverse
learning in a left-right discrimination in a Y-maze.
We tested 8 control males and 8 males which had been
exposed to 100 mg 2,4,5-T/kg on day 8 of gestation on a
Y-maze brightness discrimination for food reward. Controls
took a mean (± standard error) of 80 ± 13 trials to reach a
criterion of 10 consecutive correct responses. Six of the
2,4,5-T exposed rats acquired the task in an equivalent
number of trials (80 ± 9), but 2 failed to acquire the task
in 200 trials and were discontinued from further testing.
The remainder were tested on reversal learning. The
controls required 116 ± 4 trials to reach a reverse
criterion of 10 consecutive correct responses, while
performance of 2,4,5-T animals showed extreme reactions.
4 reversed faster than controls (mean 99 ± 4) and 2 took
more than 170 trials (distributions significantly different
Wald-Walforitz Runs test, p < 0.05). This demonstrates
significant effects of 2,4,5-T on decision making capacity
but perhaps not a simple one. Performance on the Hebb-
Williams maze was not impaired by foetal exposure to
100 mg/kg 2,4,5-T, n = 12 per group.

Teratogenic effects of 2,4-D on behaviour

     Testing for similar effects of 2,4-D on behaviour can
tell us whether the behavioural teratogenicity of 2,4,5-T is

due to the phenoxyacetic acid itself or to dioxin
contaminants, since 2,4-D is not contaminated with dioxin.
We repeated our experiments on pups born of mothers
exposed to 2,4-D on day 8 of gestation (25, 100 or 200
mg/kg); see Fig. 4.

The 25 and 100 mg/kg significantly elevated ambulation
and rearing. In contrast to 2,4,5-T, no significant
effects were obtained in the test for exploration. In the
test for fear responsiveness no significant differences
between groups were found for sniffing without entry, but
the number of entries and total time spent in the dark
box was elevated (significant for the 100 mg 2,4-D/kg dose).
Perhaps this indicates that these two related chemicals
disturb behaviour via different cellular mechanisms.
The U-shaped nature of some of the dose curves we obtained
(e.g. open field and fear responsiveness data) implies
that a masking effect of some responses is occurring at
higher doses, which means either that non-specific effects,
like general sickness may be coming into play at high doses
or that we are dealing with more than one simple cellular
mechanism. The latter would not be at all surprising given
the large number of cellular processes disturbed by the
phenoxyacetic acids; e.g. thyroid hormone metabolism
(Sjödén and Söderberg, 1978; Florsheim and Velcoff, 1962),

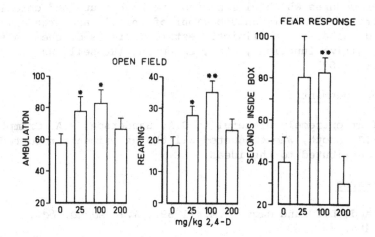

Fig.4
*Teratogenic effects of 2,4-D on behaviour. Details as in
previous figures.*

ATP utilization (Gamble, 1975), inhibition of foetal
cerebral ribonucleotide reductase when 50 mg/kg is given to
pregnant females on day 14 (Millard et al, 1973), raised
brain tryptophane and 5-hydroxyindole acetic acid levels
over an acute time cause and reduced serotonin levels 2
months later (Sjödén and Soderberg, 1978).

The shape of the dose-response relationships
demonstrates the need to use a wide range of doses. If
only the higher doses had been used, genuine behavioural
effects would have been missed. Also, the sex differences
in effects of 2,4,5-T on open field performance
demonstrate the need to test both sexes and analyse the
data separately.

Concluding remarks

Exposure of the rat foetus to doses of 2,4,5-T as low
as 6 mg/kg of maternal weight on day 8 of pregnancy
causes behavioural deformations, and this dose is some
ten to one hundred fold less than the lowest doses
reported to be morphologically teratogenic (Khera &
McKinnley, 1972). 2,4-D also is behaviourally teratogenic
at much lower doses (25 mg/kg), than previously reported
to be toxic and we have not yet tested lower doses.

Procedures which will screen for both acute and chronic
effects of chemicals on behaviour of animals are urgently
needed, as also are clinical tests for effects of chemicals
on cognitive functions, etc., in humans (Russell and
Singer, 1982).

Acknowledgements:

I am extremely grateful to C.A. Sanderson, M.A. Crampton
and P.J. Booth, who conducted all the experiments reported
and contributed to the ideas.

References

Candland, D.K. and Nagy, Z.M. (1969), *N.Y. Accad. Sci.
     Ann. 159*, 831.

Fang, S.C., Fallin, E., Montgomery, M.L. and Freed, V.H.
     (1973), *Toxicol. Appl. Pharmacol. 24*, 555.

Freeman, B.M. and Vince, M.A. (1974). "Development of the
    Avian Embryo". Chapman Hall, London.
Florsheim, W.H. and Velcoff, S.W. (1962), *Endocrinol. 71,*
    1.
Gamble, W. (1975). *J. Theor. Biol. 54,* 181.
Iversen, S.D. and Iversen, L.L. (1975). "Behavioural
    Pharmacology", Oxford University Press, U.S.A.
Khera, K.S. and McKinnley, W.P. (1972). *Toxicol. Appl.
    Pharmacol. 22,* 14.
Lagerspetz, K.Y.H. (1981). In "Current Developments in
    Psychopharmacology" (W.B. Essman and L. Valzelli eds.),
    Vol. 6, p. 1, MTP Press, U.S.A.
Loomis, T.A. (1978). "Essentials of Toxicology". Lea and
    Febiger, Philadelphia.
Millard, S.A., Hart, M.B. and Shimek, J.F. (1973), *Biochem.
    Physiol. Acta 308,* 230.
Mello, N.K. (1975). *Fed. Proc. 34,* 1832.
Norton, S. (1980). In "Scientific Basis of Toxicity
    Assessment" (H.R. Witsch, ed.), p. 91, Elsevier,
    Amsterdam.
Rogers, L.J. and Sanderson, C.A. (1982). *Science 215,* 1422.
Rogers, L.J., Drennen, H.D., Mark, R.F. (1974). *Brain Res.*
    79, 213.
Russell, R.W. and Singer, G. (1982). *Aust. Psychol. 17,*
    199.
Sanderson, C.A. and Rogers, L.J. (1981). *Science 211,* 593.
Sjödérn, P.O. and Archer, T. (1977). *Physiol. Behav. 19,*
    159.
Sjödérn, P.O. and Söderberg, U. (1972). *Physiol. Behav. 9,*
    357.
Sjödén, P.O. and Söderberg, U. (1975). *Physiol. Psychol. 3,*
    175.
Sjödén, P.O. and Söderberg, U. (1978). *Ecol. Bull.
    (Stockholm) 27,* 149.
Sjödén, P.O., Archer, T. and Carter, N. (1979). *Physiol.
    Psychol. 7,* 93.
Spyker, J.M., Sparber, S.B. and Godlberg, A.M. (1972)
    Science 177, 621.
Welker, W.J. (1957). *Psychol. Rep. 3,* 95.
Whimbley, A.E. and Denenberg, V.H. (1967). *J. Comp. Physiol.
    Psychol. 63,* 500.
Wolf, J.L. and Barnett, S.A. (1977). *Biol. J. Linn. Soc. 9,*
    73.

THE EFFECTS OF HEAVY METAL EXPOSURE ON BEHAVIOUR

A.M. Williamson,
Department of Industrial Relations,
Division of Occupational Health,
P.O. Box 163,
LIDCOMBE, N.S.W.   2141

ABSTRACT

Many of the heavy metals are neurotoxic. Our knowledge of this is from clinical evidence where in most cases high level and/or chronic exposure to the metal produces overt signs and symptoms. Recent controversies however, have singled out two metals, mercury and lead, as being particularly hazardous to the nervous system. The important questions that have arisen from this surge of interest are: at what level of exposure do these metals become neurotoxic and what specific effects do they have on the nervous system? This second concern is of greater interest to neuroscientists as it not only covers the question of toxicity, but may also provide us with some insight into how specific behaviour is moderated. We have investigated the effects of inorganic mercury on man using an information processing based battery of tests. Together with the well known motor disturbances, mercury exposure was shown to produce specific short-term memory impairment(Williamson et al,1982). Recent biochemical evidence suggests a reason for this. Injections of both organic and inorganic mercury reduced $Na+/K+$ ATP'ase levels (Gallagher et al, 1982) in the rat brain in the same manner as did ouabain. Significantly, Gibbs and Ng (1977) showed using ouabain that short-term memory is $Na+/K+$ pump dependent. We have used the same battery of tests to investigate the effects of lead exposure on adults. The results of this study also will be discussed.

That toxic substances can effect the nervous system is becoming increasingly obvious both because our techniques for assessing nervous system dysfunction are improving and because the range and usage of known and potential toxic substances is increasing. The heavy metals are not "new" toxins by any means. Clinical evidence from high level or chronic exposure to the metal tells us this.

Two metals in particular, mercury and lead, have attracted a great deal of attention, even controversy, largely due to their widespread use in the workplace and in the community at large. Increases in the incidence of clinical symptons and signs of such exposure as well as the amount of related research from the animal kingdom have reinforced our awareness that mercury and lead can be particularly hazardous to the nervous system.

This interest in the neurotoxic effects of mercury and lead has been channelled into two basic questions:

1.   At what level of exposure do these metals become neurotoxic? This is the more pragmatic problem. Both metals occur in organic and inorganic forms and in each case, the organic form is thought to be the most toxic. Nevertheless, the nervous system is a target in both forms, and clinical symptoms of neurological involvement will show up sooner or later. For example, one of the earliest observable and classic signs of inorganic mercury exposure is tremor, (Gowers, 1888; Neal and Jones, 1938), but at what exposure level does this occur? Questions like this are important for the safety of those in contact with the toxin and are becoming an integral part of the regulation of such substances particularly in the workplace. In addition, environmental exposure is being examined from this viewpoint. Levels of safe exposure to environmental lead are being reviewed on the basis of such evidence as demonstrated neuropsychological effects occurring in children with abnormally high body burdens of lead. (Rutter, 1980).

2. What specific effects do these metals have on the nervous system? This question is slowly gaining more attention, and is the primary concern of this paper. The search for an answer is often limited, however, by the methods, training and the biases of the researcher as well as the organism being observed.

TABLE 1.

Method	Exposure Effects	Possibility of Human Research
MEDICAL		
Gross morphological, clinical signs, symptoms	eg. Lead: blue line on gums(Chisholm 1971)	human testing possible
	eg.Mercury:tremor (Neal & Jones,1943)	
BEHAVIOURAL		
Changes in neuro-psychological function	eg.Lead:hyperactivity (David, 1974)	human testing possible
	eg.Mercury: psycho-motor impairment (Langolf,Whittle & Henderson, 1979)	
PHYSIOLOGICAL		
Changes in electro-physiological function (eg:EMG,EEG,ERP's)	eg.Lead: slower EMG of nerves of forearm (Seppalainen,1971)	human testing only on a small scale
	eg:Mercury:slower EMG of motor nerves (Langolf,Whittle & Henderson, 1979)	

PHYSIOLOGICAL - contd.

Method	Exposure Effects	Possibility of Human Research
Changes in fine and ultra anatomy	eg.Lead: axonal degeneration of PNS (Lampert & Schochet, 1968) eg.Mercury:demyelination of sensory fibres(Chang,1977)	Largely limited to animal studies

BIOCHEMICAL

Method	Exposure Effects	Possibility of Human Research
Changes in specific indicators	eg.Lead:increases in blood lead (Chisholm, 1974) eg.Mercury in Urine(WHO,1979)	Human testing limited
Changes in related indicators	eg.Lead:increases ALAD,ZPP(Zielhuis, 1971) eg.Mercury:not commonly used	Human testing limited
Changes in possibly related factors eg.hormones, neuro-transmitters etc.	eg.Lead:various, unresolved (Hrdina,Hanin & Dubas,1980) eg.Mercury:various unresolved(Chang, 1977)	Largely limited to Animal studies

Table 1 outlines a relatively simple division of the disciplines and their methods that are or can be used in neurotoxicology. The divisions between the disciplines are by no means clear and it is common for research to cover at least two disciplines, usually in the combination of any of

the first three and biochemistry.   It is clear however,
that the specific neurotoxic effect that will be seen and
even whether an effect is seen at all as a result of lead
or mercury exposure will be determined by the method
applied in each discipline.

This problem is further compounded by the nature of the
organism being tested. Determination of the dimensions of
neurotoxicity in the human organism can be extremely
difficult. Decisions all too obviously depend on what is,
and what can feasibly be measured in the human.
Consequently regulations for control of neurotoxins are
usually based on animal studies, as they are thought to
provide the "cleanest" evidence. The drawbacks of such
extrapolation from effects on the animal model to the
control of toxins for human usage however are obvious and
raise a great deal of controversy especially where regulatory levels are thought to be too low.

Where some human study is undertaken it often does
little to resolve controversy. For example a relatively
large number of studies of the neurotoxic effects of lead
in children have only confused, not resolved the issue due
to difficulties with experimental design and poor measurement techniques. (Needleman, 1979; Rutter, 1980). Often
the measureable neurological change which results from low
level toxic exposure in humans occurs at the behavioural
level, and is quite subtle, difficult to detect and can be
too easily dismissed as being due to other factors such as
lack of sleep or age.

Given that human testing is limited to certain accessible aspects of neurological function, it is important
that their measurement be as sensitive as possible.
Pragmatically the most accessible level of neurological
function is probably the behavioural as it is relatively
non-invasive and equipment-free. It is at this level
however that the most severe controversy rages regarding
test methods. (Valciukas and Lilis, 1980). Unfortunately
much of this criticism is entirely justified.

Surveys of the human research on lead or mercury
exposure often become discussions of methodological and
design problems most of which are due to inappropriate
test selection and standardisation. selection of tests is

frequently dependent on the researchers knowledge of the
clinical and pathological changes expected from a neurotoxic agent. For example for inorganic mercury exposure
tremor is the most obvious neurological sign, consequently
tests of behavioural change are almost exclusively psychomotor therefore neglecting the important possibility that
cognitive processes may also be affected. Some researchers
have attempted to use as broad a range of tests as possible
but with little clear rationale. Where well standardised
tests are used, they are often from intelligence test
batteries such as the Wechsler Adult Intelligence Test.
These tend to lack the subtlety required to pick-up early
behavioural change due to toxic exposure as well as
confounding specific psychological functions with one
another such as memory processes with the response
required to assess them.

In addition, other factors which may confound
performance are too often ignored. Age differences, socio-
economic status, occupational and educational differences
can all affect psychological function and may account for
any observed changes.

Despite these problems behavioural testing should not
be disregarded however. Behavioural change is often the
earliest indicator of neurotoxic effect and as our knowledge increases it can be related to underlying changes in
physiological and biochemical aspects of neurological
function. (Silbergeld, 1982).

DEVELOPMENT OF A BEHAVIOURAL TEST BATTERY

With these advantages in mind, we have designed a
battery of tests which cover the range of psychological
functions that allow the organism to process information
from its environment. (Williamson & Teo, 1982). The theory
of Information Processing predicts the way the organism
will deal with a stimulus and produce an appropriate
response to it. Figure 1 shows the general framework of
this theory. Each major aspect of Information Processing
is represented by a test in the battery, thus allowing us
to draw conclusions not only about the various performance
tests that reflect CNS damage, but also about which
specific process is affected.

Fig. 1

INFORMATION PROCESSING THEORY

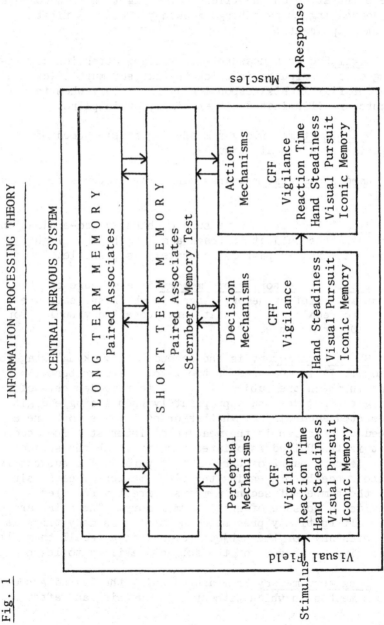

Briefly the tests were as follows:

1. <u>Critical Flicker Fusion</u> (CFF) is a measure of basic cortical arousal in which the subject is required to report the point at which the flicker of a light that is constantly decreasing in switching frequency (2Hz/sec) first becomes apparent .

2. <u>Vigilance</u> is a measure of sustained attention continuing over 20 minutes in which the subject must track the path of five lights,responding appropriately when the lights are illuminated either singly or in pairs.

3. <u>Reaction time</u> involves measuring simple speed of reaction to a visual stimulus.

4 . <u>Hand steadiness</u> measures hand tremor over a 60 second period.

5. <u>Visual Pursuit</u> is a measure of hand-eye co-ordination requiring the subject to track a moving beam of light around a circular path as accurately as possible.

6. <u>Iconic</u> or <u>Sensory store memory</u> is a measure of the first and briefest memory stage, in which subjects are asked to recall letters that were presented visually for 150, 300 or 450 msecs.

7. <u>Short term memory</u> is the second and "working" stage of memory. It is measured in two ways, the Sternberg memory test in which the subject is asked to remember sets of 2 to 5 digits then respond appropriately when a single digit is presented according to whether or not it was to be recalled. Speed of reaction is the measure of interest. The second test is the Paired Associates test in which the subject must learn 5 pairs of three letter words. The subject is tested once by presenting the first member of each pair and the number of second members correctly recalled provides a measure of short term memory. The pairs are then alternatively presented and tested as many times as is necessary for the subject to correctly recall them all. This gives a measure of the subjects ability to learn.

8. <u>Long term memory</u> is measured using the Paired Associates method in which without prior warning and after a

delay of 1.5 hrs. the subject is aksed to recall the
second member of each pair they had learned previously.

Before applying this or any test battery to a potentially neurotoxic problem, it is necessary as discussed
above to ascertain the "normal" limits of performance on
each test as well as the influence of potential confounding
factors. In an on-going project, we have gathered data on
70 "control" or non-exposed individuals of as wide a range
of characteristics as possible. This gives us an estimate
of the critical limits of performance and allows us to
place any individual in the "normal" (within ± 3 S.D.) or
affected" (outside 3 S.D.) range of performance. Possible
confounding variables have also been investigated as shown
in Table 2.

TABLE 2.

Tests which are significantly affected by Confounding
    Variables

Age	Occupation Type	Educational Level	Factors Relating to Time, Place etc.(Test-Retest)

* Vigilance
* Sensory store
  memory
* Verbal memory
  (paired assoc-
  iates short and
  long term memory)
	* Hand-eye
	co-ordination
	(visual pursuit)
		Nil	*Hand steadiness
			  (fatigue measure)
			*Vigilance
			*Long term memory
			  (paired-associates)

For a few tests, age, occupation and situational
factors can influence performance. Knowing this, we can
account for it in neurotoxicity testing by either comparing
the performance of exposed and non-exposed individuals who
are first matched on age and occupational level where
appropriate, or using post hoc statistical methods.

Other confounding factors such as medication, alcohol,
caffeine and cigarette consumption are also accounted for
by eliminating any individual who uses these drugs

excessively or who have consumed them within a significant period before the test.

Similarly, test data is not included where individuals report significant sleep debit or disruption to sleep/working routine.

USING THE TEST BATTERY TO INVESTIGATE NEUROTOXICITY

Inorganic Mercury

Occupational exposure is the most common reason for inorganic mercury neurotoxicity effects such as increased hand tremor.

Accordingly, we compared a group of 12 workers occupationally exposed to inorganic mercury, with a group of matched controls (matched on age, sex and occupation). (Williamson, Teo and Sanderson, 1982). As expected from previous research (Wood, 1973; Langolf, Whittle & Henderson, 1979) in tests where some co-ordination was required between stimulus and response in an on-going fashion, such as in the hand steadiness or visual pursuit tests, the mercury-exposed group showed significant impairment. In addition short term memory deficits were found on both types of tests. This was a true short term memory deficit since no other memory stage was affected and since neither arousal levels (CFF) nor attention (vigilance) were impaired, we know that the stimulus actually reached the stage of short term memory. Similarly, we know that simple response (measured as reaction time) was not impaired so our measurements of short term memory were not confounded by a poorer ability to simply respond to the stimulus.

Knowing that inorganic mercury exposure can produce short term memory deficits, we can postulate about the possible physiological or biochemical damage that may be responsible.

We know from experiments by Gibbs and Ng (1977) using ouabain, that short term memory is $Na+/K+$ pump dependent. It is logical to suggest then that inorganic mercury may limit this same mechanism. Significantly, Gallagher, Mitchell and Wheal (1982) found that injections of both organic and inorganic mercury reduced $Na+/K+$ ATP'ase

levels in the rat brain in exactly the same manner as did
ouabain.

TABLE 3.

SUMMARY OF BEHAVIOURAL PERFORMANCE
OF MERCURY - EXPOSED WORKERS

---

1.   Short term memory impairment(on both Sternberg &
                                            Paired Associates)

2.   No impairment of arousal or attention

3.   No impairment of simple response

4.   No impairment of sensory store memory (1st stage
          memory) or long term memory

Attempts to relate psychological function to exposure in
this study revealed that only psychomotor functions were
accounted for by the conventional exposure measures of
Mercury in Urine (Table 4) or length of exposure.

The only exposure measure to significantly account for
the deficits in short term memory was whether or not the
individual was actively using mercury at the time of test
and had increasing levels of mercury in urine. This finding
naturally raises some interesting questions about the nature
of mercury's effect on the CNS. It suggests that the effect
of mercury may be of a dynamic nature in which increasing
mercury levels may upset homeostatic mechanisms which in
turn produce the behaviour change. It is possible that
changes in mercury status, rather than absolute levels are
detrimental to the CNS.

Inorganic Lead

Similar analysis is currently being attempted to
investigate the effects of occupational exposure to lead.
Preliminary findings indicate that lead exposure involving
levels below those currently designated "safe" (70μg/100ml.
blood) appear to produce deficits at the behavioural level.

TABLE 4.

RELATIONSHIPS BETWEEN MEASURES OF EXPOSURE
AND PSYCHOLOGICAL FUNCTIONS

Test	Mercury in Urine	Total hr. Contact	Active Contact (yes - no)
Hand steadiness			
Upper time 1	0.31	ns	ns
11	0.1	ns	ns
III	0.13	ns	ns
Lower time I	0.5*	ns	ns
II	0.23	ns	ns
III	0.1	ns	ns
Upper touches 1	0.57*	ns	ns
II	0.32	ns	ns
III	0.17	ns	ns
Lower touches I	0.63**	ns	ns
II	0.48	ns	ns
III	0.43	ns	ns
Sternberg test			
Positive set	0.26	0.23	0.65*
Negative set	0.27	0.20	0.72**
Visual pursuit			
Fast (30 rpm)	-0.48	-0.55*	-0.57*
Slow (15 rpm)	-0.34	-0.18	-0.52*
Paired associates (STM)			
No. correct	-0.37	-0.26	-0.55*
Trials to criterion	0	0.08	-0.51*

*P <0.05, **P <0.01

The test results of fifty-nine lead-workers, none of whom had blood lead levels exceeding 70μg/100ml. were compared with those from our standardised test battery. The findings can be summarised as follows:

1. Critical flicker fusion thresholds (CFF) were significantly lower than normal, indicating that general arousal levels were depressed in the lead-exposed group.

2. Sensory store memory seemed to be unaffected by lead-exposure.

3. Short term memory performance on both the paired-associates and Sternberg short term memory tests was significatnly poorer in the lead-exposed group.

4. Long term memory was also significantly poorer in the lead-exposed group.

5. There were limited motor and psychomotor effects which appeared when the lead-exposed individuals were stressed during the test, such as when the Visual Pursuit required fast tracking. There was no sign of tremor.

Caution must be used in assessing these findings as the statistical analysis requires considerably more attention, particularly with respect to careful matching of lead-exposed and control groups. Nevertheless, it is clear that the profile of effects of lead exposure is unique. The effects are not the same as those seen in mercury exposure. Thus, while both heavy metals are neurotoxic, they each act upon specific psychological functions. Armed with this knowledge we can then make some informed hypotheses about the physiological and biochemical changes that each metal brings about.

R E F E R E N C E S

Chang, L.W. (1977) *Environ. Res. 14,* 329.

Chisholm, J.J.(1971) *Sci. Am.   224,* 15.

David, O. (1974) *Environ. Health Perspect. 7,* 17.

Gallagher, P.J., Mitchell, J. & Wheal, M.V. (1982)
        Toxicol. 23, 261.

Gibbs, M.E., Ng, K.T. (1977). *Bioheav. Rev. 1,* 113.

Gowers, W.R. (1888) "Diseases of the Nervous System,Vol.11"
        J. & Churchill, London.

Hrdina, P.D., Hanin, I. & Dubas, T.C. (1980). In Lead
                Toxicity" (R.L. Singh (ed.)). p. 273.
                Urban & Schwarzenberg, Baltimore.

Lampert, P.W., & Schochet, S.S. (1968).*J. Neuropath.Exptl.
        Neurol. 27,* 527.

Langolf, (D., Whittle, H.P., Henderson, R. (1979). *Arch.
        Hig. Rada. Toksikol. 30* (suppl.), 275.

Neal, P.A., & Jones, R.R. (1938). *JAMA. 110,* 337.

Needleman, H. (1979). "Final report to International Lead
        Zinc Research Organisation".

Rutter, M. (1980). *Dev. Med. Child Neurol. 22, Suppl.,* 1.

Seppalainen, A.M. (1971). *Scand. J. Clin. Lab. Invest. 27,*
        70.

Silbergeld, E.K. (1982). *TINS, Sept.,* 291.

Valciukas, J.A., & Lillis, R. (1980). *Environ. Res. 21,*275.

W.H.O., (1979). "Early detection of health impairment in
        occupational exposure to health hazards".
        Report of W.H.O. meetings, W.H.O.

Williamson, A.M., & Teo, R.K.C. (1982). *Proc. 5th Asian
        Occ. Health, Sept.*

Williamson, A.M., Teo, R.K.C., & Sanderson, J. (1982). *Int.
        Arch. Occ. Env. Health, 50,* 273.

Wood, R.W., Weiss, A.B., & Weiss, B. (1973). *Arch. Environ.
        Health 26,* 249.

Zeilhuis, R.L. (1971). *Arch. Environ. Health, 23,* 299.

THE EFFECT OF STRESS ON CENTRAL NERVOUS SYSTEM
PROTEIN PHOSPHORYLATION AND CYCLIC AMP

Peter R. Dunkley,[+*] Jill Cockburn,[*]
Peter A. Power and Maurice G. King
The Neuroscience Group, Medical Faculty[*]
and Psychology Department, University of
Newcastle, N.S.W. 2308 Australia

ABSTRACT

The effect of mild stressors on central nervous
(CNS) levels of protein phosphorylation and cyclic AMP
was assessed in rats. Uncontrollable electric footshock
significantly increased the in vitro phosphorylation of
a protein of approximate molecular weight 42,000 that had
been identified previously as the α subunit of pyruvate
dehydrogenase. This increase was not due to the stress
of handling the animal before the experiment or during
the sacrifice procedures, but may have been due in part
to exposure to a novel environment. No other phosphoprotein in the crude synaptosome fraction was significantly affected. Cyclic AMP levels were also unchanged.
The literature is discussed with special reference to
the procedures used to estimate in vivo levels of protein
phosphorylation and cyclic AMP.

INTRODUCTION

In a wide range of species, including man, stress
can be induced by either physical or psychological
stimuli. In the rat, stress causes changes in motor
activity, peripheral hormone levels, memory, emotionality
and in extreme cases frank pathology such as gastric ul-
cers (see Seyle, 1976; Anisman, 1978 for review). In

+ To whom reprint requests and correspondence should sent.

297

order to understand the consequences of stress it is necessary to understand how various stimuli lead to changes in
neuronal function in the CNS. It is well-established
that uncontrollable stress increases the activity of CNS
catecholaminergic neurons (Stone, 1975; Oei and King, 1981).
This has been documented by findings of decreased receptor
density and levels of noradrenaline, and increased levels
of tyrosine hydroxylase (Weiss et al., 1981; Stone and
Platt, 1982). The problem with estimating changes only
in the noradrenergic system is that most stressors lead
to some effect. It would be advantageous to have other
neurochemical markers that correlate with particular types
of stimuli as many other neuron types are also presumably
affected by stress.

    Protein phosphorylation is a good marker of neuronal
cell function for several reasons; specific proteins
can be assayed, the subcellular location and function of
some of the proteins is known and the release of certain
neurotransmitters is accompanied by changes in protein
phosphorylation (Dunkley, 1981; Robinson and Dunkley,
1983a; b). Cyclic AMP is a non-specific marker of cell
function, but it is known to be increased as a result of
increased release of catecholamines and its only function
is to modify the activity of protein kinase enzymes
(Greengard, 1976). Both protein phosphorylation (Williams
and Rodnight, 1977; Routtenberg, 1979) and cyclic AMP
levels (Delapaz et al., 1975; Kant et al., 1981) have
been shown to be altered by different stressors with the
extent and direction of the effect depending on the
procedures used. In the present paper the procedures
used to assess in vivo levels of protein phosphorylation
and cyclic AMP are described, and the results of experiments aimed at determining the effect of handling, exposure to a novel environment and mild electric footshock
on these neurochemical markers are presented. These
data are integrated with discussion of past literature
since significant differences in findings exist between
laboratories and these are probably due to differences
in methodology.

                        EXPERIMENTAL

Animals. Male Wistar rats, aged 90-110 days at time of
sacrifice, were used after four weeks of individual
housing with a 12 h night-day routine (light on 0600) and

regulated temperature (22 ± 1°C) and humidity. Food and water were provided <u>ad lib</u>. The following groups of animals were used.

HC Group: home cage animals remained in the holding room during the experimental period. All other animals were transferred individually to an experimental room where they were handled for two min a day for 10 days prior to treatment on the eleventh day as follows:
    H Group: handled animals were returned to the holding room for 58 min immediately after handling.
    N Group: novelty animals were placed in a clear Plexiglas box (27 x 35 x 42cm with a grid floor of stainless steel bars each 0.32cm in diameter and 0.78 cm apart) for 1 h.
    U Group: uncontrollably shocked animals were placed in the box and a mild (2mA) intermittent (10s on), scrambled electric footshock was applied for 1 h (total of 120 shocks).

Rats were then sacrificed between 1000-1300h in an experimental room away from the remaining animals. Care was taken to thoroughly clean and dry all apparatus and to remove the carcasses before sacrificing the next animal.

Protein Phosphorylation. Animals were sacrificed by whole body immersion in liquid nitrogen for 4 min and heads were stored at -70°C for up to a week. The forebrain was removed without thawing and homogenised (10gm/100ml) in 0.32 M sucrose containing 30mM Tris, pH 7.4, and 1mM EDTA. A crude synaptosome (P2) preparation was rapidly obtained and calcium-stimulated protein phosphorylation estimated (Dunkley and Robinson, 1981a; b). The results were obtained from densitometric scans of autoradiographs and are expressed in arbitrary units, representing the peak height of an individual protein/total amount of label incorporated into all proteins.

Cyclic AMP. Animals were placed head first into a plastic cylinder (30 x 10cm diam) in a microwave oven (1200 watts) and they were sacrificed by irradiation for 30s. In one experiment different sacrifice procedures were compared. Animals were either anaesthetised with ether for 2 min prior to decapitation, decapitated without anaesthesia, placed in liquid nitrogen for 4 min

or were sacrificed in the microwave oven for 15 or 45s.
After sacrifice tissue was immediately removed and placed
in liquid nitrogen for 2 min. Brains were stored for up
to two weeks at -20°C when they were homogenised in 6ml
of 6% tricholoroacetic acid (w/v). After centifugation
at 5000 rpm for 10 min the supernatant fractions were
washed 6 times with 4 vol. of water saturated ether.
Ether was removed in a stream of air. Aliquots were
reconstituted and assayed for cyclic AMP using the binding
protein assay of Brown et al. (1973).

RESULTS AND DISCUSSION

A. <u>In Vivo Levels of Protein Phosphorylation and Cyclic</u>
<u>AMP</u>.

    It is not possible to measure protein phosphorylation
or cyclic AMP levels <u>in vivo</u>. Changes in these markers
must therefore be assayed <u>in vitro</u> using procedures that
assess the actual <u>in vivo</u> levels and reliably reflect
genuine differences between control and stressed groups.

(i) <u>Protein Phosphorylation</u>. The extent of phosphorylation of an individual protein when measured <u>in vitro</u> can be
dramatically altered by the procedures used, including the
methods of sacrifice, subcellular fractionation and incubation (Dunkley, 1981). These differences must reflect
changes in the amount of substrate available, or in the
relative activity of the protein kinases and phosphatases.
Procedures which reduce protein phosphatase activity are
especially desirable when attempting to measure <u>in vivo</u>
levels of protein phosphorylation. Recent studies have
suggested that liquid nitrogen is the preferred procedure
for sacrificing animals, as enzymes were inactivated more
rapidly than with anaesthesia or decapitation and no effects on subsequent subcellular fractionation of phosphoproteins were observed (Conway and Routtenberg, 1978;
1979; Ehrlich et al., 1980; Mitrius, 1981). Subcellular
fractionation should be at 4°C and as rapid as possible.
Preincubation of tissue should be avoided as it inactivates
calcium-stimulated protein kinases and allows time for
phosphatase activity (Dunkley and Robinson, 1981a; b).

An alternative procedure is to combine <u>in vivo</u>

labelling of phosphoproteins, by injections of ^{32}P-inor-
ganic phosphate, with subsequent in vitro assays for protein phosphorylation (Perumal et al., 1977). Changes due
to phosphatase activity during subcellular fractionation
can still occur with this procedure, but they can be controlled for using^{32}P-inorganic phosphate (Perumal et al.,
1977). The phosphoprotein profiles of synaptic fractions
after injection of ^{32}P-inorganic phosphate have been
investigated (Berman et al., 1980; Mitrius et al., 1981).
The majority of the in vivo labelled phosphoproteins
comigrate with phosphoproteins that are labelled in
vitro which suggests that both procedures are reflecting
the same events. The method of choice for stress related
studies will depend on experimental aims, but both
approaches are desirable.

(ii) Cyclic AMP. A number of in vitro assays are available for cyclic AMP each of which accurately and reliably
measures levels in CNS tissue (Brown et al., 1973;
Skinner et al., 1978; Kant et al., 1981). However, the
actual tissue levels of cyclic AMP can be altered by up
to fivefold depending on the procedure used to sacrifice
the animal (Fig.1). Tissue levels of cyclic AMP are
primarily controlled by the relative activities of the
adenylate cyclase and phosphodiesterase enzymes, although
the level of protein bound cyclic AMP that is inacessible
to phosphodiesterases is also important. Sacrifice causes
anoxia and the subsequent release of neurotransmitters,
and adenosine, activates adenylate cyclase and increases
tissue cyclic AMP levels (Daley, 1979). The very high
levels of cyclic AMP found after anaesthesia/decapitation
(Fig.1) are assumed to be due to these consequences of
anoxia (Lust et al., 1973). Lower levels of cyclic AMP
can be found after inadequate exposure to microwave
irradiation as adenylate cyclase is inactivated more
rapidly than phosphodiesterase (Lenox et al., 1977). The
actual in vivo levels of cyclic AMP are therefore not
certain, although it is generally accepted that high
power (5-10Kwatt) focussed microwave instruments applied
for short times (<500ms) provide the most accurate levels
(Schneider et al., 1982), both enzymes are rapidly inactivated. One problem with the microwave procedure is that
during sacrifice animals must be restrained so that their
heads are correctly placed in the wave guide. Restraint
is known to be a powerful stressor as judged by objective
criteria such as plasma hormone levels (Lenox et al.,1980).

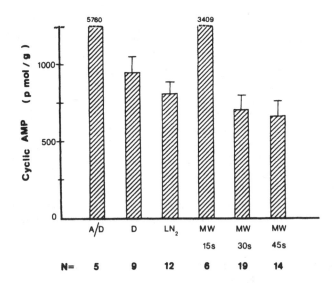

Fig.1. *The Effect of Sacrifice Procedures on CNS Levels*
of Cyclic-AMP. Rats were sacrificed by anaesthesia
decapitation (A/D), decapitation (D), liquid
nitrogen (LN$_2$) or microwave (MW) irradiation
for the times indicated. **T**; *S E M*

Also microwave irradiation lyses cell membranes allowing
diffusion of neurochemicals down concentration gradients
(Kant et al., 1979) and the extent of enzyme inactivation
differs for each CNS region (Lenox et al., 1977). Finally,
cyclic AMP levels in the CNS undergo circadian rhythms
(Kant et al., 1981; Dunkley et al., unpublished data)
and therefore experimental animals must be sacrificed
at the same time each day.

B.   The Effect of Stress on Protein Phosphorylation

(i)   Electric Footshock. A number of studies have been
undertaken to investigate the effects of electric footshock on the levels of synaptosomal protein phosphorylation (Table 1; Williams and Rodnight, 1977; Routtenberg,
1979). Gispen et al.,(1977) found that uncontrollable
footshock did not affect the level of total synaptosomal
protein phosphorylation when compared to home cage controls. Ehrlich et al., (1977) found that uncontrollable

footshock increased the cyclic AMP stimulated phosphorylation of proteins F (mol. wt approx. 47,000) and H1
(mol. wt approx. 15,000) relative to controls that had
been exposed to a novel environment. These effects were
only seen in the neostriatum and not in the cortex and
it is important to note that all animals were sacrificed
24h after exposure to the stressor. Routtenberg and
Benson (1980) found that uncontrolled footshock increased
the basal and cyclic AMP stimulated phosphorylation
of total proteins as well as phosphoprotein F2 (mol. wt
approx. 41,000) relative to handled controls. This effect was seen in the frontal cortex and again all animals
were sacrificed 24h after exposure to the stressor. In
a further study Morgan and Routtenberg (1981) found that
uncontrollable footshock did not alter basal and cyclic
AMP stimulated phosphorylation of total proteins, or of
phosphoprotein F2, relative to handled controls. On this
occasion however, rats were sacrificed immediately following exposure to the stressor.

These studies also addressed the hypothesis that
training to avoid escape from electric footshock would
increase the phosphorylation of a synaptosomal protein
(Table 1). This was found to be the case for proteins
F and F2. It should be noted that protein F (Ehrlich et
al.,1977) was comprised of more than one phosphoprotein
and protein F2 was the major constituent (Routtenberg
and Benson. 1980). Protein F2 has now been identified
as the α subunit of the mitochondrial enzyme pyruvate
dehydrogenase (Morgan and Routtenberg,1980). Morgan
and Routtenberg (1981) found that the correlation between
band F2 phosphorylation and pyruvate dehydrogenase activity was high and increased phosphorylation of pyruvate
dehydrogenase in vitro in trained animals reflected a
reduced phosphorylation in vivo. Training therefore
induced an increase in frontal cortex pyruvate dehydrogenase activity after dephosphorylation of pyruvate
dehydrogenase in vivo.

The investigations described above suggested a
number of testable hypotheses relating to the effects
of uncontrollable stress on protein phosphorylation.
Firstly uncontrollable footshock significantly decreases
the in vivo phosphorylation of pyruvate dehydrogenase.
Secondly, pyruvate dehydrogenase phosphorylation is

Table 1.   *The Effect of Stress on CNS Protein*
             Phosphorylation. *1. Gispen et al., 1977;*
2. Ehrlich et al., 1977; 3. Routtenberg and Benson,
*1980; 4.Morgan and Routtenberg, 1981. *, cerebral cortex*
was also investigated but is not reported here. A/D,
LN$_2$ as in Fig. 1 legend. W, whole brain; Neo, neostriatum;
FC, frontal cortex; Syn, synaptosomes; SynM, synaptosomal
*membranes; ** Pi labelling was in vivo, ATP labelling*
was in vitro. Groups HC, U, H and N are equivalent to
those defined in the experimental section, while Group T
are animals trained to escape or avoid the electric
footshock.

Study	1	2*	3	4
Procedure				
Species	mice	rat	rat	rat
Handling	–	1m/day 4 days	2m/day 16 days	2m/day 5 days
Sacrifice	A/D	LN$_2$(24h)	LN$_2$(24h)	LN$_2$
Region	W	Neo	FC	FC
Subcellular fraction	Syn	SynM	SynM	W
Labelling**	Pi	ATP +cyclic AMP	ATP ±cyclic AMP	ATP ±cyclic AMP
Footshock (mA)	0.3	0.5	3.4	3.4
Results for	T>U,HC	T>U>N (T>U,N)	T/U>H (T,U>H)	T>H,U
Protein	Total	H1,F (E)	F2 (Total)	F2

significantly altered only 24 h after electric footshock.
Finally, the effect of uncontrollable footshock on pyruvate dehydrogenase activity is due only to the footshock
and not to the handling or exposure to a novel environment which occurs during the experiment. These hypotheses were tested using four groups of rats (HC, H, N and
U) and the results for group U will be discussed initially.
These rats were handled for 10 days, exposed to inescap-
able electric footshock for 1 h and immediately sacrificed in liquid nitrogen. A forebrain P2 fraction was
prepared, labelled with[γ-^{32}P] ATP and the phosphoryla-
tions of individual proteins was assessed. (Fig. 2). Some
of the phosphoproteins present were readily identified by
comparison with previous studies including Greengard's
protein I (phosphoprotein 5) and the α subunit of pryuvate
dehydrogenase (phosphoprotein 12)(Dunkley 1981; Robinson
and Dunkley, 1983a). Quantitative analysis of the data
(one way ANOVA, Duncan Post Hoc comparison) indicated that
for the shocked animals in vitro phosphorylation of pryuvate dehydrogenase was significantly increased ($p < 0.05$)

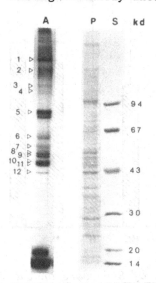

Fig. 2. *Protein and Phosphoprotein Profiles of Rat CNS
         Synaptosomes*. *Autoradiograph (A) and protein pro-
tein profile (P) are shown beside a set of molecular weight
standards (S). The approximate molecular weights are shown
on the RHS and major phosphoproteins numbered on the LHS.*

when compared with the HC controls (Fig.3) which supports
the first hypothesis outlined above. No other phosphoprotein was significantly affected by the uncontrollable
stress (Table 2). Mean levels of phosphorylation for some
phosphoproteins were altered relative to HC controls but
the differences did not reach significance. Total protein
phosphorylation did not vary significantly between the U
and HC groups which is in contrast to the results found
by Routtenberg and Benson (]980), but may reflect differences in times of sacrifice or phosphorylation procedures.
The data also suggest that 24 h is not required to observe
a difference in pyruvate dehydrogenase phosphorylation
and the second hypothesis is therefore refuted.

(ii) <u>Handling and Novelty</u>. Holmes <u>et al</u>., (]977) found
that basal and cyclic AMP-stimulated protein kinase
activities were increased in rats exposed to chronic sham

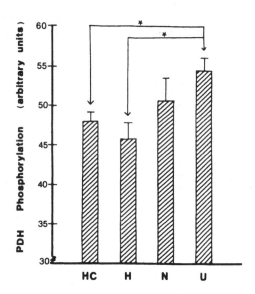

Fig. 3. The Effect of Stressors on the Phosphorylation
of Synaptosomal Pyruvate Dehydrogenase (PDH)
in vitro. Rats remained in their home cages (HC)
or were handled (H), exposed to a novel environment (N)
or were uncontrollably shocked (U). Data were analysed
using one-way ANOVAS *, P<0.05; F(3,21) = 3.71.

Table 2. *The Effect of Stressors on the Phosphorylation of Major Synaptosomal Phosphoproteins*

Phosphoprotein	Home Cage (HC) n = 7	Handled (H) n = 7	Novel Cage (N) n = 6	Electric Shock (U) n = 5
1	54.2 ± 3.0	56.1 ± 1.9	56.4 ± 2.0	55.6 ± 3.1
2	45.0 ± 2.7	47.6 ± 1.7	49.1 ± 1.6	50.3 ± 4.1
3	37.2 ± 2.2	38.3 ± 0.8	39.0 ± 0.6	38.9 ± 2.1
4	32.9 ± 1.8	33.6 ± 0.9	35.6 ± 0.3	35.1 ± 1.8
5	115.8 ± 5.6	120.1 ± 4.6	124.3 ± 2.6	116.8 ± 2.2
6	53.3 ± 1.9	54.8 ± 0.7	55.1 ± 0.9	58.1 ± 1.4
7	50.5 ± 1.3	49.1 ± 1.1	49.4 ± 2.6	52.6 ± 1.3
8	82.7 ± 4.8	81.4 ± 4.7	84.2 ± 2.9	85.6 ± 1.6
9	69.9 ± 2.2	68.5 ± 1.3	73.9 ± 3.0	73.1 ± 3.9
10	91.6 ± 5.7	95.5 ± 2.5	92.7 ± 2.8	98.1 ± 7.0
11	88.1 ± 3.7	93.5 ± 2.2	93.1 ± 2.9	99.4 ± 5.8
12	48.0 ± 1.2	45.7 ± 2.2	50.6 ± 2.5	54.4 ± 1.6

electroshock treatment, but no increase was found if the animals had been handled prior to the sham treatment. They concluded that in naive animals the anxiety accompanying an electroshock procedure (handling, restraint, placement of earclips, etc.) increased the activity of a membrane bound phosphorylating system. This did not occur if animals were habituated to handling over a 15-day period. No previous study has attempted to assess the effects of exposure to a novel environment on CNS levels of protein phosphorylation.

Analysis of variance and post hoc comparison (Duncan) showed the phosphorylation of pyruvate dehydrogenase was significantly increased ($P<0.05$) in the U group when compared to the HC and H groups, but was not different from the N group (Fig. 3). This indicates that habituation to handling does not alter the effects of electric footshock on pyruvate dehydrogenase labelling and suggests

that at least part of the footshock stress was due to
exposure to the novel cage, this finding negates the
third hypothesis. No other protein showed any significant
changes in response to handling and novelty and total
protein phosphorylation did not vary significantly between any of the groups investigated. The difference
between these results and those that would be predicted
from Holmes et al .(1977) may be due to different protein
phosphorylation conditions, but could also be due to the
increased stress of restraint in the electroshock treatment relative to exposure to a novel cage.

(iii) Other Stressors. Holmes and Rodnight (1978)
found that restraint for 10 min, but not cold stress,
significantly increased basal and cyclic AMP-stimulated
protein phosphorylation relative to handled rats exposed
to chronic sham electroshock,

C.   The Effect of Stress on Cyclic AMP.

Many groups have investigated the effects of stressors
on CNS levels of cyclic AMP, but only studies where
sacrifice was by liquid nitrogen immersion or microwave
irradiation will be considered here. Delapaz et al.
(1975) found that uncontrollable electric footshock
increased cyclic AMP levels in the septum and hippocampus
relative to home-cage controls that had been habituated
to handling.Eichelman et al. (1976) found an increase in
whole brain cyclic AMP levels if footshock was administered to fighting animals relative to non-fighting, non-
shocked controls. Skinner et al. (1978) using cryoplates
implanted in the cerebral cortex of conscious rats to
collect tissue, found that cutaneous electric shock
decreased the cyclic AMP content of the parietal cortex
relative to handling-habituated controls. We have shown
previously that no changes in CNS levels of cyclic AMP
could be detected in chronically shocked rats or animals
trained to avoid/escape electric footshock relative to
controls exposed to the novel environment (Cockburn et al.,
1981).

Handling rats for 15 days made no significant difference to forebrain cyclic AMP levels after chronic sham
electroshock when compared to home cage controls (Holmes
et al., 1977). However, others have reported differences,

Table 3. *The Effect of Stressors on CNS Levels of Cyclic AMP*

Exp.	Cyclic AMP (pmol/g)	
	1	2
Home Cage (HC)	725 ± 74	521 ± 54
Handled (H)	–	599 ± 57
Novelty (N)	659 ± 70	–
Uncontrollable footshock (U)	765 ± 64	–

including Corda et al. (1980) who found that striatal cyclic AMP levels were increased in naive rats when compared to animals habituated to the handling that precedes microwave irradiation. Skinner et al. 1978, in contrast, found that parietal cortex cyclic AMP levels were decreased in naive rats when compared to handling-habituated animals.

Open field acitivity in some respects is comparable to exposure to a novel cage in that both evoke similar stress responses and Kant et al. (1981) found no change in cyclic AMP levels in the pituitary, hypothalamus, pineal and cerebellum during 10 min open field acitivty when compared to home cage controls.

Exposure of rats to electric footshock or the Plexiglas box without shock did not alter CNS levels of cyclic AMP when compared with home cage controls (Table 3). The rats used in this initial experiment had not been habituated to handling and so a further experiment was performed which indicated that habituation to handling and/or the sacrifice procedure for microwave irradiation also had no effect on cyclic AMP levels relative to home cage controls (Table 3). Although cyclic AMP levels were not altered by any of the stressors evaluated here changes were found in other unrelated experiments.

CONCLUSIONS

1. Assessment of actual in vivo levels of protein phosphorylation is complex, while cyclic AMP levels can be

accurately and reliably assessed if appropriate procedures are adopted.

2.   Uncontrollable electric footshock increases the in vitro phosphorylation of CNS pryuvate dehydrogenase but does not alter the phosphorylation of any other synaptosomal protein. It is proposed that this increase is reflected in vivo by an increased activity of the enzyme.

3.   Exposure to a novel environment, but not the stress of handling or sacrifice, may contribute to the effects of footshock on pyruvate dehydrogenase.

4.   CNS levels of cyclic AMP are not altered by handling, novelty or mild electric footshock under the conditions used.

ACKNOWLEDGEMENTS

The NH & MRC and the Faculty of Medicine Research Committee are thanked for financial support for this project. Mrs. P. Jarvie is thanked for excellent research assistance.

REFERENCES

Anisman, M. (1978). In "Psychopharmacology of Aversively Motivated Behavior" (H. Snisman and G. Bignami, eds.) Plenum Press, N.Y.

Brown, B.L., Alban, J.D.M., Ekins, R.P. and Sgherzi, A.M. Biochem. J. 121, 561-562.

Berman, R.F., Hullihan, J.P., Kinnier, W.J. and Wilson, J.E. (1980). J. Neurochem. 34, 431-437.

Cockburn, J., Dunkley, P.R., Brown, C. and King. M. (1981). Neuroscience Letters S7, 423.

Conway, R.G. and Routtenberg, A. (1978). Brain Res. 139, 366-373.

Conway, R.G. and Routtenberg, A. (1979). Brain Res. 170, 313-324.

Corda, M.G., Biggio, G. and Gesso, G.L. (1980). Brain Res. 188, 287-290.

Daley, J.W. (1979). In "Physiological and Regulatory Functions of Adenosine and Adenine Nucleotides" (H.P. Baers and G.I. Drummond, eds.),pp.229-241. Raven Press.

Delapaz,R.L., Dickman, S.R. and Grosser, B.I. (1975).

Brain Res. 85, 171-175.

Dunkley. P.R. (1981). In "New Approaches to Nerve and Muscle Disorders. Basic and Applied Contributions" (A.D. Kidman, J.M. Tomkins and R.A. Westerman,eds.) pp. 38-51. Excerpta Medica, Amsterdam.

Dunkley, P.R. and Robinson, P.J. (1981a). Biochem. Biophys. Res. Comm. 102, 1196-1202

Dunkley, P.R. and Robinson, P.J. (1981b). Biochem. J. 199, 269-272.

Eichelman, B., Orenbe, E., Seagraves, E. and Barchas, J. (1976). Nature 263, 433-434.

Ehrlich, Y.H., Rabjohns, R.R. and Routtenberg, A. (1977). Pharmacol. Biochem. Behav. 6, 169-174.

Ehrlich, Y.H., Redd, M.V., Keen, P., Davis, L.G., Dougherty, J. and Brunngraber, E.G. (1980). J. Neurochem. 34, 1327-1330.

Gispen, W.H., Perumal, R., Wilson, J.F. and Glassman, E. (1977). Behav. Biol. 21, 358-365.

Greengard, P. (1976). Nature 260,101-108.

Holmes, H., Rodnight, R. and Kapoor, R. (1977). Pharm. Biochem. Behav. 6, 415-419.

Holmes, H. and Rodnight, R. (1978), Biochem. Soc. Trans. 6, 863-865.

Kant, G.J., Lenox, R.H. and Meyerhoff, J.L. (1979) Neurochem. Res. 4, 529-534.

Kant, G.J., Sessions, G.R., Lenox, R.H. and Meyerhoff, J.L. (1981). Life Sciences 29, 2491-2499.

Lenox, R.H., Meyerhoff, J.L., Gandhi, O.P. and Wray, M.L. (1977). J. Cyclic Nucleotide Research 3, 367-379.

Lenox, R.H., Kant, G.J., Sessions, G.R., Pennington,L.L., Moughey, E.M. and Meyerhoff, J.L. (1980). Neuroendocrinology 30, 300-308.

Lust, W.D., Passonneau, J.V. and Beech, R.L. (1973). Science 181, 280-282.

Mitrius, J.C., Morgan, D.G. and Routtenberg, A. (1981) Brain Res. 212, 67-81.

Morgan, D.G. and Routtenberg, A. (1980). Biochem. Biophys. Res. Comm. 95, 569-

Oei, T.P.S. and King, M.G. (1980). Neurosci and Biobehav. Rev. 4, 161-173.

Perumal, R., Gispen, W.H., Glassman, E. and Wilson, J.E. (1977). Behav. Biol. 21, 341-357.

Robinson, P.J. and Dunkley, P.R. (1983a). In "Molecular Aspects of Neurological Disorders" (L. Austin and P. Jeffrey eds.), Academic Press, in the press.

Robinson, P.J. and Dunkley, P.R. (1983b). J. Neurochem, in the press.

Routtenberg, A. (1979). Progress in Neurobiology 12, 85-113.

Routtenberg, A. and Benson, G.E. (1980). Behav. Neurol. Biol. 29, 168-175.

Schneider, D.R., Felt, B.T. and Goldman, H. (1982). J. Neurochem. 38, 749-752.

Selye, H. (1976). In, "Stress in Health and Disease", Butterworths, London.

Skinner, J.E., Welch, K.M.A., Reed, J.C. and Nell, J.H. (1978). J. Neurochem. 30, 691-698.

Stone, E.A. (1975). In "Catecholamines and Behavior" (A.J. Freidhoff, ed.), Vol.2, Plenum Press, N.Y.

Stone, E.A. and Platt, J.E. (1982). Brain Res. 237, 405-414.

Weiss, J.M., Goodman, P.A. Losito, B.G., Corrigan, S., Charry, J.M. and Bailey, W.H. (1981) Brain Res. Rev. 3, 167-205.

Williams, J. and Rodnight, R. (1977). Progress in Neurobiology 8, 183-250.

IV. Neuromuscular Pathology

PHYSIOLOGICAL MECHANISMS FOR THE REGULATION OF PROTEIN BALANCE IN SKELETAL MUSCLE

D.J.MILLWARD,P.C.BATES,J.G.BROWN,D.HALLIDAY,
B.ODEDRA,P.W.EMERY & M.J.RENNIE.

Clinical Nutrition and Metabolism Unit
Department of Human Nutrition
London School of Hygiene and Tropical Medicine
4 St Pancras Way   LONDON NW1 2PE

Rates of human muscle protein synthesis and degradation
have been studied with measurements of a-v differences of 3
methyl histidine(3MH) across the leg and with 13C leucine
incorporation into muscle protein in vivo.These studies
show that in most disease states protein synthesis is
markedly depressed with degradation also depressed. This
finding shows that measurements of urinary 3MH are
unreliable indices of muscle protein turnover.The role of
insulin, glucocorticoids and T3 in regulating the
translational phase of protein synthesis , ribosome content
and protein degradation is discussed in the light of animal
experiments.In addition recent studies on the role of
calcium, prostaglandins and branched chain amino and keto
acids in the regulation of protein balance are reviewed.

INTRODUCTION

The impact of neuromuscular pathology on skeletal
muscle usually results in not only a functional defect but
also often has an effect on protein balance in the muscle.
In the adult this is perceived as a wasting while in the
younger patient the result is a slowing down or even a
cessation of growth. These effects may involve the disease
state directly affecting either protein synthesis or
degradation, or may be a secondary response to loss of
function. This is because, the maintenance of normal

315

contractile activity is essential for the maintenance of normal growth and protein balance (See Booth et al 1982).Of course the actual mechanisms by which most neuromuscular pathologies manifest themselves are unknown,but the continuous turnover of muscle proteins means that a change in balance can be achieved by any combination of changes in protein synthesis and degradation. At the moment it is a fact that very little is known in detail about changes in protein metabolism in human muscle in diseased states. However evidence is accumulating about the sites of the defects in terms of protein synthesis or degradation.This paper reviews current knowledge about changes in protein turnover in human disease states in the light of what is already established about normal physiological regulation which has largely come from animal studies.

PROTEIN SYNTHESIS AND DEGRADATION IN NORMAL AND DISEASED HUMAN MUSCLE

Although studies of protein turnover were undertaken soon after the discovery of stable isotopes (Schoenheimer et al 1939,Sprinson and Rittenburg 1949), information has been largely limited to studies of whole body protein turnover(see Waterlow et al 1978). The use of radioactive isotopes, which has enabled investigation in animals,is of limited use in man (although in certain patients some studies with 14C can and have been undertaken, with important results: see Garlick & Clugston 1981 ,Clague 1981). However two methods have been developed which are proving of great value in human studies, the first involving 3-methyl histidine (3MH), and the second involving amino acids labelled with the stable isotope of carbon (13C).

3MH occurs exclusively in actin and some species of myosin heavy-chain as a result of a post-translational modification, and since it is not metabolised in man (see Young & Munro 1978) it is excreted in the urine at a rate which only reflects the degradation rate of these two proteins. On a meat- free diet this will only include contractile proteins in the tissues. Since creatinine excretion can be determined as an index of muscle mass (Graystone 1968), the 3MH/creatinine ratio has been taken to indicate the fractional rate of skeletal muscle protein degradation. This method has been very widely adopted and values for the 3MH excretion rates reported for many of the neuromuscular diseases (see Warnes et al 1981)

The main inference from these studies is that muscle pathology is usually associated with increased muscle protein degradation,since the 3MH/creatinine ratio is usually increased. The first observation was that of McKeran et al (1977) who reported an increase in the ratio in Duchenne muscular dystrophy. Since then the accumulation of a large number of disorders exibiting this phenomenon has strenthened the not unreasonable assumption that increased degradation is a common pathological change.

We have been unhappy about the validity of one of the assumptions in this method for some time and these worries have recently been confirmed in studies on patients.

Our concern has involved the assumption that most of the urinary 3MH originates from skeletal muscle (Millward et al 1980a, 1982, Rennie & Millward 1983). We showed that in the rat the turnover of 3MH in skeletal muscle was so slow that the observed rate of excretion could only be explained by significant non-muscle sources. Although the amounts of actin in tissues other than skeletal muscle is small (it is present in smooth muscle and to a limited extent in all cells), rapid turnover in these tissues would mean that they would produce disproportionate amounts. Smooth muscle of the intestine is one obvious source, and Wassner & Li (1982) have shown that in the rat the perfused intestine produces 3MH at a rate equivalent to two thirds of that arising from perfused skeletal muscle. Our own recent measurements of the rate of 3MH turnover in intestinal muscle show that the rate is nearly 20 times faster (at 26%/d) than in skeletal muscle (Millward & Bates 1983) . When account is taken of the relative pool sizes intestine alone would account for over a quarter of the excretion,with skeletal muscle accounting for one half and the rest presumably arising from other smooth muscle sources (e.g. blood vessels) and non muscle cells.

TABLE 1.RELEASE OF 3-METHYL HISTIDINE FROM HUMAN LEG
(nmol/min per 100g)

Well nourished patients	(n=7)	1.92(0.40)
Acutely ill patients	(n=8)	0.93(0.32)
Malnourished patients	(n=6)	0.31(0.15)
Cachectic cancer patients	(n=20)	0.33(0.45)

Results of Lundholm et al (1982)

Not unexpectively these results have proved particularly controversial (see Munro 1982) and are not universally accepted but our concern for the method is gaining support by new human data. One report involves a less equivocal use of 3MH. This is a study of a-v differences of amino acids including 3MH across leg muscle in acutely ill patients and those losing muscle protein as a result of cancer and malnutrition (Lundholm et al 1982).As shown in table 1 in the acutely ill patients and especially in the malnourished and cancer patients, the efflux of 3MH out of muscle was lower than in the well nourished patients, even though muscle wasting was occuring judging by increased tyrosine efflux.This is an unequivocol indication of decreased muscle protein degradation. In the most recent studies (Lundholm ,Rennie & Emery in preparation) these decreased outputs of 3MH were also observed in patients with increased urinary 3MH following acute abdominal surgery.

These studies showed a remarkably consistant response to these catabolic states, namely a fall in the rate of contractile protein degradation. Any wasting of muscle which occured could only have been achieved by a very marked reduction in the rate of protein synthesis.

The availability of 13C-labelled amino acids such as 13C-(carboxl) leucine,and of mass spectrometric techniques for their detection in muscle sampled by needle biopsy has enabled the direct measurement of the rates of protein synthesis in vivo (see Halliday & Rennie 1982, Rennie et al 1982a,b).

Table 2 shows results of such measurements on 7 normal adults in the fed and fasted state, 14 patients with muscular dystrophy and in individual patients with cancer, and hypothyroid myopathy. Also shown is the urinary 3MH/creatinine ratio for all but the last two patients. In the normal adult the rate of protein synthesis in muscle is so rapid(equivalent to a turnover rate of about 3.6%/day or a half life of 19 days) that muscle accounts for about half the rate of protein synthesis in the whole body (Rennie et al 1982a). The marked fall after an overnight fast shows a remarkable sensitivity of protein synthesis in muscle which is consistent with what we have observed in animal experiments (Millward & Waterlow 1978).

In all of the patients protein synthesis in muscle was markedly reduced. Since most of the dystrophic patients were young boys who would normally have faster rates than in adults (Millward 1980a), the extent of the reduction was

TABLE 2 PROTEIN SYNTHESIS IN NORMAL AND DISEASED MUSCLE

SUBJECTS		PROTEIN SYNTHESIS (%/hour)	3MH/CREATININE (molar ratio) (x100)	MUSCLE MASS (%normal)
NORMAL adults	(7)			
fed		0.198(.055)	19.0(2.4)	96(12)
fasted		0.098(.043)	17.6(1.9)	
DUCHENNE boys	(9)	0.055(.033)	49.1(8.5)	31(16)
LIMB GIRDLE adult(1)				
quadriceps		0.120	26.2	57
calf		0.020		
MYOTONIA adults	(4)	0.081(.033)	27.2(7.8)	58(21)
HYPOTHYROID MYOPATHY		0.105		
CANCER CACHEXIA		0.044		

Results of Rennie et al(1982a,b),Griggs et al(1983) & Rennie (unpublished).

probably more marked than the 75% fall indicated in comparison with the adult values.

The most suprising feature of these findings is the contrast between the fall in the rate of protein synthesis measured by this direct method and what we could expect from the changes in 3MH excretion. In the Duchenne patients the 3MH/creatinine ratio was more than twice the value observed in the normal adults in line with the several previous reports (McKeran et al 1977, Ballard et al 1979, Warnes et al 1981). These changes had previously been interpreted by most workers including ourselves (Rennie et al 1982c), as indicating increased protein degradation in muscle. In these particular patients although their muscle mass is markedly reduced, there is probably not an actual wasting,but rather a failure to grow so that the rates of protein synthesis and degradation cannot be very different from one another. Thus according to the measurements of protein synthesis, protein degradation must be reduced. On the other hand according to the measurements of 3MH excretion there is increased degradation so that protein synthesis must also be increased and clearly these two conclusions are discrepant.

We believe that the 3MH excretion rates in these patients do not indicate what is occurring in the muscle.

It should be appreciated that although the 3MH/creatinine ratio is increased the actual 3MH excretion is depressed because of the marked reduction in muscle mass. As shown in the table it was only 30% of the normal value. Thus the fall in 3MH output was not as great as the reduction in creatinine output. Clearly if there is a part of the urinary excretion which originates from non-muscle sources then as the muscle mass is reduced as in these patients, the non-muscle sources become a larger proportion of the total and the 3MH/creatinine ratio will increase and the larger the component of the urinary 3MH excretion which originates from non-muscle sources, the greater the discrepancy. In the case of the results for the boys with Duchenne dystrophy the measurements of whole-body protein-turnover coupled with the measurements of muscle mass and turnover indicate that non-muscle tissues may actually be turning over faster than usual (Rennie et al 1982b), so that non-muscle sources of 3MH may be disproportionately increased in these patients. This would make the problem even greater and has lead us to conclude that the measurement of 3MH excretion in these patients is of little if any value.

It would appear then that the major problem in these patients with specific muscle wasting diseases as with malnourished and cancer patients is that protein synthesis is severly depressed and that protein degradation, if changed at all, is also depressed. Thus as we have argued elsewhere (Millward et al 1980b Rennie et al 1982b), any therapy should be aimed at stimulating synthesis rather than suppressing protein degradation.

THE REGULATION OF PROTEIN SYNTHESIS IN MUSCLE

General Considerations.

It appears that there are two main types of influences that affect protein synthesis in muscle, namely the extent of use and hormones.The first of these two factors has recently been reviewed (Booth et al 1982) where it was concluded that the great majority of reports indicated that changes in protein synthesis (rather than protein degradation) were responsible for either the atrophy following disuse or any hypertrophy subsequent to increased use.Certainly our own studies on work-induced growth of muscle indicated very marked increases in protein synthesis

(Laurent et al 1978a, Millward 1980a).

When use-induced changes in protein synthesis occur a pattern of response is seen which is very similar to that observed when muscle growth or atrophy is induced by nutritional intervention or by hormonal treatment.There are usually changes in ribosome content as judged by tissue RNA content as well as changes in the translational phase of protein synthesis as indicated by what we term the RNA activity i.e.the rate of protein synthesis per unit RNA (see Millward and Waterlow 1978,Millward et al 1981). The importance of use in regulating muscle protein balance is indicated by the observation that in the absence of both food and hormonal support increased muscle activity in rats can induce growth of the individual muscle (see Goldberg 1968).Given the fact that increased muscle activity can activate all the anabolic processes neccesary for growth i.e. DNA synthesis, RNA synthesis, protein synthesis in the muscle cells as well as protein synthesis in the connective tissue cells which make collagen (Laurent et al 1978a, b, Millward 1980a) activity must be accepted as a major "pleiotypic activator" for the tissue. Furthermore this pleiotypic activation is most likely not just associated with increased activity but is probably a continuous function of the use of each muscle, to the extent that the size and functional characteristics of muscles largely reflects their history of use (see Booth et al 1982).

As far as hormonal regulation is concerned, the characteristic of muscle is its extreme sensitivity to hormones (see Millward et al 1981). It is most likely that its response to the nutritional state is mediated through dietary-induced hormonal changes.It has been suggested that the atrophy induced by disuse is a result of increased sensitivity to glucocorticoid hormones (Dubois and Almon 1980), thus linking the roles of activity and hormones although this link is disputed by others(Booth et al 1982). In what follows the way in which these factors affect protein synthesis in muscle will be reviewed in terms of the regulation of the RNA activity and the RNA content in muscle as the two principal determinants of the overall rate.

Hormonal Regulation of Ribosome Activity and Content.

Our own work has concerned the role of three hormones which we consider to be important in regulating protein balance in muscle, insulin, glucocorticoid hormones (cortisol in man or corticosterone in the rat) and tri iodothyronine, T3, the active thyroid hormone. Specific myopathies are associated with excessive steroid hormone levels and with thyroid abnormalities, whereas in diabetes the other consequences of insulin deficiency tend to overshadow any abnormalities of muscle growth.Clearly there are other hormones involved of which growth hormone is the most obvious omission from our studies.The reason for this is the uncertainty about the extent to which this hormone is directly involved in regulation or is active via the somatomedin peptides (Salmon & Daughaday 1957,Schoenle et al 1982).A peptide with insulin-like activity (insulin-like growth factor II) has been reported to have specific mitosis-inducing effects on muscle cells in culture (J.R.Florini personal communication). However the extent to which these hormones are involved in the regulation of protein balance is still to be determined.

Ribosome activity. In a recent review (Millward et al 1981) we examined the relative importance of these three hormones in regulating RNA activity in muscle, but in the light of subsequent findings we can reexamine the conclusions we reached then.
Insulin and Triiodothyronine. We concluded that insulin was an independent activator of RNA activity but might not be obligatory in the presence of elevated levels of T3. Certainly in the diabetic rat the RNA activity is as low as ever observed and the addition of insulin will restore it to normal (Millward et al 1976, Odedra et al 1982). These effects have been known since the pioneering work of Wool in the 60's (Wool et al 1968) and subsequent work has shown that initiation is the most likely site of action of insulin (see Jefferson 1980). However we observed that in hypophysectomised rats treated with T3 protein synthesis was stimulated in muscle in part through increased RNA activity even though the very low insulin levels, a feature of these rats,remained with the treatment (Brown et al 1981). We thought that the high levels of T3 were replacing insulin as a stimulus for normal RNA activity. This suggestion appeared to be supported by subsequent experiments in which we observed in rats maintained on very high, catabolic doses of thyroid hormones that although the insulin levels were very low, the RNA activities were well maintained (Brown and Millward 1983).Further work has shown that we were premature in our suggestion that T3 could replace insulin entirely.

TABLE 3 RESPONSE OF MUSCLE PROTEIN SYNTHESIS IN DIABETIC
RATS TO T3 TREATMENT (soleus muscle)

	Protein synthesis (%/day)	RNA activity (g protein/day per g RNA)
CONTROL	17.3(3.4)	14.5(2.5)
DIABETIC	9.1(2.1)	8.1(1.9)
DIABETIC +T3	10.6(1.1)	7.2(1.1)

Brown, van Beuren & Millward 1983

We have examined the effect of treatment with T3 in
diabetic rats in which we can be sure of the absence of
insulin. After 7 days treatment with T3 the translational
defect remained in terms of reduced RNA activity (see table
3).Interestingly the treatment did partially restore the
reduced RNA levels in the diabetic animals showing the
importance of T3 in regulating RNA synthesis (as discussed
below, table 5). We have to conclude therefore that in the
absence of insulin,T3 cannot stimulate translation. However
in the absence of T3 or in markedly hypothyroid states the
correlation between the RNA activity and the insulin level
is much more marked than in euthyroid animals (Brown and
Millward 1983).

    These results suggest that whilst insulin and T3 can
both regulate the rate of translation (which we observe as
changes in the RNA activity), insulin has the primary role,
being obligatory, with T3 having a secondary role. This
would tend to confirm the suggestion (Pain & Clemens 1980)
that initiation, the putative site of insulin action,is the
rate limiting step in protein synthesis, and also fits with
the proposal that T3 acts on the elongation phase
(Mathews et al 1973).

    We have recently approached the problem by examining
the response to refeeding in 4-day fasted rats as a more
physiological situation. As already shown (table 1) the
synthesis rate in muscle falls markedly on fasting in man
(Rennie et al 1982a) as well as in the rat (Millward and
Waterlow 1978).The recovery is remarkedly rapid on
refeeding, the rate doubling over the first hour with
increases apparent at 40 minutes (see fig 1). Such a rapid
response is only measurable with the large dose method of
Garlick et al (1980) which allows accurate measurements

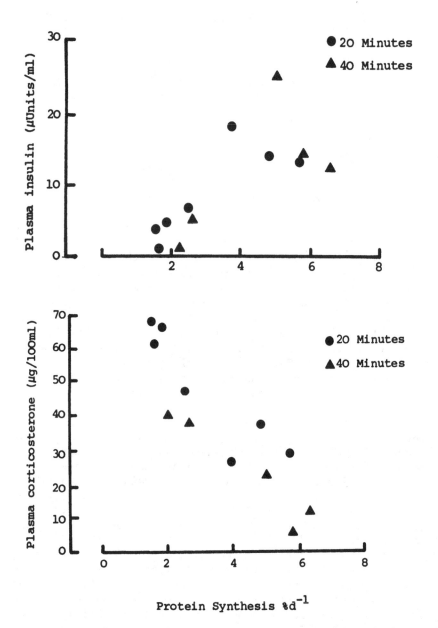

Fig 1 increase in muscle protein synthesis(measured with a
flooding dose of phenylalanine) in respons to refeeding in
4 day fasted rats in relation to the increase in insulin
(top 1a) and the fall in corticosterone (bottom 1b).

TABLE 4 RESTORATION OF MUSCLE PROTEIN SYNTHESIS ON
         REFEEDING 4-DAY FASTED RATS (gastrocnemius muscle)

	Protein synthesis (%/day)	insulin (uunits/ml)
Well fed	15.7 (1.5)	32.8(8)
A.4-day fasted	4.3 (1.0)	4.3(2)
60-min refed	8.0 (0.5)	25 (8)
60-min refed + corticosterone	6.3 (0.7)	12.7(4)
B.4-day fasted	2.2 (0.7)	1.6(1)
60-min refed	4.9 (1.1)	19.7(9)
6o-min refed + anti-insulin serum	3.5 (0.3)	ND

Bates, Odedra & Millward (unpublished results).

over 10 minutes. There is no doubt of the importance of
insulin in mediating these responses since the recovery of
protein synthesis correlates absolutely with the rise in
insulin levels (see fig 1a) and if this is blocked by
administering anti-insulin serum prior to the refeeding,the
restoration of protein synthesis is partially blocked (see
table 4,experiment B).We have yet to find out why the anti-
insulin serum does not completely block the increase in
protein synthesis.
     Glucocorticoid hormones. However there are occasions
when the response to insulin can be blocked and this
appears to be an important feature of the role   of
glucocorticoid hormones. While the catabolic effects of
these hormones on muscle has long been known (see Munro
1964),and while an inhibitory action on protein synthesis
was demonstrated many years ago(see Young 1970) the actual
mechanism by which they achieve their effects on muscle is
poorly understood.In reviewing the role of corticosterone
in the rat (Millward et al 1981), we concluded that
corticosterone was an independent suppressor of protein
synthesis, will override insulin's stimulatory effect, but
was not obligatory for the shut down of protein synthesis
in starvation These conclusions were based on our
experiments on corticosterone-treated rats in some of which
we independently manipulated the insulin levels (Odedra and
Millward 1982).These experiments showed that large doses of
corticosterone inhibited muscle growth through suppressing

protein synthesis even though the insulin concentrations were markedly elevated (hyperinsulinemia is a well documented response to glucocorticoid treatment Perley & Kipnis 1966).

Further evidence of the inhibitory action of corticosterone over the stimulation by insulin of RNA activity in muscle came from experiments examing the acute response to infused insulin in diabetic rats (Odedra et al 1981). In these experiments it was observed that the restoration of protein synthesis to normal took between 6 and 24 hours of insulin administration suggesting an insulin resistance.However this was not observed in adrenalectomised diabetic rats. They responded within the first hour of insulin infusion. Since the level of corticosterone was high in these diabetic rats and since the insulin resistance was also observed in the adrenalectomised rats treated with corticosterone prior to the infusion, we postulated that the insulin resistance in diabetes reflected the elevated corticosterone levels.

We have recently extended these studies of the interaction of corticosterone and insulin in our fasting refeeding experiments. In addition to the increase in insulin on refeeding there is a very dramatic fall in the corticosterone concentration observable in the first 30 minutes (see fig1b).As can be seen,in the same way that the recovery of protein synthesis correlates with the increase in insulin (fig 1a) there is a remarkable correlation with the fall in corticosterone. However if the fall in corticosterone is blocked by injecting corticosterone prior to the refeeding, the restoration of protein synthesis at 60 minutes is only half that seen in the untreated refed rats.

There are several important implications of these results The first is that corticosterone does inhibit the stimulatory effect of insulin on muscle protein synthesis but this is only a partial effect. The reduction in RNA activity following corticosterone treatment (Odedra & Millward 1982) is never as marked as that seen in the diabetic rat (Odedra et al 1981). The second is that this effect of corticosterone is a very rapidly reversible one and this is important as far as the nature of the mechanism of action of corticosterone is concerned. Thus any action of corticosterone which involves interaction with cytoplasmic receptors and subsequent translocation into the nucleus to modify gene expression (see Thompson and Lippman 1974) is unlikely to be reversed as quickly as the observed recovery of protein synthesis on refeeding.It is much more likely therefore that this aspect of the role of corticosterone involves either some direct action on protein synthesis or a direct inhibition of the stimulatory effect of insulin. The likelihood that the action is at the same site as insulin is indicated by the report of Rannels et al (1978) that initiation is inhibited by dexamethasone in rat muscle.In any case the suggestion that glucocorticoid hormones act by inhibiting the stimulatory effects of insulin has been around for some time, since Munck(1971) suggested that inhibition of glucose uptake was the primary event in glucocorticoid action on the peripheral tissues. From our results we would propose that corticosterone has two somewhat separate actions on muscle protein synthesis, one as just described, the second one being a primary regulator of ribosome levels through its inhibitory action on ribosomal RNA synthesis.

TABLE 5 REGULATION OF MUSCLE RNA CONTENT
-role of thyroid and glucocorticoid hormones

	RNA/protein (x1000)	free T3 pg/ml
1 Well fed rats (gastroc.muscle)		
Control	7.7(1.1)	
Thyroidectomised (5 days)	4.9(0.5)	
Thyroidectomised (22 days)	3.2(0.5)	
Thyroidectomised (T3 treated)	5.2(1.1)	
2 Diabetic rats (soleus muscle)		
Control	14.3(0.7)	
Diabetic	10.8(1.3)	
Diabetic+T3	14.7(1.2)	
3 Malnourished adx rats (gastroc.muscle)		
3 days low protein diet	9.0(0.4)	5.3
9 days low protein diet	5.9(0.4)	3.6
+ 1mg corticosterone/day	6.0(0.4)	7.2
+ 2mg corticosterone/day	5.6(0.8)	10.4
+10mg corticosterone/day	5.8(0.8)	9.7
+ 2mg corticosterone/day (food restricted)	4.2(0.6)	7.5

Results of Brown et al (1980)
& Brown,Odedra & Millward (unpublished)

Ribosome Content

The changes in muscle ribosome content appear to be separately regulated from the RNA activity. Although much less is known about this aspect of regulation it would appear that the two hormones which play a key role are T3 and glucocorticoids (see table 5). The role of T3 is indicated by the fact that following thyroidectomy in the rat a loss of muscle RNA is observed before any other change is apparent and this loss of T3 is reversed by T3 treatment (Brown et al 1980,). These effects of T3 are consistant with very early observations of the way in which thyroid hormones work (Tata and Widnell 1966) as well as more recent reports by others (e.g. Flaim et al 1978).Thus T3 appears to regulate the overall capacity for protein synthesis in muscle.The fact that this aspect of regulation in muscle is quite independent from regulation of translation is confirmed by some of our recent observations on the effect of T3 on diabetic rats. The reduced RNA content in muscle (and liver) is largely restored to normal by T3 treatment,suggesting that there is little requirement for insulin to maintain muscle RNA (Brown,van Bueren and Millward in preparation).

The physiological importance of this role of thyroid hormones would appear to be to relate the level of protein turnover in muscle to the overall metabolic rate. Thus since there is a reduction in free T3 (the active thyroid hormone) in undernutrition (Cox et al 1981) the marked fall in the rate of protein synhesis is not supprising.However an increase in the concentration of glucocorticoids also occurs in undernutrition and this will also induce a loss of ribosomes. Corticosterone treatment in rats markedly reduces RNA levels (Odedra and Millward 1982) by reducing the rate of rRNA synthesis (Goodlad & Onyezeli,1981) so T3 and corticosterone will interact in regulating RNA levels in muscle.

Recently we examined this interaction in adrenalectomised rats which were fed a protein deficient diet and treated with various levels of corticosterone. The effect of this treatment was to increase the T3 levels possibly as a result of the increased food intake. Thus the fall in free T3 which occured in the untreated malnourished rats did not occur in the steroid treated rats. Indeed there was an increased level in the group treated with moderate doses of corticosterone (i.e.2mg/100g see table 5) However the fall in muscle RNA observed in the untreated

rats was equally apparent in the corticosterone-treated,
hyperthyroid rats.The most pronounced loss of RNA was
observed in the rats fed a restricted amount of food which
did not achieve such a marked increase in T3 levels. These
results indicate two things.Firstly since RNA was lost from
the adrenalectomised rats it is clear that corticosterone
is not obligatory for the reduction in RNA levels and this
confirms our observation that fasted adx rats also lose RNA
The fall in T3 presumably mediates the response in each
case (see Millward et al 1981).Secondly when corticosterone
levels are elevated as in the treated rats this induces the
loss of RNA even when T3 levels are normal or even elevated
and even when translation is well maintained by insulin (as
it was in this case,compare with the synthesis rates in fig
2).Thus the inhibitory effect of corticosterone on muscle
RNA synthesis is dominant to the stimulatory efect of T3.

REGULATION OF PROTEIN DEGRADATION IN MUSCLE.

General Considerations

The distinctive feature of protein degradation in
muscle is the fact that paradoxical changes in the rate of
degradation can occur, with increases during growth and
decreases during wasting (see Millward et al 1980b) The
observation that degradation in muscle can change in any
direction including a decrease in catabolic states and an
increase in anabolic states prompted us to suggest that the
changes could usefully be classified as'anabolic', for
those changes which occur during growth and 'catabolic',
for those changes which occur during atrophy or growth
failure. In these terms the measurements on the patients
with Duchenne muscular dystrophy (Rennie et al 1982) and
cancer patients (Lundholm et al 1982), indicate that in
each case there are 'catabolic' decreases in
degradation. Such changes have been reported for children
fed protein-deficient diets (Holmgren 1974) and are
observed in malnourished rats (e.g. Millward et al 1975)
and in fasted adults judging by the fall in the excretion
of 3MH (see Young and Munro 1980).
In trying to account rationally for the changes
observed, the anabolic increase in degradation is most
difficult to explain, but because of the fact that it is
always observed (see Millward 1980a, Goldspink et al 1983),
we have suggested that it is necessary to allow the

architectural changes of the contractile apparatus which occur during growth as well as allowing the alterations in the pattern of cytoplasmic proteins associated with development.We believe that because muscle is a relatively slow turning over tissue, major changes in the type and arrangement of its proteins can only be achieved quickly by increasing turnover rates.Whatever the explanation,if there is a need for this increased degradation any attempt to limit it as therapy in disease states may well be misplaced (Millward et al 1980b, Rennie et al 1982c).

The catabolic decrease in degradation can be more logically accounted for by postulating that it is an adaptive response, serving the purpose of limiting the losses of protein which would otherwise occur because of the reduction in the rate of protein synthesis.

Hormonal Regulation of Protein Degradation

There is good evidence that many of the changes in degradation in response to altered nutritional state reflect the thyroid status. In the same way that T3 regulates the capacity for protein synthesis, it also regulates the capacity for proteolysis (De Martino and Goldberg 1978,Millward et al 1980b).When the thyroid status in rats is manipulated the rate of degradation varies directly with the T3 level (Millward et al 1981, Brown and Millward 1983).

This relationship between T3 and protein degradation in malnutrition is well illustrated in our recent experiments already referred to (table 5-3). Fig 2 shows rates of muscle protein synthesis and degradation (measured as the differance between synthesis and growth) in the protein deficient rats treated with varying amounts of corticosterone. Treatment with replacement (1mg) or moderate (2mg) doses of corticosterone did not affect protein balance but did result in higher rates of protein turnover than in the untreated malnourished rats. Rates of protein synthesis were better maintained (because of the higher food intakes and insulin levels) and the higher rates of degradation reflected the elevated T3 levels. However when protein synthesis was impaired by restricting the intake of the low protein diet, or by treating with catabolic doses of the steroid, muscle protein was lost even though the impairment of synthesis was not as great as in the untreated rats. This inability to lower degradation to match synthesis was a failure of

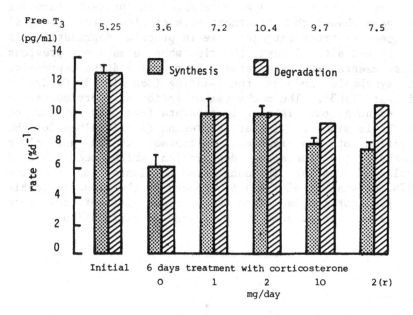

Fig 2 Role of thyroid and glucocorticoid hormones in adaptive changes in muscle protein turnover in malnutrition

adaptation which we feel may be relevant to real situations of marginal malnutrition.Thus environmental stress in terms of infection or altered patterns of activity could induce the hormonal changes which would prevent the adaptive matching of rates of degradation with barely adequate rates of protein synthesis.

Although the results presented here have emphasised the reduced rates of degradation in diseased states and malnutrition there is no doubt that increased degradation can occur in muscle. In response to hyperthyroidism degradation is increased particularly in oxidative postural muscles (Millward et al 1981, Brown & Millward 1983). A catabolic increase in degradation also occurs after prolonged fasting in young animals (Millward and Waterlow 1978) and as an initial response to diabetes (Albertse et al 1980).In rats several authors have reported increased 3MH excretion after treatment with large doses of glucocorticoid hormones (see Munro 1982) although we (Millward et al 1976,Odedra and Millward 1982) and others (Rannels and Jefferson 1980) have been unable to observe any changes in degradation. We have resolved this by

following the time course of changes in protein turnover
and have showed that treatment with corticosterone (10mg/d)
induces a transient increase in protein degradation in
muscle,but after 5 days, the time when we made our previous
measurements, the rate returns to normal and the depression
in synthesis induces the wasting (see fig 3 Odedra &
Millward 1983). The mechanism of action of corticosterone
is unknown but is clearly separate from its effect on
synthesis since the latter suppresion is maintained for the
duration of the treatment. Furthermore it is not clear
whether the increased degradation which occurs after
prolonged fasting in young rats (Millward and Waterlow
1978, Goodman et al 1981) is induced by the elevated levels
of glucocorticoids since the increase in corticosterone
occurs well in advance of any change in degradation.

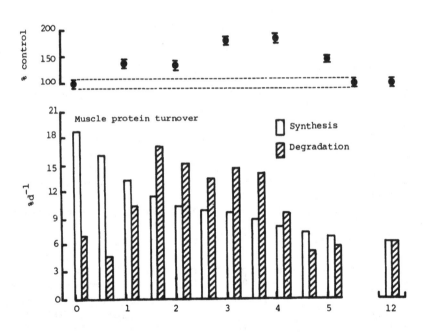

Fig 3 Time course of changes in protein synthesis and
degradation in muscle and 3MH excretion in rats treated
with catabolic doses of corticosterone

TABLE 6   CHANGES   IN RNA   ACTIVITY   IN   DUCHENNE   MUSCULAR
           DYSTROPHY

	Protein synthesis (%/day)	RNA activity (g protein /day per g RNA)
NORMAL fed	4.75(1.32)	21.8 (7.2)
fasted	2.35(1.03)	10.58(0.4)
DUCHENNE	1.30(0.67)	3.84(1.9)

Rennie et al (1982 a&b)

INTRACELLULAR REGULATORY MECHANISMS AND POTENTIAL DEFECTS

     The way in which hormones and/or usage effect changes
in protein synthesis or degradation in muscle is not
understood in any great detail, other than through the
already mentioned changes in the levels of ribosomes and
lysosomal   proteinases. This almost certainly involves
transcriptional regulation of the appropriate genes by the
hormones involved (e.g.glucocorticoid and thyroid hormones
acting competitively on the rRNA gene and thyroid hormones
additionally regulating the expression of the proteinase
genes). The regulation of translation is poorly understood
but the involvement of the protein kinase system (e.g.see
Czech 1981) would be consistent with the phosphorylation-
dephosphorylation cyle which regulates initiation (see
Clemens et al 1982).It is clear however that in Duchenne
muscular dystrophy it is the translational phase which is
depressed.As shown in table 6 the RNA activity is much
lower than observed in fed or fasted normal adults.
     As for potential defects in regulatory mechanisms,
changes in calcium concentrations have been proposed as
mediating changes in protein turnover in muscle   in
pathological states. When intracellular calcium levels are
increased in incubated muscles by means of ionophores which
increase   calcium   transport   across   membranes   (e.g.
A23187), net catabolism is increased (e.g. Kameyama &
Etlinger 1979, Lewis et al 1982, Rodemann et al 1982).
     Increased calcium levels in muscle have been reported in
several pathological states such as Duchenne muscular
dystrophy (see Emery & Burt 1980), possibly resulting from
defective mechanisms of sequestration of calcium into the

sarcoplasmic reticulum(SR). These observations have been
developed into the theory that structural abnormalities
resulting in failure to regulate calcium levels are the
primary reason for the functional deterioration and wasting
of muscle in a range of pathological states (e.g. see
Duncan 1978).

The main problem in assigning a role to calcium at the
moment is the inconsistency of the reports about the effect
of increased calcium on protein turnover in muscle.
Kameyama & Etlinger (1979) reported that increased
calcium levels were catabolic with increased rates of
protein synthesis as well as protein degradation. Rodemann
et al (1982) reported similar increases in degradation in
response to treatment with A23187, but they did not observe
an increase in protein synthesis. When they attempted to
increase intracellular calcium levels by depolarising the
muscle with high K concentrations however degradation was
increased but on this occasion synthesis was depressed.

In contrast to these reports Lewis et al (1982) showed
a catabolic response in muscles incubated with the
ionophore which was mediated by a fall in synthesis with no
change in degradation. However local anaesthetics, caffeine
and thymol, all agents which increase intracellular
calcium, resulted in a decrease in synthesis but did
increase degradation.

Although all these reports showed a net catabolic
effect, the discrepant changes in synthesis and degradation
do raise serious problems in assessing their physiologial
relevance. If the studies of Lewis et al (1982) showing
decreased rates of synthesis as the primary effect are
correct then the case for an important role for calcium in
muscle wasting becomes more persuasive since as we have
shown above depressed synthesis is the main change in most
wasting states.However there is no obvious reason why the
results of this study should be more acceptable than the
others, apart from the fact that the preparations of Lewis
et al (1982) are generally nearer to a balance between
synthesis and degradation than the others.

However the emphasis of the Lewis study on synthesis as
the target for increased calcium raises a serious problem
in assessing the work on the role of the
prostaglandins. This is because the studies of Rodemann et
al (1982) not only emphasise increased degradation as the
target for calcium but provide a mechanism for this effect
through the action of prostaglandins. PGE2 was shown by
Rodemann & Goldberg (1982) to stimulate protein

degradation in muscle by a mechanism involving stimulation of lysosomal thiol proteinases. These findings were a logical extension of the fact that the synthesis of PG is rate limited by a calcium-dependent enzyme, phospholipase A. Thus because treatment with the ionophore A23187 increased PGE2 synthesis and because the increase in degradation induced by the ionophore was reduced if PGE2 synthesis was suppressed, they concluded that the calcium effect was mediated by PGE2.

A suprising feature of these studies relates to the role of the calcium-activated protease (CAP) which has generally been thought to be responsible for mediating any calcium induced increases in degradation in pathological states (see Millward 1980b). The enzyme is present in muscle in two forms, one requiring high concentrations of calcium (250uM), the other requiring much lower concentrations (20uM Waxman 1980). Because the stimulation of degradation by the ionophore was not affected by an agent which blocks the CAP, they concluded that increased calcium induced an increase in degradation not through the CAP, but through a PGE2 stimulation of lysosomal proteinases.

The problem for us in interpreting these results in the light of our findings that decreased synthesis rather than increased degradation is the main change in muscle wasting states is that there is little evidence that any PG mediated effects of calcium involve a decrease in synthesis In fact according to Rodemann & Goldberg (1982) another prostaglandin PGF2 stimulates protein synthesis in muscle. Thus although prostaglandins may play a part in mediating the increased turnover which could well occur in muscle as part of the generalised increase in whole body protein turnover in fever (see Waterlow & Tomkins 1981) a role for these compounds in the reduced turnover in diseased states does not yet firmly exist, and the calcium-induced decreases in protein synthesis reported by Lewis et al (1982) must be mediated by an as yet unknown mechanism. However it would be premature to rule prostaglandins out entirely since in one study in which muscles were incubated with increased levels of K (to increase calcium) there was a marked increase in PG synthesis and a fall in protein synthesis (Rodemann et al 1982). However, the authors did not connect the two responses, and if they are connected there is no evidence as to how the effects would be achieved.

Leucine and its Keto Acid. The provision of substrates

and amino acid supply in particular has been extensively studied as a regulatory influence over protein synthesis particularly in cultured cell systems (see Pain & Clemens 1980).In pathological states in muscle if the transport of substrates into muscle was predudiced then it might be supposed that this would result in an inability to sustain protein synthesis. Certainly there is evidence that amino acid transport in muscle is reduced in atrophic states (see Goldberg et al 1978) Furthermore there have been reports that some amino acids, particularly leucine, can stimulate protein synthesis in incubated muscles (see Goldberg & Tischler 1981, Morgan et al 1981). However whilst the provision of amino acids is a neccesary precondition for protein synthesis, we are unconvinced of a specific regulatory role for amino acids in muscle.

It should be recognised that amino acids are generated continuously intracellularly, and in muscle and most extra-hepatic tissues where amino acid oxidation is minimal the only fate of these amino acids is resynthesis into protein or efflux from the tissue.Thus a shortage of amino acids in wasting states is highly unlikely.The branched chain amino acids are an exception to this since they can be oxidised in muscle. Thus it is possible that their concentrations could be depressed as a result of increased oxidation and they could have a regulatory role.

However no effect of increasing amino acid or leucine concentrations on muscle protein synthesis per se has ever been observed in vivo. The injection of large doses of leucine into either fed or fasted rats has no effect on protein synthesis in muscle (McNurlan et al 1982). This really is not surprising since the concentration of leucine and most of the rate limiting amino acids is actually increased in muscle in catabolic states (e.g. Millward et al 1976).

According to our measurements of leucine oxidation in vivo, the activation of the BCAA dehydrogenase which increases leucine oxidation appears to be linked to an activation of protein synthesis, since leucine oxidation increases with feeding and falls on fasting (Rennie et al 1982a) contrary to the established wisdom from in vitro studies (see Goldberg & Tischler 1981).Thus it is not at all suprising to find that concentrations of leucine are actually depressed in muscle when protein synthesis is stimulated (Jefferson et al 1974).

There is a large body of work which suggests that leucine or its keto acid can regulate protein degradation.

This originally arose from studies on incubated or perfused muscles (see Goldberg and Tischler 1981,Morgan et al 1981) but is also supported by studies in vivo in man (see Walser et al 1981,Stewart et al 1982) In this case the evidence appears to point to an inhibitory effect of the keto acid of leucine (keto isocaproate, KIC) on protein degradation (Tischler and Goldberg 1979). Added support comes from in vivo studies reporting a nitrogen-sparing effect of KIC when given to fasted adults (Mitch et al 1981), and a reduction in 3MH excretion when given to patients with Duchenne muscular dystrophy (Stewart et al 1982)

Clearly the latter report is very important giving physiological relevance to the in vitro studies. However given our arguments above that the 3MH in these patients originates largely from non muscle sources, and that the rate of degradation is already very low then we would conclude that it is the release of 3MH from non-muscle tissues which is being reduced by the treatment. In any case our own studies on the effect of exercise on muscle protein balance show opposite effects to these. During exercise when leucine oxidation is increased, KIC levels in plasma fall, but increase markedly after the exercise has stopped (Rennie et al 1981,Millward et al 1982b). However the urinary 3MH/creatinine ratio falls during the exercise, returning to normal when the exercise has ceased, an opposite effect to that expected from the results of the above mentioned studies. Thus as far as we are concerned an important physiological role for KIC in the regulation of protein balance in skeletal muscle has yet to be demonstrated.

CONCLUSIONS

Because of our experience based on observations of actual changes in protein turnover in vivo in animals and humans, our perspective on the cause of muscle wasting as reflected in this review is differant from that held by those with more experience of in vitro studies and we fully recognise this. We do not dismiss the large body of work showing that protein degradation in muscle in vitro is a very labile process increasing markedly in response to lack of hormonal and nutritional support in the same way as it does in other tissues in vivo (see Millward 1980b).Furthermore we have reported here conditions when degradation does increase in vivo as part of a catabolic response. Nevertheless in an increasing number of situations muscle protein degradation does appear to be depressed in wasting states. We would propose two possible explanations for the difference between our findings and those based on the in vitro studies.The first is to do with the time course of any changes in protein degradation. All studies in vitro are necessarily concerned with acute responses (in terms of a few hours at the most).In vivo acute changes are extremley difficult to measure even in animals and although reliable reports do not indicate acute increases even in complete fasting (see Millward and Waterlow 1978,Goodman et al 1982 Rennie et al 1982a) we cannot be sure that they do not occur.If they do occur for very short periods then it is unlikely that they are physiologically important.

The second explanation is that although several reports have pointed out the problems associated with incubated muscle systems (e.g.Garber et al 1978,Seider 1980),some of the preparations used in current studies are far from ideal as evident by the marked negative balance even in the presence of hormonal and nutritional support. This may be one reason for the lack of consistency between superficially similar experimental approaches as discussed above.Clearly since protein synthesis is so sensitive in muscle the study of its regulation can only sensibly be performed when it is operating maximally and has the potential for responding to regulatory influences.

Acknowlegements
These studies are part of a collaborative programme with the Dept of Medicine at University College Hospital (Rennie & Emery) where we recognise the enthusiastic support of Prof.R.H.T.Edwards, and with the MRC Clinical Research Center at Northwick Park (Halliday) where we recognise the dedication of Walter Read and Charles Ford.We also recognise the wider collaboration with Dwight Matthews in St Louis USA and Kent Lundholm in Gothenburg, Sweden.The work was possible because of generous support from the Muscular Dystrophy Group of Great Britain, The British Diabetic Association, the Medical Research Council and the Wellcome Trust. DJM is grateful to Adam Osborne and Wordstar for the preparation of this manuscript.

REFERENCES

Albertse,E.C.,Pain,V.M. & Garlick,P.J.(1980) Proc. Nut. Soc. 39, 19A

Booth,F.W.,Nicholson,W.F.,& Watson,P.A. (1982) Exercise Sport Sci.Rev.II

Ballard,F.J.,Tomas,F.M.& Stern L.M. (1979) Clin.Sci.56,347-352

Brown, J.G. & Millward,D.J. (1983) Biochim. Biophys. Acta. (in the press)

Brown,J.G.,Bates,P.C.,Holliday,M.A. & Millward,D.J. (1981) Biochem.J. 194, 771-782.

Clague,M.B. (1981). In "Nitrogen Metabolism in Man" (J.C.Waterlow & J.M.L.Stephen ed.) 525-540 Applied Science Publishers London

Clemens,M.J., Pain,V.M., Wong,S-T,& Henshaw,E.C. (1982) Nature 296,93-94

Cox,M.D., Dalal,S.S.,& Heard C.R.C.(1981) Proc.Nut,Soc. 40,39A

Czech,M.P. (1981) Am.J.Med. 70 142-150.

DeMartino,G.N. & Goldberg,A.L. (1978) Proc.Natl.Acad.Sci. 75,1369-1373.

DuBois,D.C.& Almon,R.R.(1980) Endocrinol. 107,1649-1651

Duncan,C.J. (1978) Experientia 34,1531-1535.

Emery,A.E.H. & Burt D. (1980) Br.Med.J.280 355-357

Flaim,K.E., Li.J.B. & Jefferson L.S.(1978) Am.J.Physiol 235,E231-237

Garber,A.L.,Karl,I.E. & Kipnis,D.K. (1976) J.Biol.Chem. 251 826-835

Garlick,P.J. & Clugston, G.H. (1981) In "Nitrogen Metabolism in Man" (J.C.Waterlow & J.M.L.Stephen ed.) 303-322 Applied Science Publishers London

Garlick,P.J., McNurlan,M.A. & Preedy,V.R. (1980) Biochem. J. 192, 719-723

Goldberg,A.L.(1968) Endocrinol.83,1071-1073.

Goldberg,A.L. & Tischler,M.C. (1981) In"Metabolism & Clinical Implications of the Branched Chain Amino & Keto Acids" (M.Walser & J.R.Williamson eds) 205-216. Elsevier/North-Holland

Goldberg,A.L., Jablecki,C. & Li J.B. (1978) Ann.N.Y. Acad.Sci. 228,190-201.

Goldspink,D.F., Garlick,P.J. & McNurlan,M.A.(1983) Biochem. J. 210, 89-98.

Goodlad,G.A.J.& Onyezali,F.N. (1981) Biochem.Med. 25,34-47.

Goodman,N., McElaney,M.A. & Ruderman N.B.(1981) Am. J. Phys. 241,E321-327.

Graystone,J.E. (1968) In "Human Growth" (D.B.Cheek,ed.) p192 Lea and Febiger Philadelphia.

Halliday,D. & Rennie,M.J. (1982) Clin.Sci. 63,485-496.

Holmgren,G.(1974) Nutr, Metab.,16,223-228

Jefferson,L.S. (1980) Diabetes 39,487-496.

Jefferson,L.S., Rannels,D.E., Munger,B.L. & Morgan, H.E. (1974) Fed Proc 33,1098-1111

Kameyama,T., & Etlinger,J.D. (1979) Nature 279, 344-346.

Laurent,G.J.,Sparrow,M.P., & Millward,D.J. (1978a) Biochem J.176,407-417

Laurent,G.J.,Sparrow,M.P.,Bates,P.C.& Millward (1978b) Biochem.J. 176,419-427.

Lewis,E.M., Anderson, P. & Goldspink, D.F.(1982) Biochem.J. 204 257-264.

Lundholm,K. Bennegard,K. Eden,E. Svaninger,G. Emery,P.W. & Rennie,M.J. (1982) Cancer Res. 42,4807-4811.

Mathews,R.W.,Oronsky,A. & Haschemayer,A.E.(1973) J. Biol. Chem., 248, 1329-1333

McKeran,R.O., Halliday,D. & Purkiss,P. (1977) J. Neurol. Neuros. Psych. 40,979-981.

McNurlan,M.A., Fern,E.B. & Garlick,P.J.(1982) Biochem.J.204 831-838

Millward,D.J.(1980a) In "Degradative Processes in Heart & Skeletal Muscle" (K.Wildenthal ed.) 161-169 Elsevier/North-Holland Oxford

Millward, D.J. (1980b) Comprehen. Biochem. 19b 153-232

Millward,D.J. & Bates,P.C. (1983) Biochem.J. In the press

Millward,D.J. & Waterlow,J.C.(1978) Fed.Proc.37, 2283-2290.

Millward,D.J.,Garlick,P.J.,Stewart,R.J.C.Nnanyelugo,D.O. & Waterlow,J.C.(1975) Biochem.J.150,235-243

Millward,D.J.,Garlick,P.J., Nnanyelugo,D.O.& Waterlow,J.C. (1976) Biochem.J.156, 185-188

Millward,D.J.,Bates,P.C., Grimble. G.k.,Brown,J.G. Nathan, M. & Rennie,M.J. (1980a) Biochem J.190, 225-228.

Millward,D.J., Bates,P.C., Brown,J.G., Rosochacki,S.R. & Rennie, M.J. (1980b) in"Protein Degradation in Health and Disease" Ciba Symposium No 75 307-329

Millward,D.J.,Brown,J.G.& Odedra B.(1981) In "Nitrogen Metabolism in Man (J.C.Waterlow & J.M.L. Stephen eds) 475-494 Applied Science Publishers London.

Millward,D.J.,Bates,P.C.,Broadbent,P & Rennie,M.J.(1982) In "Clinical Nutrition 81" (R.I.C.Wesdorp ed) 190-203 Churchill-Livingstone Edinburgh

Millward,D.J., Davies,C.T.M., Halliday,D., Wolman,S.L., Matthews,D.& Rennie,M.J.(1982) Fed Proc. 41, 2686-2691.

Mitch,W.E.,Walser,M.& Sapir,D.G. (1981) J.Clin.Invest.67,

553-562

Morgan,H.E.,Chua,B.H.,Boyd,T.A. & Jefferson L.S.(1981) In Metabolism & Clinical Implications of the Branched Chain Amino & Keto acids(M.Walser & J.R.Williamson eds) 217-226.Elsevier/North-Holland Oxford.

Munck,A.(1971) Perspect.Biol.Med. 14,265-289.

Munro,H.N. (1964) In "Mammalian Protein Metabolism" (H.N.Munro &J.B.Allison eds) Vol 1 382-482 Academic Press N.Y.& London

Munro,H.N. (1982) In "Clinical Nutrition 81" (R.I.C. Wesdorp ed) 181-189 Churchill-Livingstone Edinburgh.

Odedra,B. & Millward,D.J. (1982) Biochem.J 209,663-672.

Odedra,B. & Millward,D.J. (1983) Biochem.J.(in the press)

Odedra,B., Dalal,S.D. & Millward, D.J.(1982) Biochem.J. 202, 363-368.

Pain,V.M.& Clemens,M.J.(1980)in Comprehen.Biochem.19b 1-76.

Perly,M.& Kipnis,D.M. (1966) N.Eng.J.Med.,274,1237-1241.

Rannels,S.R. & Jefferson L.S.,(1980) Am.J.Physiol.238 E564-572.

Rannels,S.R.,Rannels,A.E. Pegg,A.E. & Jefferson,L.S.(1978) Am.J.Physiol 235 E134-139.

Rennie,M.J., Edwards,R.H.T., Krywawych,S., Davies, C.T.M., Halliday,D. Waterlow,J.C. & Millward,D.J. (1981) Clin. Sci. 61, 627-639

Rennie,M.J. & Millward,D.J. (1983) Clin Sci (in the press).

Rennie,M.J. Edwards, R.H.T.,Halliday,D.,Matthews,D.E., Wolman,S.L.& Millward,D.J.(1982a) Clin.Sci. 63,519-523

Rennie,M.J.,Edwards,R.H.T., Millward,D.J. Wolman,S.L. Halliday,D.& Matthews,D.E.(1982b) Nature 296, 165-167

Rennie,M.J.,Edwards,R.H.T. & Millward,D.J. (1982c) Muscle & Nerve 5,85-86

Rodemann,H.P. & Goldberg, A.L. (1982) J Biol Chem 257 1632-1638

Rodemann,H.P., Waxman, L. & Goldberg, A.L.(1982) J. Biol. Chem. 257 8716-8723

Salmon,W.D. & Daughaday,W.H. (1957) J.Lab.Clin.Med. 49 825-836.

Schoenheimer,R. ,Ratner,S. & Rittenberg,D. (1939) J.Biol. Chem., 127,333-344.

Schoenle,E.,Zapf,J.,Humbel,R.E & Froesch,E.R. (1982) Nature 296 252-253.

Seider,M.J., Kapp,R., Chen,C-P. & Booth,F.W. (1980) Biochem. J . 188 247-254

Sprinson, D.B. & Rittenberg, D. (1949) J.Biol.Chem., 180, 707-726

Stewart,P.M., Walser,M. & Drachman,D.B. (1982) Muscle Nerve
    5 197-201.

Tata,J.R. & Widnell,C.C.(1966) Biochem.J.98 604-610.

Thompson,E.B. & Lippman,M.E.(1974) Metabolism, 23,159-202.

Walser,M.,Sapir,D.G.,Mitch,W.E.&   Chan,W.   (1981)   in
    Metabolism & Clinical Implications of Branched Chain
    Amino & Ketoacids (M.Walser&J.R.Williamson) 291-300
    Elsevier/North-Holland Oxford

Waxman, L (1982) Methods Enzymol. 80, 664-680

Warnes,D.M., Tomas,F.M. & Ballard,F.J. (1981) Muscle &
    Nerve 4,62-66.

Wassner,S.J. & Li J. (1982) Am.J Physiol. 243,E293-297

Waterlow,J.C. ,Garlick,P.J. & Millward,D.J. (1978) Protein
    Turnover in Mammalian Tissues and in the Whole Body
    North Holland, Oxford.

Waterlow,J.C.& Tomkins,A.M. (1981) In "Nitrogen Metabolism
    in Man" (J.C.Waterlow & J.M.L.Stephen eds) 541-548
    Applied Science Publishers.

Wool.I.G.,Stirewalt,W.S.,Kurihara,K.,Low,R.B.,Bailey,P.   &
    Oyer,D.(1968) Rec Prog Horm.Res.,24,138-208

Young,V.R.   (1970)   in "Mammalian Protein Metabolism"
    (H.N.Munro ed) vol4 586-674 Academic Press N.Y. London

Young,V.R. and Munro, H.N. (1978) Fed. Proc. 37, 2291-2300.

Young,V.R,& Munro,H.N.(1980) in "Degradative Processes in
    Heart & Skeletal Muscle"(K.Wildenthal ed) 271-294
    Elsevier/North Holland Oxford

THERAPEUTIC STRATEGIES FOR PROTEIN WASTING STATES

Peter M. Stewart

Royal Prince Alfred Hospital

Missenden Road, Camperdown 2050, NSW Australia

Mackenzie Walser

Daniel G. Sapir

Daniel B. Drachman

Johns Hopkins Medical Institutes

Baltimore MD 21205   U.S.A.

ABSTRACT

The ketoanalogue of leucine, αketoisocaproate (ketoleucine) has significant protein sparing effects in fasting man. Studies designed to test its therapeutic potential in the post operative period and in patients with Duchenne muscular dystrophy were performed. Post operative patients were randomised to receive either glucose, leucine, keto-leucine in equivalent amounts. Leucine infusions had no effect on nitrogen balance, 3methylhistidine excretion or the plasma levels of prealbumin and retinol binding protein compared with glucose. On the other hand, keto-leucine resulted in a less negative nitrogen balance, and reduced 3methylhistidine excretion. Plasma prealbumin and retinol binding protein concentrations at the end of the study were significantly higher in the ketoleucine group compared with the glucose group. Thus ketoleucine reduces nitrogen loss, myofibrillar breakdown and hepatic

protein synthesis in postoperative patients. Leucine is
without effect. In Duchenne muscular dystrophy,
administration of the ornithine salt of ketoleucine
along with the ornithine salt of the ketoanalogue of
isoleucine and valine brought about a small (14%) but
highly significant fall in net protein degradation as
measured by 3methylhistidine excretion.

     Protein wasting states are manifest by an excess of
protein degradation over synthesis. Net protein degradation can be estimated by nitrogen (N) balance, the
difference between nitrogen intake and excretion. Protein
wasting states are characterised by a negative N balance.
Growth can be regarded as a state of positive N balance.
Fasting, (Adibi, 1971) post surgery, (Nehauser, 1980)
trauma and sepsis (Long, 1981) are examples of acute
protein wasting states in man. More chronic examples
include cancer (Dewy, 1980), liver (O'Keefe, 1980) and
renal disease (Grodstein, 1980). Finally muscular dystrophy typifies failure of normal protein accumulation in
muscle over a protracted period (Walton, 1974).
     This negative N balance with the inevitable depletion
of lean body mass that occurs, contributes to the
morbidity and mortality associated with this disorder.
Post operative morbidity measured by hospital stay and
complication rate can be correlated with both pre-
operative nutritional state and post operative nutritional
therapy (Collins 1978). An early feature of protein
wasting is impairment of cell mediated immunity (Chandra,
1983). This is seen particularly frequently in trauma
and sepsis because of the very rapid rate of loss of body
protein that occurs in these conditions. There is also a
high incidence of impaired immune function in liver
(O'Keefe, 1980) and renal disease (Kopple, 1978). This is
likely to contribute to the high incidence of infection
seen in these disorders.
     The major site of protein wasting in these conditions
is skeletal muscle as this is the major protein store in
the body. There is usually preservation of cardiac, brain
and hepatic protein until later in the illness (Moore,
(1959). Consequent upon protein wasting are loss of
muscle bulk and strength. A similar situation occurs in
muscular dystrophy.
     Protein balance in the whole animal is determined by
interplay between genetic, endocrine and nutritional
factors and it is by manipulation of these factors that

therapeutic strategies for protein wasting may be designed. Potential for growth is genetically determined. This potential is susceptible to genetic manipulation, as was recently shown by the insertion of rat growth genes into the mouse (Palmitier, 1982). However, it is unlikely that such techniques could have widespread application in the immediate future.

Endocrine factors exert potent effects on both protein synthesis and degradation. Insulin is the major anabolic hormone(Tischler, 1981). Infusion of this hormone can blunt the catabolic response to trauma (Woolfson, 1979). Under some circumstances glucagon, thyroxine and catecholamines have a catabolic action (Tischler, 1981). Furthermore prostaglandins seem to play a major role in the catabolic response to fever (Baracos, 1983). Anabolic steroids have been used widely in veterinary practice but their role in clinical medicine has yet to be defined (Heitzman, 1980).

Nutritional manipulation is another potentially effective method for improving protein balance. For example, feeding will increase protein synthesis over two-fold compared with prefed values (Millward, 1983). On the other hand fasting can bring about a significant reduction in protein loss during the course of a fast although it cannot reduce net protein loss to zero (Adibi,1971). In individual tissues such as liver, heart and skeletal muscle amino acid supply can reduce protein loss from these tissues (Ballard, 1982).

Of particular interest is the effect of branched chain amino acids in combination, or leucine alone, on protein balance in muscle. Leucine accelerates the rate of protein synthesis and reduces the rate of protein degradation (Buse, 1975). A similar effect can be seen in liver (Poso, 1982). As can be seen in Figure 1, Tischler et al have further clarified this effect on protein turnover in vitro and found that stimulation of protein synthesis can be attributed to the parent amino acid (Tischler 1982). In the whole animal, leucine does not stimulate protein synthesis when this is measured directly (McNurlan, 1982).

On the other hand, the effects on protein breakdown are due to a product of leucine catabolism (Tischler, 1982). Thus an alternative explanation may be that leucine through a metabolite reduces protein degradation. It is therefore likely that the ketoanalogue of leucine, αketoisocaproate may be as, or more effective than the parent amino acid. The negative nitrogen balance of fasting can be attenuated

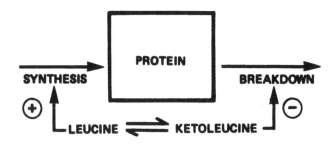

Figure 1. Effects of leucine and ketoleucine on protein synthesis and breakdown.

by ketoleucine. Leucine at three times the dose does not have this effect (Mitch, 1981). This paper describes the results of the use of this compound in other protein wasting states, in particular post surgery and Duchenne muscular dystrophy.

The studies described were performed at Johns Hopkins Medical Institutes and were approved by the Committee on Clinical Investigation. Informed consent was obtained from participants in the studies.

Methods for plasma amino acids and total nitrogen determination have been reported (Mitch, 1981). Creatinine, electrolytes, uric acid, glucose, albumin and CK were determined by automated methods in the clinical chemistry laboratory. Serum insulin was measured by radio-immuno-assay. Urinary 3 methylhistidine (3MeH) was measured on a Glenco MM70 amino acid analyser. Serum prealbumin and retinol binding protein were determined by radial immuno-diffusion. Blood acetoacetate and 3 hydroxybutyrate were determined enzymatically.

Keto acids were purchased from SOBAC, Paris, France. Ornithine salts of keto acids were synthesised as described previously (Herlong, 1980). Data were compared by analysis of variance and Wilcoxon's rank sum test.

Effects of Ketoleucine and Leucine on Nitrogen Metabolism

in Post-operative Patients

In the early post surgery period, patients have a markedly

negative N balance and elevated protein degradation as
measured by 3MeH excretion. In addition decreased levels
of the short life proteins such as prealbumin and retinol
binding protein are found (Large, 1980), suggesting
possible impairment of hepatic protein synthesis. In this
study the effect of leucine and its ketoanalogue αketoisocaproate on these parameters was investigated (Sapir,
1983).

Twenty one patients undergoing major abdominal surgery
were allocated randomly to 3 groups. Randomisation was
successful for sex, height and weight. The group that
received ketoleucine was significantly younger. Each
group received an infusion over a 12 hour period, immediately post surgery and on each of the following 4 days
one of the following solutions: 10 g glucose + 70mmol
NaHCO$_3$, 70 mmol of leucine + 70 mmol NaHCO$_3$, 70 mmol
sodium ketoleucine. Before surgery, all patients were
maintained on a meat-free diet for at least 2 days in
order that 3MeH excretion could be used as an index of
endogenous production. During the study period, no other
energy-containing fluids were administered. N excretion
(which equalled N balance in all groups except in the
leucine treated group) was calculated as the sum of the
urinary and gastric nitrogen losses.

The daily creatinine excretion varied widely between
patients due to a large variation in lean body mass
(creatinine 0.7g to 2.3 g/day). Therefore results for N
excretion, N Balance and 3MeH excretion were normalised
per g creatinine. Results were compared with and without
this correction.

Median total nitrogen excretion in the 3 groups
(glucose, leucine and ketoleucine respectively) was 7.29,
7.62 and 4.57 g/day. N balance was less negative than
total N excretion in the leucine infused group, -6.64 g/day,
by virtue of the nitrogen contained in the infused amino
acid. Total N excretion and N balance was significantly
less negative in the ketoleucine group compared with the
glucose infused group, whether or not it was corrected for
creatinine ($p < 0.05$). The results did not differ between
the leucine and control groups. As can be seen in Fig. 2,
there is no time trend in the data.

Urinary 3MeH excretion was lower in the keto leucine
infused group than in the glucose infused group (225 µmol/
day vs 424 µmol/day, $p = 0.02$). When results were corrected
for creatinine excretion, 3methylhistidine production was
lower in the ketoleucine group, than either of the groups

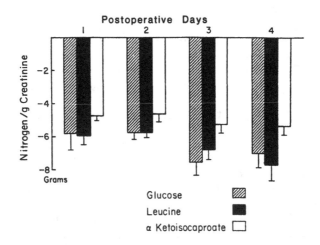

Figure 2. Time course of daily N balances during infusions. Results are expressed per gm of urinary creatinine to allow for differences in muscle mass between patients.

given leucine (p<0.02) or glucose (p<0.01). There was no difference between the glucose and leucine groups. Figure 3 shows the median daily 3MeH excretion expressed per g. creatinine. There was no time trend in 3MeH excretion.

Table 1 shows the plasma protein concentrations on the 5th post operative day. The values fell in all 3 groups over the time of the study. However, ketoleucine infusion attenuated the fall in both prealbumin and retinol binding protein compared with glucose infusion. There was no difference in the concentrations of these proteins between the leucine and glucose infused groups. Albumin concentrations were not significantly different.

In Table 2 it can be seen that total ketones, hydroxybutyrate and acetoacetate were higher in the ketoleucine infused group compared with glucose treatment. Acetoacetate was also higher in the leucine group than in the glucose infused group. There was no difference in the ratio of hydroxybutyrate to acetoacetate. There was no other difference in the compounds measured between the three groups.

Thus ketoleucine diminishes the negative nitrogen balance post surgery while leucine in an equivalent dose does not. There are several possible pathways by which

Table 1. Plasma albumin, prealbumin and retinol binding protein concentrations on the fifth post-operative day (median and range, n=7).

	Infusion		
	glucose	leucine	ketoleucine
albumin gm/L	34	33	37
	(32-42)	(26-39)	(29-40)*
prealbumin mg/L	108	90	138*
	(93-135)	(66-153)	(117-200)
retinol binding protein mg/L	17	21	26*
	(12-24)	(12-24)	(21-37)

(* significantly different from values obtained in glucose infused patients, $p<0.03$).

Table 2. Blood ketone concentrations on the fifth post operative day (median and range n=7).

	Infusion		
	glucose	leucine	ketoleucine
acetoacetate mM	0.7	0.9*	1.3*
	(0.5-0.8)	(0.8-1.3)	(0.9-1.7)
3 hydroxybutyrate mM	1.1	1.4	2.2*+
	(0.9-1.6)	(0.6-2.2)	(1.3-3.1)
total ketones	1.7	2.3	3.9*
	(1.6-2.8)	(0.7-3.5)	(2.3-4.2)

*   significantly different from values in glucose infused groups $p<0.03$.
+   significantly different from values obtained in leucine infused group $p<0.05$.

this compound could exert its metabolic effect.

The reduction in myofibillar protein degradation as measured by 3 MeH excretion would be more than adequate to explain the improvement in N balance (Young, 1978). Besides these effects on muscle protein turnover, keto-leucine may have affected either the rate of synthesis or breakdown of hepatic proteins. Both prealbumin and retinol binding protein were higher in the ketoleucine infused group suggesting that these processes may have been affected. As there was no change in the concentration of albumin, it is unlikely that redistribution of the proteins would explain the observed differences.

The exact mechanism to account for the metabolic effects of ketoleucine was not identified in this study. Ketoleucine itself has been shown to improve net protein balance in muscle (Tischler, 1982). However another

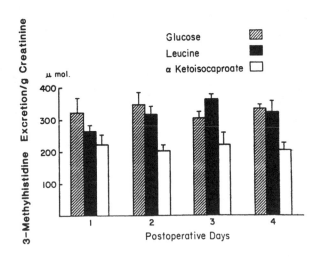

Figure 3. Time course of urinary 3MeH excretion during infusions, plotted as in figure 2.

striking metabolic effect resulting from the infusion of this compound was greatly increased concentrations of ketone bodies. The compound 3 hydroxybutyrate has been identified as having nitrogen sparing properties in some studies (Sherwin, 1975).

Reduction of Muscle Protein Degradation as Measured by 3MeH Excretion in Duchenne Muscular Dystrophy (Stewart, 1982)

Duchenne muscular dystrophy (DMD) is an X-linked progress-ive disorder of muscle. An indirect measure of protein breakdown is 3MeH excretion which is greatly increased in this disorder suggesting that myofibrillar protein break-down is greatly accelerated (Ballard, 1979). However a recent study using stable isotope methodology suggests that in the human disease the opposite may be the case; muscle protein turnover is depressed (Rennie, 1982). Whatever the rate of protein turnover, if a small reduction in the rate of protein degradation could be achieved without any change in protein synthetic rate, this must favourably influence net protein loss from muscle in this disorder.

Nine boys with a definitive diagnosis of DMD were entered into the study. They were hospitalised for 11 days and placed on a diet similar in protein and energy intake

Table 3. *Changes in the excretion rates of creatinine and 3MeH in nine dystrophic boys during administration of ketoacids.*

	Creatinine (μmole/day)	3MeH (μmole/day)	3MeH/Creatinine
Control	1640+210	643+5.5	0.042+.004
Drug	1600+180	550+ 4.3	0.364+0.003
Change	-40+48	-93+3.6[*]	-0.006+0.002[*]

p <0.01 by analysis of variance

to their usual diet but meat-free to remove any source of
exogenous 3MeH. After a 3 day equilibration period, 24
hour excretion rates of total nitrogen, creatinine and
3MeH were made on 2 consecutive 4 day periods. Total
nitrogen excretion in the two 4 day pooled stool samples
was also measured. The first 4 day period was to determine
control 3MeH and N balance. During the second 4 day
period, ornithine salts of αketoisocaproate, αketoiso-
valerate and αketo-B-methylvalerate in the proportion 4:1:1
at a dose of 0.45 gm/kg body weight/day were administered
in divided doses. Protein intake was reduced by an amount
iso-nitrogenous with the administered mixture.

There was no significant difference in creatinine
excretion rates during the treatment periods. The total
excretion rates were considerably lower than in normal
boys (Ballard, 1979). As can also be seen in Table 3 there
was a significant fall in mean 3MeH excretion either as a
daily output or expressed as molar ratio to creatinine.
The molar ratio of 3MeH to creatinine fell during therapy
in 8 of the 9 patients (Fig. 4). Nitrogen balance during
the control period showed a mean value of +1.4 $\pm$ 0.3 gm/day.
Mean nitrogen balance during the treatment period was +1.2
$\pm$ 0.2, not significantly different from the control period.
Plasma creatine kinase levels did not change with therapy.
Plasma amino acids did not change significantly except for
the presence of allo isoleucine which invariably occurs
during ketoisoleucine administration (Walser, 1981).

From this study, it appears that protein degradation
rates can be reduced acutely by 14%. Such a reduction without any alteration in the rate of muscle protein synthesis
would lead to a net accumulation of 3 g/day of muscle
protein. This would improve nitrogen balance by 0.48 g/day,
an amount not able to be detected by methods employed. It
has been estimated that a reduction in the net rate of
muscle protein degradation of only 4% would result in a
normal muscle growth in these children provided there was
no change in the rate of synthesis (Ballard, 1979).

SUMMARY

The keto analogue of leucine is a potent N sparing compound.
Its efficacy has been demonstrated both in fasting and post
surgery patients. It can also acutely reduce protein
degradation as measured by 3MeH excretion in Duchenne
muscular dystrophy. An evaluation of its therapeutic

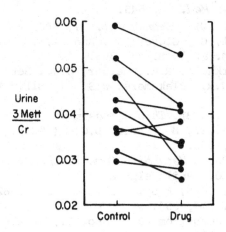

Figure 4. Molar ratio of 3MeH to creatinine excretion in each of the nine patients before and during keto acid administration.

efficacy in more serious disorders such as severe trauma and sepsis that are characterised by an uncontrolled and greatly increased rate of protein breakdown **seems warranted.**

REFERENCES

Adibi, S.A. (1971).*J. Lab. Clin. Med. 77, 278.*

Ballard, F.J., Tomas, F.M. Stein, L.M. (1979). *Clin. Sci. Mol. Med. 56, 347.*

Ballard, F.J., Gunn, J.M. (1982). *Nutr. Rev. 40, 33.*

Baracos, V., Rodemann, H.P., Dinarello, C.A., Goldberg, A.L. (1983). *New Engl. J. Med. 308, 553.*

Buse, M.G., Reid, S.S. (1975). *J. Clin. Invest. 56,* 1250.

Chandra, R.K. (1983). *Lancet I, 688.*

Collins, J.P., Oxby, C.B., Hill, G.L. (1978). *Lancet I, 788.*

De Whys, W.D. (1980). *J. Am. Med. Assoc. 244, 374.*

Grodstein, G.P., Blumerkrantz, M.J., Kopple, J.D. (1980). *Am. J. Clin. Nutr. 33, 411,*

Heitzman, R.J. (1980). *In Hormones and Metabolism in Ruminants.* (Forbes, J.M. and Lomax, M.A. eds.), p129 Agricultural Research Council, London.

Herlong, H.F., Maddrey, W.C., Walser, M. (1980).
    Ann. Intern. Med. 93, 545.

Kopple, J.D. (1978). *Kidney Int. 14,* 340.

Large, S., Neal, G., Glover, J., Angkul, O., Olson, R.E.
    (1980). *Br. J. Nutr. 43,* 393.

Long, C.L., Birkhalm, R.H., Geiger, J.W., Betts, J.E.,
    Schiller, W.R., Blakemore, W.S. (1981). *Metabolism
    30,* 765.

Millward, D.J. (1983). *This symposium.*

Mitch, W.E., Walser, M., Sapir, D.G. (1981). *J. Clin.
    Invest. 67,* 553.

Moore, F.D. (1959). *Metabolic Care of the Surgical Patient*
W.B. Saunders Co., Philadelphia.

McNurlan, M.A., Fern, E.B., Garlick, P.J. (1982).
    Biochem. J. 204, 553.

Neuhauser, M., Bergstrom, J., Chao, L., et al (1980)
Metabolism 29, 1206.

O'Keefe, S.J., El-Zayodi, A.R. Carraher, T.E., Dorus, M.,
    Williams, R. (1980). *Lancet 2,* 615.

Palmetier, R.D., Brinster, R.L., Hammer, R.E., et al
    Nature 300, 611.

Poso, A.R. West Jr., J.J., Mortimore, G.E., (1982)
    J. Biol. Chem. 257, 12114,

Rennie, M.J., Edwards, R.H.T., Millward, D.J. Wolman, S.L.,
Halliday, D. (1982). *Nature 296,*165

Sapir, D.G., Stewart, P.M., Walser, M., et al (1983)
    Lancet. In press.

Sherwin, R.S., Hendler, R.G., Felig, P. (1975). *J. Clin.
    Invest. 55,* 1382.

Stewart, P.M., Walser, M., Drachman, D.B. (1982). *Muscle
    and Nerve 5,* 197.

Tischler, M.E., (1971). *Life Sciences 28,* 2569.

Tischler, M.E., Desautels, M., Goldberg, A.L. (1982).
    J. Biol. Chem. 257, 1613.

Walser, M., Sapir, E.G., Mitch, W.E., Chan, W. (1981).
    *In Metabolism and Clinical Implications of Branched
    Chain Amino and Keto Acids* (Walser, M. and Williamson,
    J.R. eds.,) p291, Elsevier/North Holland, New York.

Walton, J.N., Gardner-Medwin, D. (1974). *In Disorders of
    Voluntary Muscle 3rd ed.* (Walton J.N. ed.) p561
    Churchill Livingstone, Edinburgh.

Woolfson, A.M.J., Heatley, C.V., Allison, S.P. (1979).
    New Engl. J. Med. 300, 14.

Young V.R., Munro, H.N. (1978), *Fed. Proc. 37,* 2291.

SKELETAL MUSCLE FIBRE BUNDLES FOR THE STUDY OF PROTEIN TURNOVER IN NORMAL AND DYSTROPHIC MOUSE TISSUE

LYNDA BUTCHER and JOHN K. TOMKINS

Neurobiology Unit, School of Life Sciences,
The N.S.W. Institute of Technology,
Westbourne St. GORE HILL NSW 2065 AUSTRALIA

ABSTRACT

An *in vitro* mouse skeletal muscle preparation, the teased fibre bundle, has been investigated as a means of study of protein turnover. The repsonse of this preparation to nutrient supply is reported and compared with the results of other *in vitro* skeletal muscle preparations from rodents.

Using the preparation, we have observed, in agreement with other studies, that the rate of protein degradation in mouse dystrophic muscle is significantly elevated. The effects of various protease inhibitors have been tested in this system and one, leupeptin, showed a significant and consistent effect in decreasing protein degradation in normal and dystrophic tissue.

INTRODUCTION

Muscle protein is being continuously degraded and resynthesised. Changes in the rates of these processes will be reflected in muscle growth or the atrophy observed in some pathological states. *In vivo* methods for the evaluation of protein metabolism are complex and subject to a variety of artefacts such as the influence of physiological status, whereas *in vitro* systems can be used for studying protein turnover in carefully controlled conditions. These include the use of rodent whole muscle preparations such as the extensor digitorum longus (EDL), soleus (Goldberg *et al*, 1977; Goldspink, 1976) and dia-phragm (Fulks *et al*, 1975).

Two *in vitro* muscle preparations have been under con-sideration by our laboratory for their suitability for clinical metabolic studies. The first utilizes a tissue slice technique (Tomkins *et al*, 1982) and the second a teased fibre preparation. If these *in vitro* preparations are to be of value in understanding protein metabolism in normal and pathological muscle, they must respond, at least qualitatively, in a manner similar to that seen by muscle *in vivo*. While it has been found that skeletal muscles *in vitro* are in a state of negative nitrogen balance, some factors known to influence protein synthesis and degradation *in vitro* are recognised to be important *in vivo* (Goldberg *et al*, 1977; Goldberg and Odessey, 1973). These include (i) hormones, such as insulin, which is pro-bably the most important factor regulating protein balance in skeletal muscle, (ii) nutrient supply, (iii) levels of contactile activity and (iv) calcium. However, there is a difference in the directional response of protein turn-over to some factors *in vitro* compared to *in vivo*. It has been observed that stretching muscle *in vivo* increases the rate of protein degradation (Goldspink, 1977) whereas others have observed a decrease in the rate of protein degradation in stretched muscles *in vitro* (Goldberg and Odessey, 1973). Also, direct stimulation by leucine of protein synthesis in muscle tissue *in vitro* has been dem-onstrated (Buse and Reid, 1975; Fulks *et al*,1975) whereas, *in vivo*, protein synthesis was not stimulated by the admin-istration of leucine to fed or starved rats (McNurlan *et al*, 1982).

In our laboratory, we wished to develop an *in vitro* method that could be used to clarify conflicting results that have been reported with regard to protein turnover in Duchenne muscular dystrophy (DMD). Rennie *et al* (1982) used *in vivo* stable isotope methods to examine protein turnover in DMD and reported that in patients the synthetic rate (and by implication the degradative rate) was depres-sed. Their result appeared at variance with a number of previous reports: (i) the 3-methyl histidine to creatin-ine ratio, as a measure of degradation rate, is elevated in DMD (Warnes *et al*, 1981). The discrepancy of this result compared with the conclusions of Rennie *et al* may

be explained by the substantial non-muscle sources of
3-methyl histidine (Millward *et al*, these proceedings);
(ii) the majority of muscle proteinases and peptide hyd-
rolases active in the acid, neutral and alkaline pH range
are elevated in human muscular dystrophies (Kar and
Pearson, 1978). Marked early rises in cathespin D and
dipeptidylpeptidase IV suggest their role is important.
In addition, two sarcoplasmic proteinases, the Ca++
activated proteinases and group specific chymotrypsin-
like serine proteinases may be involved in the Duchenne
type of dystrophy; (iii) measurement of several animal
models of DMD have indicated increased protein synthesis
in the dystrophic animal (Hilgartner *et al*, 1981; Garber
et al, 1980).

     This paper describes the development of an *in vitro*
system using the dystrophic mouse, C57BL dy^{2J}/dy^{2J}.   In
the development of the method, we have examined the ways
that the *in vitro* preparation can be modified while still
maintaining the characteristics expected with respect to
protein turnover. As we wish to apply these methods to
human muscle, the modifications of the preparation were
carried out in light of the limitations imposed by use of
muscle obtained from human biopsy material.

MATERIALS AND METHODS
     Mice used for these studies were C57BL/6J strain and
the dystrophy studied was due to the autosomal recessive
mutation dy^{2J} (Macpike and Meier, 1976). The mice were
obtained either directly from the Jackson Laboratories,
Bar Harbor, Maine, or bred from Jackson Laboratory stocks.
Normal mice were genetically C57BL/6 J +/+ and dystrophic
mice were C57BL dy^{2J}/dy^{2J}. At all times mice had free
access to food and water and those of approximately 3
months of age were used.

     For the teased fibre bundle preparation, the tibialis
anterior was removed and, under the dissecting microscope,
fibres were cut close to the tendon and fibre bundles
stripped away. About 10mg of tissue containing bundles
of approximately 0.5 to 2mm were used. All preparations
were made at or above $25^{\circ}C$. The tissue preparations were
placed in Krebs Ringer phosphate buffer saturated with a
95% O_2:5% CO_2 gas mixture. Incubation of tissue was at
$37^{\circ}C$. Unless otherwise stated, the incubation medium
contained radioactive tyrosine precursor (L-$[3,5-^3H]$

tyrosine, $3\mu Ci\ ml^{-1}$, 0.35 mM), glucose (8.25mM), and a
mixture of 17 L-amino acids at plasma concentration.

Protein turnover was determined by the method of
Fulks et al, 1975. Briefly, protein synthesis (nmol
tyrosine incorporated/mg muscle/2hr) was determined by
measuring the rate of incorporation of labelled tyrosine
into muscle protein after correcting for intracellular
specific activity of tyrosine. Degradation (nmol tyrosine
released/mg muscle/2hr) was determined independently of
synthesis by measuring the release of tyrosine into the
medium and muscle pool from tissue incubated in the presence of puromycin (125 mg/ml) to prevent reutilization of
amino acids.

The processing of tissue for determination of isotope incorporation was by a filter paper disc technique
(Weinstein et al, 1975). Determination of tyrosine in
muscle pools or released into the medium was made fluor-
metrically (Waalkes and Udenfriend, 1957).

For studies of protease inhibitors the following
inhibitors were used; leupeptin (2.5×10^{-5}M), pepstatin
2.5×10^{-5} M), ξ-amino caproic acid (ξACA 5×10^{-3} M) and
trans-4-aminomethyl (cyclohexane)-1-carboxylic acid (AMCHA
1×10^{-4} M). The first two of these inhibitors were dissolved in 0.5% dimethyl sulphoxide).

All measurements of protein turnover are means from
replicate samples of up to six animals. Two way analysis
of variance was applied to all data and F-values were calculated.

RESULTS
Protein synthesis was measured using radioactive
tyrosine as precursor since it is neither synthesised nor
degraded by skeletal muscle (Odessey and Goldberg, 1972).
Also, it has been reported that when skeletal muscle was
incubated in the presence of tyrosine, there was rapid
equilibration between intracellular pools and the medium
and that the intracellular pool of tyrosine served as a
precursor for protein synthesis (Li et al, 1973). In our
teased fibre bundle preparation, tyrosine equilibration
between the intracellular pools and the medium occurred
within 30 min of incubation (Fig. 1), with a ratio of
intracellular to extracellular specific activity of 0.6.

Using the intracellular specific activity to calculate protein synthesis ^{3}H-tyrosine was incorporated at a linear rate of up to 2.5 hrs (Fig. 1). Since the intracellular specific activity remained constant, the fall in tyrosine incorporation after 2.5 hrs reflected a depression in protein synthesis. In subsequent experiments the teased fibre bundle was preincubated for 30 mins to permit equilibration of tyrosine between muscle pools and the medium, then incubated for 2 hrs to measure protein synthesis.

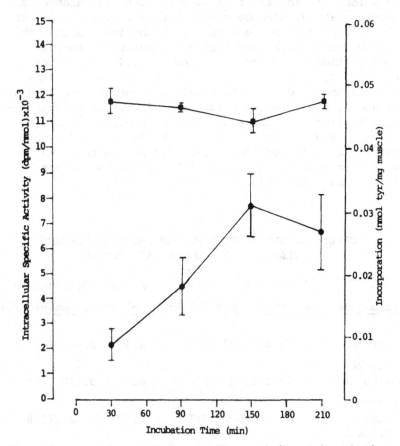

FIGURE 1:   *Intracellular specific activity (■) and time course of incorporation (●) of tyrosine into muscle using a teased fibre bundle preparation incubated in unsupplemented Krebs Ringer bicarbonate buffer. Values are the mean ± SEM for at least three animals.*

Protein degradation was measured independently of synthesis by incubating tissue in the presence of puro-mycin. When the rate of degradation was compared to the rate of synthesis, the teased fibre bundle preparation was observed to be in a state of negative nitrogen balance, degradation exceeding synthesis by a factor of 17 (Table 1).

Goldberg et al, (1977) reported that the addition of nutrients and hormones improved the overall nitrogen balance by altering the rates of protein synthesis and degradation. In an effort to improve nitrogen balance in the preparation, glucose and a mixture of amino acids or 0.5 mM leucine were added to the incubation medium. The addition of glucose plus leucine stimulated tyrosine incorporation and glucose plus amino acids or leucine inhibited tyrosine release (Table 1). Since the intra-cellular specific activity remained constant when leucine was added, the observed stimulation in tyrosine incorporation reflected an increased rate of protein synthesis. However, when a mixture of amino acids were added, the specific activity of the protein did not increase in comparison to control; this was probably due to the observed fall in the intracellular specific activity.

TABLE 1

EFFECT OF NUTRIENT SUPPLY ON PROTEIN TURNOVER
IN TEASED FIBRE BUNDLE PREPARATIONS

Conditions of Incubation	Protein Synthesis (nmol tyr/mg muscle/2hr)	Protein Degradation (nmol tyr/mg muscle/2hr)
No addition	0.02 ± 0.002 (5)	0.39 ± 0.019 (6)
Glucose + amino acids	0.03 ± 0.002 (5)	0.33 ± 0.017 (6)*
Glucose + leucine (0.5 mM)	0.04 ± 0.005 (5)"	0.29 ± 0.020 (5)#

Numbers of animals are given in parenthesis.

* $0.025 < p < 0.05$ # $0.01 < p < 0.025$ " $p < 0.01$

Using the *in vitro* teased fibre bundle preparation, protein degradation was found to be significantly increased (by 115%) above normal when dystrophic mice were compared to normal controls (Table 2). This is due to an elevation in both free tyrosine in muscle tissue and an increase in tyrosine released into the medium during incubation (Table 2). When two-way analysis of variance was applied to the data, a significant interaction between normal and dystrophic groups was obtained, indicating that some dystrophic individuals had rates of protein degradation within normal levels. The overlap of degradation rates between normal and dystrophic mice was due particularly to a large range of values in the dystrophic group.

Several protease inhibitors were examined for their ability to return the elevated rate of protein breakdown in mouse dystrophic tissue to normal levels. Whilst two inhibitors, leupeptin and AMCHA inhibited protein degradation, the rate of protein breakdown was still significantly higher than normal (Table 3). Pepstatin and ξACA had no effect on the rate of protein degradation. Leupeptin inhibited protein breakdown in both normal and dystrophic muscle by approximately 19%, but the inhibitory effect of AMCHA appeared specific for the dystrophic tissue. However, there is a significant interaction between AMCHA and the subject tested, with some dystrophic individuals displaying no inhibition of protein degradation in response to this inhibitor.

The results for the two dystrophic groups in Table 3 were found to be significantly different. This was attributable to a difference in slope of the tyrosine assay standard curves.

DISCUSSION

it is usual that intact mammalian skeletal muscles are used in *in vitro* preparations. Goldberg *et al*, (1975) reported that metabolism in an intact rat diaphragm preparation *in vitro* closely approximated the metabolic characteristics of the *in vivo* diaphragm. In a preparation with ribs removed from the diaphragm, the levels of creatine phosphorylcreatine, ATP and inorganic phosphate fell during a 90 min incubation. They suggested that some fibres were damaged upon removal of the ribs and leaked metabolites into the medium. Seider *et al* (1980) ob-

TABLE 2

PROTEIN DEGRADATION IN NORMAL AND DYSTROPHIC
TEASED FIBRE BUNDLE PREPARATIONS

Phenotype	Tyrosine in muscle pools (nmol/mg muscle)	Tyrosine in medium (nmol/mg muscle)	Degradation (nmol/mg muscle/2hr)
Normal (C57BL/6J +/+)	0.07 ± 0.010	0.36 ± 0.035	0.42 ± 0.037
Dystrophic (C57BL/6J dy^{2J}/dy^{2J})	0.29 ± 0.042	0.63 ± 0.047	0.91 ± 0.069*

Values are the mean and SEM from 11 animals.

* p < 0.001

TABLE 3

EFFECT OF PROTEASE INHIBITORS ON PROTEIN DEGRADATION
IN TEASED FIBRE BUNDLE PREPARATIONS
FROM NORMAL AND DYSTROPHIC SKELETAL MUSCLE.

Conditions of Incubation	Protein Degradation (nmol tyr/mg muscle/2hr)	
	NORMAL	DYSTROPHIC
Control	0.48 ± 0.063 (6)	0.76 ± 0.072 (5)
+ Leupeptin	0.39 ± 0.073 (5)*	0.61 ± 0.093 (5)✱
+ Pepstatin	0.52 ± 0.054 (6)N.S.	0.72 ± 0.121 (5)N.S.
Control	0.36 ± 0.016 (5)	1.03 ± 0.100 (6)
+ ξACA	0.35 ± 0.021 (5)N.S.	1.04 ± 0.076 (6)N.S.
+ AMCHA	0.32 ± 0.020 (5)N.S.	0.89 ± 0.077 (6)#

Numbers of animals are in parenthesis.
Levels of significance of treated compared with control preparations.
*$0.01 < p < 0.025$ ✱$p < 0.005$ #$0.005 < p < 0.01$
N.S. Not significant.

served an altered rate of protein synthesis and degradation
and a fall in the concentration of high energy phosphate
when muscle fibres were cut. For most studies of *in vitro*
preparations, therefore, whole muscles are selected that
are thin enough to ensure that adequate amounts of nutrient
and tracer reach all fibres in the absence of a circulatory
system (Goldberg et al, 1975).

While preparations containing cut muscle fibres exhibited several changes, it became apparent that these
changes were restricted to the early stages of incubation.
Diaphragm incubated without ribs were able to actively
transport amino acids and cations, synthesise protein and
respond to hormones such as insulin (Goldberg et al,1975).
Teased fibre preparations from human tissue also incorporated amino acids into protein, exhibited active transport
mechanisms and initiated and terminated peptide formation
(Lundholm et al, 1975). When fibres were sealed off at the
cut ends, damage appeared to be restricted to the area
immediately adjacent to the ties, contractile properties
were maintained and high energy phosphate compounds were
well preserved (Moulds et al, 1977).

The teased fibre bundle preparation used in these
studies incorporated radioactive tyrosine precursor into
muscle protein at a linear rate for up to 2 hours, but this
preparation appeared less stable in terms of maintaining
protein synthesis than a similar preparation reported by
Lundholm et al (1975). Protein synthesis provides a
sensitive index of energy supply and viability, and such
differences in viability are possibly due to differences
in fibre integrity. Teased fibres isolated from human
biopsy material by Lundholm et al were approximately 20mm
in length. In the murine studies reported here, fibres of
about 5-8mm in length were used. Therefore the length of
intact fibre was greater in the human muscle preparation.
Seider et al (1980) demonstrated that whilst a single cut
through the intact soleus does not alter the rate of protein degradation, a second cut significantly increased
protein breakdown. Thus the extent of injury to muscle
during preparation affects the maintenance of the tissue
in vitro.

Amino acids have been reported to promote protein
synthesis and inhibit protein degradation in skeletal
muscle *in vitro*, in particular the branded chain amino

acids (Fulks *et al*, 1975; Tischler *et al*, 1982). While the
teased fibre bundle appears also to be regulated by amino
acids in this fashion (Table 1), it was unexpected that
plasma levels of amino acids (including leucine) did not
stimulate protein synthesis in the preparation where 0.5mM
leucine (5x plasma level) did. The requirement for elevated amino acid supplement *in vitro* has been reported for
a perfused skeletal muscle preparation (Li and Jefferson,
1978). The decrease in intracellular specific activity
of free tyrosine in cut fibre preparations when amino acids
were added to the medium (not observed with leucine) would
provide reason for this unexpected observation.

A major difficulty in the use of *in vitro* systems is
that the cells and tissue are in a catabolic state - such
is the situation with the teased fibre preparation reported
in this study (Table 3). Such problems can be alleviated
in these preparations, particularly by the use of protein
anabolic agents (Stirewalt and Low, 1983).

Despite the difficulties, *in vitro* experiments have
several advantages. First, the specific radioactivity of
the precursor can be readily controlled and remains constant during the experiment. Secondly, by increasing the
amino acid concentration in the incubation medium, it is
possible to produce complete equilibration of amino acids
between the extracellular and free intracellular pools. A
third advantage is the use of a defined medium that allows
evaluation of the effects of various nutritional and metabolic functions.

The nature of the changes in protein metabolism in
dystrophic muscle are still not clear. Alterations in
muscle volume, precursor pools and the shift in the proportion of red and white muscle fibres (Fowler *et al*,1977)
must be borne in mind when analyzing changes in dystrophic
muscle. Kitchen and Watts (1973) reported that, whilst
muscle protein degradation was not significantly different
in dystrophic muscle, a few dystrophic individuals displayed an extremely rapid loss of label, particularly if
the disease was well advanced. Hence the stage of the
disease may be associated with the direction of change in
protein metabolism in dystrophic mice. Studies of protein
metabolism are further complicated by the heterogeneous
turnover rates of muscle protein. Any change in bulk
turnover may be a consequence of alterations in the turn-

over rates of one or more proteins (Goldberg and St. John, 1976;Koizumi, 1974). Monckton and Marusyk (1975) using autoradiography demonstrated a marked drop in the uptake of ^{3}H-leucine into myofibrils and an increased incorporation into sarcoplasmic protein from dystrophic mouse muscle.

The association of extensive loss of sarcoplasmic and contractile proteins from dystrophic muscle with a significant elevation in a number of proteases has resulted in the screening of protease inhibitors for their ability to slow or prevent the muscle wasting process. In our study, the release of tyrosine from the skeletal muscle preparations of dystrophic mice was significantly elevated when compared to normal. This confirms the work of Goldberg et al (1977) and of Garber et al (1980) who reported that significantly greater amounts of alanine and glutamine were released from mouse dystrophic muscle. The attempts to inhibit degradation showed that it was not possible to restore the increased rate of degradation in mouse muscular dystrophy to normal. Similar results were reported by Riebow and Young (1980) and implied by studies of Libby and Goldberg (1980). This may be due to several factors: these agents were unable to enter the cells or were inactivated within the cells, the proteases susceptible to these agents were not important in protein breakdown; proteolytic activity is not directly related to the elevated rate of protein degradation.

An overall decrease in protein degradation of 20% in both normal and dystrophic muscle by leupeptin,it would seem,was not due to a non-specific toxic effect since it has been reported that protein synthesis in leupeptin treated muscles was not changed (Libby & Goldberg, 1978). This indicates a role for proteases sensitive to leupeptin in overall protein breakdown. Reibow and Young (1980) have observed that leupeptin only inhibited soluble not myofibrillar protein degradation in chicken muscle cell cultures and concluded that the muscle proteases that are specifically inhibited by leupeptin seem to have no major role in initiating myofibrillar protein turnover. If an elevation in protein degradation in dystrophic muscle is due to an elevation in myofibrillar degradation (Simon et al, 1962), the inability of leupeptin to restore degradation rates to normal may reflect the inhibition of proteases that are not important to the increase of protein breakdown in murine muscular dystrophy.

Leupeptin has been reported to inhibit cathepsin B with a high degree of selectivity (Aoyagi et al, 1969). In addition, Azanza et al (1979) have shown that leupeptin completely inhibits the activity of Ca^{2+}-activated neutral protease that has been postulated to be a major enzyme in disassembly and degradation of myofibrillar proteins (Dayton et al, 1976). Based on these observations, leupeptin would be expected to inhibit the turnover of myofibrillar proteins.

The physiological function of a protease in vivo in normal and diseased stated is unclear. Whilst protease activity has been correlated with rates of protein degradation in vitro (Libby & Goldberg, 1980) and in vivo (Millward et al, 1981) an elevation in proteolytic activity is not necessarily reflected in an increased rate of protein degratation (Crie et al, 1981). Proteases may serve other physiological roles within cells besides catabolism of endogenous protein, such as the maturation of secreted proteins or the hydrolysis of internalized extracellular proteins. Differences in protease activity in intact cells and cell-free systems may result from lack of appropriate in vitro conditions, cellular of subcellular compartmentation of proteases or release of endogenous inhibitors. In addition, different proteolytic activities may be associated with changes in cell population, Intact muscle preparations contain cells of many types(e.g., myocytes, fibroblasts, mast cells, adipocytes, etc.), which together constitute about half of the cells in some muscles. In dystrophic tissue the proportion of infiltrating cells increases. The protease inhibitors ξACA and AMCHA inhibit proteases secreted by macrophages (Brosnan et al, 1980), and the selective beneficial effect of AMCHA on dystrophic muscle may be a reflection of inhibition of proteases secreted by infiltrating mast cells in dystrophic tissue. The variation in the effect of AMCHA may correspond to the degree of infiltration of muscle by other cell types and subsequent levels of secreted proteases. This inhibitor may provide a useful probe for assessing the contribution of other cell types to proteolytic activity in muscle homogenates.

ACKNOWLEDGEMENTS
This work was supported by donations of private funds, in particular, Dick Smith Electronics Pty Ltd.

REFERENCES

Aoyagi, T., Takeuchi, T., Matsuzaki, A., Kawamurra, K.,
   Kondo, S., Hamada, M., Maeda, K. and Umezawa, H.
   (1969). *J. Antibiot. 22*, 283.
Azanza, J., Raymond, J. Robin, J., Cottin P. and
   Ducastaing, A. (1979). *Biochem J. 183*, 339.
Brosnan, C.F., Cammer, W., Norton, W.T. and Bloom, B.R.
   (1980). *Nature 285*, 235.
Buse, M.G. and Reid, S.S. (1975). *J. Clin. Invest. 56*,
   1250.
Crie, J.S., Millward, D.J., Bates, P.C., Griffin, E.D. and
   Wildenthal, K. (1981). *J. Mol. Cell. Cardiol. 13*, 589.
Dayton, W.R., Reville, W.J., Gall, D.E. and Stromer, M.H.
   (1976). *Biochem. 15*, 2159.
Fowler Jr., W.M., Taylor, R.G., Franti, C.E. and Hagler,
   A.N. (1977). *J. Neurol. Sci. 32*, 277.
Fulks, R.M., Li, J.B. and Goldberg, A.L. (1975). *J. Biol.
   Chem. 250*, 290.
Garber, A.J., Schwartz, R.J., Seidel, C.L., Silvers, A.
   and Entman, M.L. (1980). *J. Biol. Chem. 255*, 8315.
Goldberg, A.L., Griffin, G.E. and Dice Jr., J.F. (1977).
   "Pathogenesis of Human Muscular Dystrophy" (L. P.
   Rowland, Ed.) p.376. Excerpta Medica, Amsterdam.
Goldberg, A.L. and Odessey, R. (1973). *"Exploratory
   Concepts in Muscular Dystrophy"* (A. T. Milhorat, Ed.)
   p. 187. Excerpta Medica, Amsterdam.
Goldberg, A.L., Martel, S.B. and Kushmerick, M.J. (1975).
   Methods Enzymol. 39, 82.
Goldberg, A.L. and St. John, A.C. (1976). *Ann. Rev.
   Biochem. 45*, 747.
Goldspink, D.F. (1976). *Biochem. J.* 156, 71.
Goldspink, D.F. (1977). *J. Physiol. 264*, 267.
Hillgartner, F.B., Williams, A.S., Flanders, J.A., Morin,
   D. and Hansen, R.J. (1981). *Biochem. J. 196*, 591.
Kar, N.C. and Pearson, C.M. (1978). *Muscle Nerve 1*, 308.
Kitchin, S.E. and Watts, D.C. (1973). *Biochem. J. 136*,1017.
Koizumi, T. (1974). *J. Biochem. 76*, 431.
Libby, P. and Goldberg, A.L. (1978). *Science 199*, 534.
Libby, P. and Goldberg, A.L. (1980). *Biochem. J. 188*, 213
Li, J.B., Fulks, R.M. and Goldberg, A.L. (1973). *J. Biol.
   Chem. 248*, 7272.
Li, J.B. and Jefferson, L.S. (1978). *Biochem. Biophys.
   Acta 544*, 351.
Lundholm, K., Bylund, A-C., Hol, J., Smeds, S. and
   Schersten, T. (1975). *Eur. Surg. Res. 7*, 65.

Macpike, A.D. and Meier, H. (1976). *Proc. Soc. Exp. Biol. Med. 151,* 670.

McNurlan, M.A., Fern, E.B. and Garlick, P.J. (1982). *Biochem. J. 204,* 831.

Millward, D.J., Brown, J.G. and Odedra, B. (1981). *"Nitrogen Metabolism in Man"* (J.C. Waterlow and J.M.L. Stephen, Eds.) p. 475, Applied Science Publishers, London and New Jersey.

Moulds, R.F.W., Young, A., Jones, D.A. and Edwards, R.H.T. (1977). *Clin. Sci. Mol. Med. 52,* 291.

Odessey, R. and Goldberg, A.L. (1972). *Am. J. Physiol. 223,* 1376.

Rennie, M.J., Edwards, R.H.T., Millward, D.J., Wolman, S.L. Halliday, D. and Matthews, D.E. (1982). *Nature 296,* 165.

Riebow, J.F. and Young, R.B. (1980). *Biochem. Med. 23,* 316.

Seider, M.J., Kapp, R., Chem, C-P. and Booth, F.W. (1980). *Biochem. J. 188,* 247.

Simon, E.J., Gross, C.S. and Lessell, I.M. (1962). *Arch. Biochem. Biophys. 96,* 41.

Stirewalt, W.S. and Low, R.B. (1983). *Biochem. J. 210,* 323.

Tischler, M.E., Desautels, M. and Goldberg, A.L. (1982). *J. Biol. Chem. 257,* 1613.

Tomkins, J.K., Collins, S.P., De C. Baker, W., Kidman, A.D. (1982). *J. Neurol. Sci. 54,* 59.

Waalkes, R.P. and Udenfriend, S. (1957). *J. Lab. Clin. Med. 50,* 733.

Warnes, D.M., Tomas, F.M. and Ballard, F.J. (1981). *Muscle Nerve 4,* 62.

Weinstein, B.I., Bhardwaj, N. and Li, H-C. (1975). *Anal. Biochem. 68,* 62.

THE EFFECT OF THE LOSS OF WEIGHT-BEARING FUNCTION ON THE

ISOMYOSIN PROFILE AND CONTRACTILE PROPERTIES OF RAT

SKELETAL MUSCLES

J.F.Y. HOH AND C.J. CHOW

DEPARTMENT OF PHYSIOLOGY, UNIVERSITY OF

SYDNEY, SYDNEY, N.S.W., 2006, AUSTRALIA

ABSTRACT

We tested the hypothesis that the continuous reflex
neural activity of slow-twitch motor units during normal
weight-bearing function is instrumental in maintaining
their slow characteristics. Three-week-old rats were
suspended by the tail so that their hindlimbs were relieved
of their normal weight-bearing function. Six weeks later
the isometric twitch contraction time for the slow-twitch
soleus muscles, measured *in vitro* at 35°C, was significantly
reduced compared with controls. These muscles also showed
post-tetanic potentiation and cooling potentiation of the
isometric twitch, properties which are found only in fast-
twitch and intermediate muscle fibres. The fast-twitch
extensor digitorum longus (EDL) did not show significant
differences in physiological properties compared with
controls. Myosin extracted from control solei and analysed
by pyrophosphate gel electrophoresis, consisted of 88% slow
isoenzyme with 12% intermediate isoenzyme. The myosin of
solei from suspended rats contained only 44% slow isoenzyme,
the rest being intermediate isomyosin. Only minor changes
in myosin isoenzyme distribution were detected in the EDL.
Thus, the imposed change in the pattern of muscle use had
affected the physiological characteristics and myosin
isoenzyme profile of the antigravity soleus muscle,
suggesting that the gravity-induced physiological
stimulation of the soleus muscle through the stretch reflex
is important in maintaining the slow myosin isoenzyme and

the slow-contracting characteristics of the soleus muscle.

INTRODUCTION

There is now considerable evidence that the kinetic properties of the myosin molecule limits the rate of energy transduction from ATP to mechanical work (Close, 1972; Hoh, 1975; Hoh, 1979; Loiselle, Wendt and Hoh, 1982). Skeletal myosin exists in a wide range of isoenzymic forms differing in structure and ATPase activities. The phenotypic expression of specific isomyosins in muscle fibres allows them to be classified into a number of histochemical types according to their myosin ATPase characteristics, each type being associated with distinctive contractile properties.

The extensor digitorum longus (EDL) muscle of the rat is made up principally of fast-twitch motor units (Close, 1967) which correspond to Type IIB fibres. In addition, there are also intermediate motor units and Type IIA fibres. The isomyosin profile is comprised of three fast components together with an intermediate component and a trace of slow myosin (Hoh, Kwan, Dunlop and Kim, 1980). The isometric tension of this muscle is markedly enhanced by a preceeding tetanus (Close and Hoh, 1968a) as well as by a fall in temperature (Close and Hoh, 1968b). These characteristics of fast twitch muscles are referred to as post-tetanic potentiation (PTP) and cooling potentiation respectively.

The rat soleus (SOL) muscle is composed predominantly of slow-twitch motor units which are Type I histochemically. This muscle also contains 15% of Type IIA fibres, corresponding to motor units with intermediate contractile characteristics (Close, 1967; Kugelberg, 1976). The isomyosin profile of this muscle consists of a predominant slow component and a minor intermediate component (Hoh et al., 1980). In contrast to the EDL, the isometric twitch tension of this muscle is reduced by a preceding tetanus (Close and Hoh, 1969) as well as by cooling the muscle below body temperature (Close and Hoh, 1968b).

Isomyosin composition (Bárány and Close, 1971; Hoh, 1975; Hoh et al., 1980) and the contractile characteristics (Close, 1969; Close and Hoh, 1969; Hoh, 1974; Davey, Dunlop, Hoh and Wong, 1981) of skeletal muscles in mature

animals can be altered experimentally by a number of
neural interventions such as nerve cross-union and
cordotomy. These experiments provide evidence that the
nerve supply to the muscle has a specific influence on
muscle gene expression, in particular, the expression of
the myosin phenotype. The regulatory signal through which
nerves influence the expression of muscle genes is thought
to be the pattern of electrical stimulation received by
the muscle. Stimulating a fast-twitch muscle continuously
at 10 Hz, a pattern thought to be characteristic of the
slow-twitch muscle, converts a fast-twitch muscle to a
muscle which expresses the slow myosin phenotype (Salmons
and Sreter, 1976) whereas stimulating a slow-twitch
muscle with infrequent bursts of high frequency leads to the
acquisition of fast-twitch properties (Lomo, Westgard and
Engebretsen, 1980).

The apparent plasticity of skeletal muscle fibre
types in response to experimental neural interventions
suggests that muscle fibres may be able to undergo adaptive
changes in response to altered patterns of use. Indeed,
rearing rats in a centrifuge at 2 g for 3 months results
in solei with 100% Type 1 fibres (Martin and Ormond, 1975).
Since the rat soleus is tonically active when the animal is
in a normal gravitational field (Fischbach and Robbins,
1969), it may be postulated that the normal reflex activity
associated with weight-bearing provides the necessary
stimulus to maintain the anti-gravity muscles in their
slow state. In this study we find support for this concept
by demonstrating that relieving the weight-bearing function
of the hindlimbs of rats causes significant changes in the
isomyosin profile and contractile properties of the soleus
muscle towards those characteristic of fibres of intermediate speed of contraction.

METHODS

The experiments were done on 3-week-old Wistar rats.
By this age the differences in properties between the EDL
and SOL muscles have become well established (Close, 1964).
Rats were suspended by the tail in such a way that only
their forelimbs rested on the floor of the cage. Their
hindquarters were lifted up so that their hindlimbs could
not reach the floor of the cage and thus were relieved of

their normal weight-bearing function. A hook was attached
to the base of the tail using a piece of elastic tape. To
this was attached a wire hanging from a pulley which ran
along a horizontal bar situated at the top of the cage.
This arrangement allowed the rat to move about within the
cage and to have free access to food and water. In order
to permit the rat to rotate about the point of suspension,
a fisherman's swivel was incorporated into the suspension
wire. Rats were suspended for 6 weeks. Control animals of
the same age were kept in similar cages for the same
duration. All animals were 9 weeks old at the time their
muscles were studied.

The techniques and equipment used for recording
isometric contraction, PTP and cooling potentiation were
the same as previously described (Davey *et al.*, 1981)
except that muscles were stimulated directly *in vitro*.
This modification greatly simplified the experimental
procedures but introduced the problem of fatigue. However,
stimulation was kept to a minimum. Fatigue did not affect
contraction time. It may reduce the post-tetanic twitch
tension, hence reducing the measured PTP, but could hardly
affect the observed qualitative change from post-tetanic
depression to PTP in the experimental SOL muscle. After
physiological analyses, muscles were kept in 50% v/v
buffered glycerol at -20°C, pending isomyosin analysis.

The techniques for the extraction of myosin and the
analysis of isomyosins by pyrophosphate gel electrophoresis
have been described previously (Hoh, McGrath and White,
1976).

RESULTS

During the period of suspension by the tail, the rats
were observed to use their hindlimbs in a number of ways.
The most frequent movements were free kicking movements as
if to balance themselves in their attempts to move on the
forelimbs alone. Occasionally, the hindlimbs were used to
scratch the region of the head and the forequarters. The
experimental rats were retarded in growth rate compared
with controls. Their mean body mass at the time of muscle
experiment was 161 ± 21 g (n=6) compared with 263 ± 18 g
(n=9) for controls. In order to compare their muscle

Table 1: Muscle mass per unit body mass for normal (N-SOL, N-EDL) and tail-suspended (S-SOL, S-EDL) soleus (SOL) and extensor digitorum longus (EDL) muscles. The difference between the solei are statistically significant (P < 0.005, t-test). Values given are means ± S.E.

Muscle	Muscle mass (mg/g body mass)
N-SOL (n=7)	0.46 ± 0.04
S-SOL (n=7)	0.25 ± 0.05
N-EDL (n=7)	0.50 ± 0.01
S-EDL (n=6)	0.51 ± 0.04

masses, these masses were expressed as mg per g body mass in Table 1. It can be seen that there had been a marked atrophy of the solei of the tail-suspended rats (S-SOL), whereas the EDL of the tail-suspended rats (S-EDL) remained unchanged with respect to muscle mass relative to body mass

Contractile Properties

Representative isometric twitches in response to direct stimulation *in vitro* of SOL and EDL muscles from control and tail-suspended rats are shown in Fig. 1. It can be seen that the time course of the twitch for the soleus of tail suspended rat (S-SOL) is intermediate between that for the normal EDL (N-EDL) and normal soleus (N-SOL) whereas there is no apparent difference between the time courses for the normal and suspended EDL (S-EDL) muscles. In response to tetanic stimulation, N-EDL and S-EDL showed post-tetanic potentiation of the isometric twitch (PTP) while the twitch of N-SOL was depressed. In contrast to N-SOL, S-SOL showed significant PTP (Fig. 2). Associated with the observed differences in the response to tetanic stimulation were the differences in the pattern of response of these muscles to a change in temperature. N-EDL responded to a fall in temperature of 10 degrees C with a large increase in twitch tension, whereas N-SOL responded with a significant fall. While S-EDL was similar to N-EDL in showing cooling potentiation, S-SOL differed

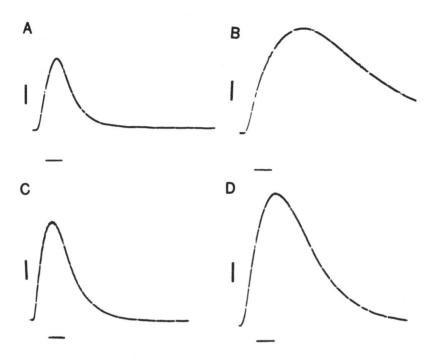

Figure 1: Records of isometric twitches at 35°C of muscles from normal and tail-suspended rats. (A) N-EDL, (B) N-SOL, (C) S-EDL, (D) S-SOL. Horizontal bars represent 10 ms. Tension calibrations for A-D are respectively 9.8, 5.0, 0.98 and 0.4 mN.

from N-SOL by having acquired cooling potentiation (Fig. 3). Table 2 summarizes these properties of normal and experimental muscles. The differences between the mean values of the three contractile parameters for N-SOL and S-SOL are all significant (P < 0.0005, t-test) whereas those between N-EDL and S-EDL are not statistically significant.

Isomyosin distribution

Fig. 4 shows isomyosins from control and experimental muscles separated on pyrophosphate gels. The profiles of isomyosins of N-SOL (Fig. 4A) and N-EDL (Fig. 4E) confirmed

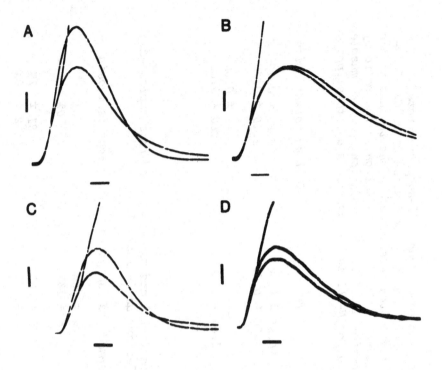

Figure 2. Superimposed records of isometric twitches at 35°C of muscles from normal and tail-suspended rats showing post-tetanic effects on the twitch. (A) N-EDL, (B) N-SOL, (C) S-EDL, (D) S-SOL. In each case except for (C), the lower trace represent the pre-tetanic twitch. The tetanic record can be seen going off the top of the screen. The post-tetanic twitch was applied 10 s after the end of the tetanus of 1 s duration at 200 Hz. Time calibrations: 10 ms. Tension calibrations for A-D are respectively 6.0, 5.0, 1.2 and 0.7 mN.

previous findings outlined in the introduction. The profile for S-SOL (Fig. 4C) showed a marked increase in the amount of intermediate isomyosin so that this component was approximately the same in amount as the slow myosin. Intermediate myosin could be seen to be composed of a major and a faster migrating minor component. This minor component could also be seen in the N-SOL when the gel was

Table 2: *Contractile properties of muscles from normal and tail-suspended rats. Contraction time is the time from onset of contraction to peak tension at 35°C. Post-tetanic potentiation (PTP) is the ratio of the twitch tension before the tetanus to the twitch tension 10 s after the end of the tetanus. Cooling potentiation is the ratio of the twitch tension at 25°C to the twitch tension at 35°C. Abbreviations for the muscles are the same as in Table 1. Note: PTP data for N-EDL is not available due to slipping of many muscles during tetanus.*

Muscle	Contraction time (ms)	PTP	Cooling potentiation
N-SOL (n=6)	32.7 ± 2.0	0.95 ± 0.04	0.80 ± 0.10
S-SOL (n=10)	21.9 ± 3.0	1.20 ± 0.10	1.10 ± 0.10
N-EDL (n=6)	11.8 ± 1.8	---	1.80 ± 0.30
S-EDL (n=11)	13.0 ± 1.1	1.50 ± 0.10	1.80 ± 0.05

Table 3: *Isomyosin profiles of muscles from normal and tail-suspended rats expressed as % of total myosin. Abbreviations for muscles are as in Table 1.*

Muscle	Slow isomyosin	Intermediate isomyosin	Fast isomyosin
N-SOL (n=6)	88 ± 5%	12 ± 5%	0%
S-SOL (n=11)	44 ± 13%	56 ± 13%	0%
N-EDL (n=6)	4 ± 1%	15 ± 8%	81 ± 7%
S-EDL (n=10)	7 ± 3%	21 ± 7%	72 ± 9%

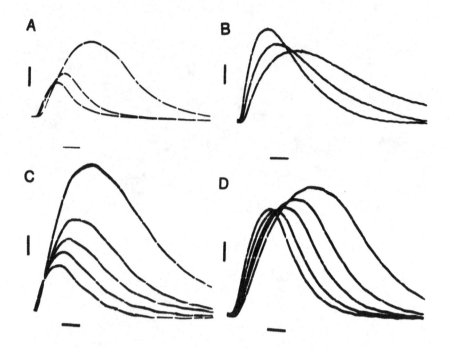

Figure 3: Superimposed records of isometric twitches of muscles from normal and tail-suspended rats showing the effects of temperature. (A) N-EDL, (B) N-SOL, (C) S-EDL and (D) S-SOL. In each case, the record with the slowest time-course was taken at 25°C, the record with the fastest time-course was taken about 10 minutes later at 35°C, the muscle was allowed to be warmed up gradually between these records. Representative contractions at intermediate temperatures are also shown. Time calibrations: 10 ms. Tension calibrations for A-D are respectively 20, 5.0, 2.0 and 0.5 mN.

heavily loaded with myosin. Mixtures of S-SOL myosin and N-SOL (Fig. 4B) and N-EDL (Fig. 4D) showed clearly that the intermediate myosin of S-SOL co-migrated with that from normal muscles. The isomyosin profile of the S-EDL was very similar to that of N-EDL. Table 3 summarizes the isomyosin distribution of normal and experimental muscles. It can be seen that the proportion of slow isomyosin in the S-SOL is half that in N-SOL, the proportion of intermediate

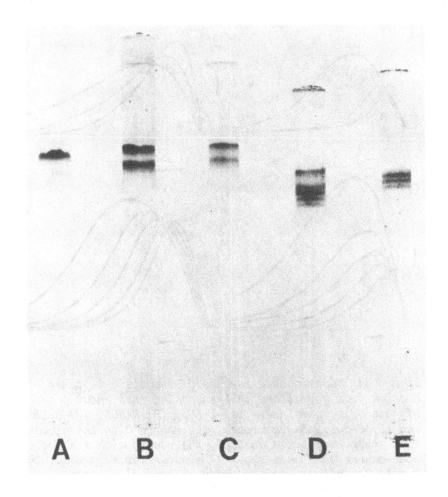

*Figure 4: Electrophoretic analysis by pyrophosphate gels
of myosins extracted from muscles of normal and tail-
suspended rats. (A) N-SOL, (B) mixture of N-SOL and S-SOL,
(D) mixture of S-SOL and N-EDL, (E) N-EDL.*

isomyosin being correspondingly increased. These differences in the profile of isomyosins are highly significant
(P > 0.0005). Interestingly, S-EDL showed a small but
significant increase (P > 0.01) in slow isomyosin associated
with a decrease in fast isomyosins (P > 0.025) compared
with N-EDL.

DISCUSSION

The experiments reported here demonstrate that relieving the hindlimbs of the rat of their weight-bearing function leads to drastic changes in relative muscle mass, physiological and biochemical properties of the anti-gravity soleus muscle, whereas these properties of the fast-twitch muscle undergo little or no change. The changes in contractile properties and isomyosin profile in the S-SOL are reminiscent of similar changes in the solei of cross-reinnervated or cordotomized rats (Hoh, 1974, 1975; Hoh et al., 1980; Davey et al., 1981). There are, however, some noteworthy differences. The mean value of the contraction time of solei of cross-reinnervated and cordotomized rats was about 14 msec in contrast to the much higher value of about 22 msec for S-SOL. This value for S-SOL is within the range for motor units of inter-mediate speed of contraction found by Close (1967). This difference in speed of contraction betwen S-SOL and cross-reinnervated or cordotomized SOL is correlated with a difference in their isomyosin profile. Whereas increase in the intermediate isomyosin was the principal feature in S-SOL, the solei of cross-reinnervated and cordotomized rats showed varied amounts of fast isomyosins which, in some cases, dominate the isomyosin profile. The change in isomyosin in S-SOL is consistent with the interpretation that there has been an increase in the number of inter-mediate motor units. Muscle fibres of intermediate speed of contraction in the mouse have been found to have the property of PTP, though the magnitude of PTP was found to be significantly lower than that in fast-twitch muscle fibres (Luff, 1981). The modest PTP found in S-SOL is consistent with this finding.

Although the electrical activity of the muscles was not monitored, it is reasonable to assume that it was reduced in the S-SOL compared with control muscles. It is unlikely to be abolished, in view of the observed limb movements. This contrasts with the situation in the cordotomized rats in which spontaneous movements were not observed. This difference in the level of activity is correlated with the presence of fast isomyosin in the solei of the more quiescent cordotomized rats. In view of the fact that continuous stimulation at 10 Hz is capable of converting a fast-twitch muscle into a slow-twitch muscle (Salmons and Sreter, 1976) or of maintaining a denervated

slow-twitch muscle in the slow state (Lomo, Westgard and
Engebretsen, 1980), the loss of slow isomyosin in the
soleus of tail-suspended, cross-reinnervated and cordotomized rats suggests that the normal impulse activity due
to the gravitational stimulation of the stretch reflex
associated with the maintenance of normal posture is
necessary for sustaining the slow-twitch characteristics
of the soleus muscle. The small increase in the slow
isomyosin in the S-EDL, too small to be detected physiologically, may be due to gravitational stimulation on this
muscle in the suspended position.

The concept that .the normal impulse activity
associated with postural reflexes provides the necessary
stimulus for maintaining the slow-twitch muscle characteristics effectively ensures that muscle fibres used for
postural function have slow-twitch characteristics. This
auto-regulatory function would ensure that the slow
isomyosin, which is energy efficient for the development
of isometric tension (Goldspink, Larson and Davies, 1970),
is synthesized in muscle fibres which receive constant
gravitational stimulation through the stretch reflex. It
follows from this concept that in zero g environment, such
as encountered in spaceflight, where impulse activity to
postural muscles would be expected to be reduced or
abolished, changes in physiological and biochemical
characteristics of postural muscles similar to those
described in this paper would take place. An opportunity
to test this hypothesis is available in NASA's Spacelab 4,
to be flown in 1985.

The concept of auto-regulation of slow-twitch fibres
has relevance to muscle pathology. It may explain the
observation that there is a general shift of isomyosins in
the direction of slow isomyosin in Duchenne muscular
dystrophy (Fitzsimons and Hoh, 1981) and murine muscular
dystrophy (Fitzsimons and Hoh, 1983). In these diseases,
the impulse activity due to the gravitational stimulus may
be channelled onto the few surviving muscle fibres, causing
a greater proportion of them to express slow-twitch
characteristics than in normal muscles.

Auto-regulation of anti-gravity muscles may have
played a significant role in the evolution of mammals. In
quadrupeds, which use all four limbs for locomotion, limb
extensor muscles are used for postural function, and these

:nus:les are rich in slow-twitch muscle fibres. Alternative
:esponses to the challenge of living in a gravitational
field have been explored by mammals during evolution, for
example, in the development of the erect posture and the
adaptation to arboreal life. These developments would
necessitate changes in the distribution of muscle tone.
Auto-regulation of slow-twitch fibres would ensure the
presence of slow-twitch fibres in the new anti-gravity
muscles. It may be predicted that slow-twitch fibres would
be abundant in limb flexors of arboreal mammals such as
the sloth, in which flexor muscles assume a postural role.
The postulated ability of mammals to auto-regulate the
expression of slow-twitch muscle genes would probably have
played an important role in their evolution by permitting
them to adapt easily to a wide range of habitats involving
novel solutions to the problem of living in a gravitational
environment

REFERENCES

Bárány, M. and Close, R.I. (1971). *J. Physiol. 213*, 455-474.

Close, R. (1964). *J. Physiol. 174*, 74-95.

Close, R. (1967). *J. Physiol. 193*, 45-55.

Close, R. (1969). *J. Physiol. 204*, 331-346.

Close, R.I. (1972). *Physiol. Rev. 52*, 129-197.

Close, R. and Hoh, J.F.Y. (1968a). *J. Physiol. 197*, 461-477.

Close, R. and Hoh, J.F.Y. (1968b). *Nature 217*, 1179-1180.

Close, R. and Hoh, J.F.Y. Hoh (1969). *Nature 221*, 179-181.

Davey, D.F., Dunlop, C., Hoh, J.F.Y. and Wong, S.Y.P. (1981).
    Aust. J. Exp. Biol. Med. Sci. 59, 393-404.

Fischbach, G.D. and Robbins, N. (1969). *J. Physiol. 201*,
    305-320.

Fitzsimons, R.B. and Hoh, J.F.Y. (1981). *J. Neurol. Sci. 52*,
    367-384.

Fitzsimons, R.B. and Hoh, J.F.Y. (1983). *J. Physiol.*, in
    press.

Goldspink, G., Larson, R.E. and Davies, R.E. (1970).
    Z. Vergleich, Physiol. 66, 389-397.

Hoh, J.F.Y. (1974). *Exp. Neurol. 45*, 241-256.

Hoh, J.F.Y. (1975). *Biochemistry 14*, 742-747.

Hoh, J.F.Y. (1979). *In* "Cross-bridge Mechanisms In Muscle
    Contraction" (H. Sugi and G.H. Pollack, eds), p. 489-
    498. University of Tokyo Press, Tokyo.

Hoh, J.F.Y., McGrath, P.A. and White, R.I. (1976). *Biochem.
    J. 157*, 87-95.

Ich, J.F.Y., Kwan, B.T.S., Dunlop, C. and Kim, B.H. (1980).
    In "Plasticity of Muscle" (D. Pette, ed.), p. 339-352.
    Walter de Gruyter, Berlin/New York.
Kugelberg, E. (1976). *J. Neurol. Sci. 27,* 269-289.
Loiselle, D.S., Wendt, I.R. and Hoh, J.F.Y. (1982).
    J. Musc. Res. Cell. Motil. 3, 5-23.
Lomo, T., Westgaard, R.H. and Engebretsen, L. (1980).
    In "Plasticity of Muscle" (D. Pette, ed.), p. 297-309.
    Walter de Gruyter, Berlin/New York.
Luff, A.R. (1981). *J. Physiol. 313,* 161-171.
Martin, W.D. and Ormond, E.H. (1975). *Exp. Neurol. 49,*
    758-771.
Salmons, S. and Sreter, F.A. (1976). *Nature 263,* 30-34.

ACKNOWLEDGEMENT

This work was supported by a grant from the National
Health and Medical Research Council.

LIPOPROTEINS IN PLASMA OF DUCHENNE MUSCULAR DYSTROPHY

PATIENTS AND FEMALE CARRIERS

L. Austin, H. Arthur, R. Iannello, P.L. Jeffrey

Department of Biochemistry, Monash University,

Clayton 3168, Victoria

ABSTRACT

Ultrastructural studies of plasma lipoproteins
isolated from Duchenne muscular dystrophy patients revealed
marked size variations in both very low density lipoproteins
and low density lipoproteins; the former being smaller than
control samples whilst the latter were larger. No significant variations were observed in high density lipoproteins.
Plasma lipid levels and the activities of lipoprotein lipase
and lecithin:cholesterol acyltransferase were comparable in
dystrophic patients and controls and also in carrier females
and controls. Although plasma vitamin A levels were comparable in all samples, significantly reduced levels of
β-carotene and tocopherols were found in dystrophic samples
compared with controls. The present results support the
proposal that the transport function of the plasma lipoproteins may be impaired in Duchenne patients.

INTRODUCTION

During the past decade, a large body of evidence has
been produced in support of the proposal that Duchenne
muscular dystrophy (DMD) is manifested as a membrane
abnormality wherein membrane composition and function are
altered (Kakulas, 1973; Rowland, 1977; Appel and Roses,
1978). Recent findings in this laboratory suggest that
the plasma lipoproteins may be the site of the lesion in DMD

and that as a result, the transport function of the
lipoproteins may be impaired in DMD patients (Arthur et al.,
1983). The plasma lipoproteins play an important role in
the transport of lipids which are essential for the
maintenance of membrane integrity (Nelson, 1972; Smith et
al., 1978). In addition, these lipoproteins function as
carriers of carotenoids and tocopherols (McCormick et al.,
1960; Kayden and Bjornson, 1972; Bjornson et al., 1976).
The tocopherols are known to be potent biological anti-
oxidants and it is generally considered that one of their
major functions is to prevent lipid peroxidation of highly
unsaturated fatty acids in membrane phospholipids (Machlin,
1980). Hence the tocopherols could be expected to contribute substantially to the maintenance of the optimum
degree of membrane fluidity required for proper enzyme
function.

In view of the possible role of the plasma lipoproteins
in DMD, studies were undertaken to examine ultrastructural
aspects of the individual lipoproteins [very low density
(VLDL), low density (LDL) and high density (HDL); the
activities of two major lipolytic enzymes involved in plasma
lipoprotein metabolism, lipoprotein lipase and lecithin:
cholesterol acyltransferase; and the function of the lipoproteins as carriers of the tocopherols, β-carotene and
vitamin A.

METHODS

Samples: Blood samples (10-20 ml) were collected by veni-
puncture after a 12-14 hour fasting period and the plasma
separated by low speed centrifugation (500 g, 15 min, 4°C).
In the course of experimentation, samples were collected
from dystrophic patients and carrier females, together with
age- and sex-matched controls. Lipoprotein components were
fractionated by density gradient ultracentrifugation as
described previously (Arthur et al., 1983).

Electron Microscopy: Isolated lipoprotein fractions were
negatively stained with 2% sodium phosphotungstate, pH 7.2
(Forte et al., 1968) and examined in a Jeol 100S at an
accelerating voltage of 50 kV. Histograms were constructed
with the aid of a Leitz ASM image analyzer.

Lipoprotein Lipase (LPL): LPL activities were determined according to the method described by Korn (1959). Experimental conditions were standardized using post-heparin plasma. However, in view of the physical condition of the dystrophic patients, subsequent experiments were carried out without administration of heparin.

Lecithin:Cholesterol Acyltransferase (LCAT): LCAT measurements were made using Merck System Cholesterol Enzymatic Kits (Dieplinger and Kostner, 1980). This method was also utilized to determine initial free cholesterol levels.

Plasma Lipid Analyses: Lipids were extracted with chloroform:methanol (2:1, v/v) according to the method of Folch et al. (1957). Lipid samples were applied to SII Chromarods, developed in dichloroethane:chloroform:acetic acid (92:8:0.1, v/v) and analyses performed using an Iatroscan equipped with a flame ionization detector and integrator. Cholesterol acetate was used as an internal standard and values are expressed as Internal Standard Units (ISU = Area under unknown peak/Area under internal standard peak).

Tocopherol Assays: Estimation of tocopherol levels in plasma and erythrocyte membranes was performed spectrofluorometrically (Taylor et al., 1976). Preparation of erythrocyte membranes has been described previously (Austin et al., 1983). Tocopherol recoveries were estimated using D-α-[^{3}H]-tocopherol.

β-Carotene and Vitamin A Assays: The micromethod of determination as described by Neeld and Pearson (1963) was utilized in these assays.

Plasma Absorption Spectra: Plasma samples were first diluted 1:6 with physiological saline and absorption profiles recorded over the range 380 to 550 nm with a Varian spectrophotometer.

Protein Determinations: Plasma and erythrocyte protein concentrations were measured using a modified method of Lowry et al. (1951). With lipoprotein samples, the method of Kashyap et al. (1980) was used when necessary.

RESULTS AND DISCUSSION

Previous analyses of lipoprotein fractions separated
from plasma obtained from DMD patients and carriers of the
disease showed significant decreases in LDL absorbance at
435 nm when compared with controls. Alterations in HDL
absorbance profiles were also observed (Arthur et al., 1983).
Since carotenoids are major contributors to absorbance at
this wavelength, absorption spectra of plasma samples were
prepared over the range 380-550 nm. In DMD plasma, absorbance in the range 420-425 nm was reduced with a marked
decrease also being observed in the 440-480 nm region
(Fig. 1). Authentic β-carotene in petroleum ether displays
absorbance maxima at approximately 420, 450 and 480 nm
(Bjornson et al., 1976). Since agarose gel electrophoresis
of isolated lipoproteins showed abnormal migration characteristics for LDL fractions from DMD patients (Arthur et al.,
1983), these results could be indicative of decreased carry-
ing capacity of the LDL from dystrophics.

Electron microscopic examination of isolated lipoproteins showed variations in both VLDL and LDL in DMD
samples when compared with controls. VLDL particles from
controls displayed a larger distribution area than did
DMD particles, with the latter being noticeably smaller in
the major peak area (Fig. 2). In contrast, the LDL particles from DMD samples were found to be larger overall;
again the control distribution covered a larger class range
(Fig. 3). Although some shift towards smaller HDL molecules
was observed in particles isolated from DMD patients, no
significant size variation was found (Fig. 4).

To eliminate the possibility of there being an underlying enzymatic cause for the variations observed, the
major lipolytic enzymes involved in lipoprotein metabolism
were examined. No significant differences in LPL activities were found in DMD patients and carriers and their
respective controls (Table 1). It was noted, however,
that there was an increase in activity with increasing age
of the subject. In addition, in the same age brackets,
activities observed in females were invariably lower than
those observed in males. The other major enzyme involved
in lipoprotein metabolism which was examined was LCAT. In
view of the fact that levels of free cholesterol are
intimately related to the activity of this plasma enzyme,

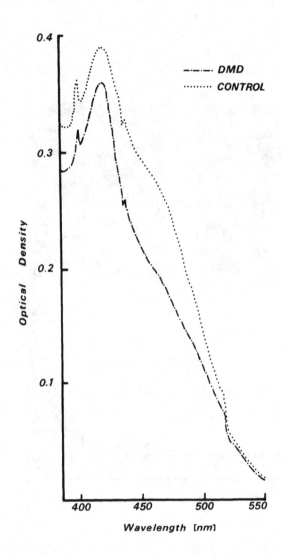

Figure 1: *Absorption spectra of DMD and control plasma*
samples. Plasma was first diluted 1:6 with physiological
saline.

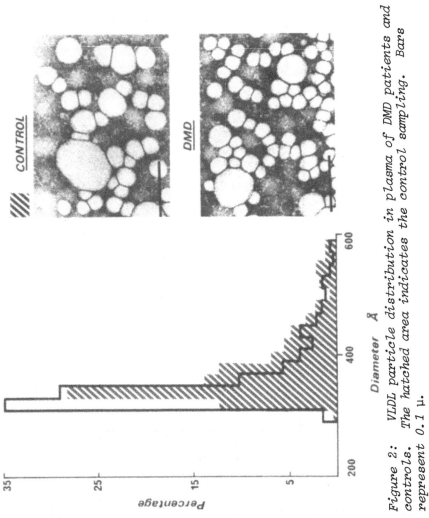

Figure 2: VLDL particle distribution in plasma of DMD patients and controls. The hatched area indicates the control sampling. Bars represent 0.1 μ.

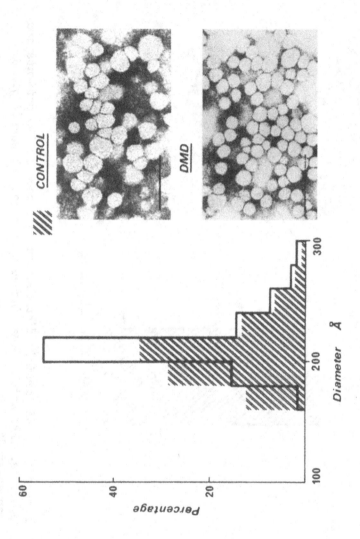

Figure 3:   *LDL particle distribution in plasma of DMD patients and controls. The hatched area indicates the control sampling. Bars represent 0.1 μ.*

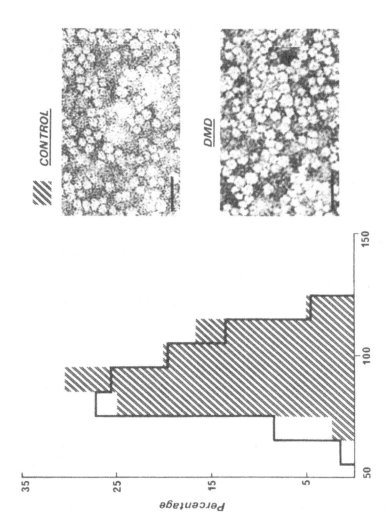

Figure 4: HDL particle distribution in plasma of DMD patients and controls. The hatched area indicates the control sampling. Bars represent 250 A.

these levels were first determined and subsequent results
expressed in terms of initial free cholesterol. No significant differences were seen in either free cholesterol
levels (Table 2) or total lipid (Table 3). LCAT assays
also showed no significant variations in DMD patients,
carriers or controls (Table 4). These results indicate
that any abnormalities observed in lipoprotein absorbance
profiles cannot be attributed to lipolytic enzymes but
rather to some other factor.

The structural variations observed in VLDL and LDL
particles could therefore be indicative of an alteration
in transport ability of the lipoproteins in DMD. Whilst
no significant differences were observed in plasma vitamin
A content, significantly reduced levels of β-carotene and
tocopherols were seen in DMD plasma compared with controls.
A significant reduction in erythrocyte tocopherol was also
observed in DMD samples (Table 5). The values obtained in
these experiments are in reasonable agreement with previously published normal values (Neeld and Pearson, 1963;
Mino et al., 1979). It is well documented that nutritional muscular dystrophy can be induced in many animal
species by feeding a diet deficient in tocopherols (Scott,
1980; Machlin, 1980). This condition can, however, be
reversed with supplementation of the vitamin. Conversely,
human sufferers of muscular dystrophy do not respond to
treatment with elevated levels of tocopherols (Rowland,
1977; Scott, 1980). This inability to alleviate the
symptoms of muscular dystrophy with supplementation of
tocopherols could be explained if it were an impairment of
the transport system rather than an inadequate supply of
the vitamin. Since all known membrane abnormalities
observed in DMD can be explained on the basis of a deficiency in tocopherols (Machlin, 1980), our results suggest
that a defective transport system for tocopherol may be
the underlying metabolic cause in DMD. Furthermore, since
the LDL are the major transport system for tocopherols
(McCormick et al., 1960; Kayden and Bjornson, 1972;
Bjornson et al., 1976), it appears that it may be the
protein moiety of the LDL which is predominantly affected.
These results suggest that the primary protein defect
which results from the mutation leading to DMD is apo-
lipoprotein B.

Table 1.   Plasma Lipoprotein Lipase Activities in DMD Patients, Carriers and Controls.

Age (Years)	No. of Subjects	Activity (nmoles glycerol/ml/min)	
		DMD	Control
4-8	3	1.78 ± 1.25	1.98 ± 0.84
11-12	6	2.70 ± 0.90	2.11 ± 0.85
17-22	3	5.19 ± 2.24	4.15 ± 1.53
Total	12	3.09 ± 0.73	2.57 ± 0.62
		Carrier	Control
21-42	11	1.95 ± 0.40	2.00 ± 0.57

T-Test Analysis: P >0.05

Table 2.   Plasma Free Cholesterol Levels in DMD Patients, Carriers and Controls.

Age (Years)	No. of Subjects	Cholesterol (mM)	
		DMD	Control
4	3	0.87 ± 0.18	0.92 ± 0.05
6-8	6	0.86 ± 0.17	0.82 ± 0.16
11-12	8	0.71 ± 0.07	0.76 ± 0.08
17-22	6	0.66 ± 0.09	0.68 ± 0.07
Total	23	0.76 ± 0.06	0.76 ± 0.05
		Carrier	Control
21.42	6	1.17 ± 0.17	0.98 ± 0.03

T-Test Analysis: P >0.05

Table 3. Lipid Analyses of Plasma Samples Collected from DMD Patients, Carriers and Controls.

Lipid Component	DMD (12)* ISU/mg Protein	%	Control (12)* ISU/mg Protein	%
CE	3.88 ± 0.45	21.6	3.17 ± 0.28	19.9
C	0.94 ± 0.08	5.2	0.91 ± 0.13	5.7
PL	13.16 ± 4.50	73.2	11.85 ± 4.18	74.4
	Carrier (5)*		Control (5)*	
CE	5.76 ± 1.25	25.0	4.24 ± 1.16	18.0
C	1.14 ± 0.40	5.0	0.94 ± 0.17	4.0
PL	16.10 ± 6.40	70.0	18.33 ± 6.19	78.0

* Number of subjects. T-Test Analysis: P >0.05

Table 4. Plasma LCAT Activities in DMD Patients, Carriers and Controls.

Sample	No. of Subjects	Activity/Initial Cholesterol (μM/hr/mM)
DMD	23	83.56 ± 14.67
Control	23	97.38 ± 19.15
Carrier	6	45.70 ± 9.89
Control	6	46.73 ± 16.93

T-Test Analysis: P >0.05

Table 5. *Vitamin and Carotenoid Assays on Samples
Collected from DMD Patients and Controls.*

	DMD	Control
Tocopherols		
Plasma (μg/ml)	***7.62 ± 1.0 (10)[a]	13.04 ± 1.6 (10)
Erythrocyte membranes (μg/mg protein)	**0.304±0.005 (16)	0.458±0.009 (19)
β-Carotene		
(μg/ml plasma)	*2.74 ± 0.37 (12)	3.35 ± 0.24 (14)
Vitamin A		
(μg/ml plasma)	0.188±0.095 (12)	0.246±0.971 (12)

[a] Number of subjects
*** $P < 0.001$
 ** < 0.01
  * < 0.05

ACKNOWLEDGMENTS

This project was supported by grants from the National
Health and Medical Research Council and the Victorian
Muscular Dystrophy Association. In addition, we thank
Stephen Morton and Barry Veitch for their excellent
technical assistance.

REFERENCES

Appel, S.H., and Roses, A.D. (1978). *In* "The Metabolic
    Basis of Inherited Disease: (J.B. Stanbury, J.B.
    Wyngaarden and D.S. Fredrickson, eds.), p.1260,
    McGraw-Hill Book Co., New York.
Arthur, H., de Niese, M., Jeffrey, P.L., and Austin, L.
    (1983). *Biochem. Int. 6,* 307.

Austin, L., Katz, S., Jeffrey, P.L., Shield, L., and
    Arthur, H. (1983). *J. Neurol. Sci.* (in press).
Bjornson, L.K., Kayden, H.J., Miller, E., and Moshell, A.N.
    (1976). *J. Lipid Res.* *179*, 343.
Dieplinger, H., and Kostner, G.M. (1980). *Clin. Chim.
    Acta.* *106*, 319.
Folch, J., Lees, M., and Sloane Stanley, G.H. (1957).
    J. Biol. Chem. *226*, 497.
Forte, G.M., Nichols, A.V., and Glaeser, R.M. (1968).
    Chem. Phys. Lipids, *2*, 396.
Kakulas, B.A. (ed.), (1973). "Basic Research in Myology",
    Excerpta Medica, Amsterdam.
Kashyap, M.L., Hynd, B.A., and Robinson, K. (1980).
    J. Lipid Res. *21*, 491.
Kayden, H.J., and Bjornson, L.K. (1972). *Ann. N.Y. Acad.
    Sci.* *203*, 127.
Korn, E.D. (1959). *Metd. Biochem. Anal.* *7*, 145.
Lowry, O.H., Rosebrough, N.J., Farr, A.L., and Randall,
    R.J. (1951). *J. Biol. Chem.* *193*, 265.
Machlin, L.J. (ed.), (1980). "Vitamin E : A Comprehensive
    Treatise", Marcel Dekker Inc., New York.
McCormick, E.C., Cornwell, D.G., and Brown, J.B. (1960).
    J. Lipid Res. *1*, 221.
Mino, M., Nishida, Y., Kijima, Y., Iwakoshi, M., and
    Nakagawa, S. (1979). *J. Nutri. Sci. Vitaminol.* *25*, 505.
Neeld, J.B., Jr., and Pearson, W.N. (1963). *J. Nutr.*
    79, 454.
Nelson, G.J. (ed.), (1972). "Blood Lipids and
    Lipoproteins : Quantitation, Composition, and
    Metabolism", Wiley-Interscience, New York.
Rowland, L.P. (ed.), (1977). "Pathogenesis of the Human
    Muscular Dystrophies", Excerpta Medica, Amsterdam.
Scott, M.L. (1980). *Fed. Proc.* *39*, 2736.
Smith, L.C., Pownall, H.J., and Gotto, A.M. Jr. (1978).
    Ann. Rev. Biochem. *47*, 751.
Taylor, S.L., Lamden, M.P., and Tappel, A.L. (1976).
    Lipids, *11*, 530.

TROPHIC INFLUENCES OF NERVE ON SKELETAL MUSCLE SARCOLEMMA

Peter L. Jeffrey

Biochemistry Department, Monash University

Clayton, Victoria, Australia

John A.P. Rostas

Neuroscience Group, Faculty of Medicine
University of Newcastle

New South Wales, Australia

Wing Nang Leung

Biochemistry Department,
Chinese University of Hong Kong

Shatin, N.T. Hong Kong

ABSTRACT

Following surgical denervation, the combined effects
of the absence of neural impulse activity and neurotrophic
(non-impulse) factors are responsible for the changes
reported in muscle metabolism. This study attempts to
evaluate the relative contributions of these factors by
comparing the effects of denervation and the blockage of
neural impulse activity on various biochemical parameters
of mixed muscle sarcolemma. Muscle paralysis was induced
by repeated injection of Tetrodotoxin (TTx) to the sciatic
nerve. After seven days of inactivity the isolated sarcolemma was analyzed for protein and glycoprotein composition,

Na^+/K^+ ATPase activity, Concanavalin A binding to intact
sarcolemma and to carbohydrate components separated in
SDS-polyacrylamide gels and sialyl and galactosyl transferase activity.

The results have shown that following muscle inactivity
all of the parameters except glycosyl transferases changed
in a similar manner but to a lesser degree than denervation.
It is concluded that trophic factors in addition to neural
impulse activity play a role in the regulation of a number
of surface membrane properties. These results are compared with other membrane parameters which are known to be
under a similar control.

                        INTRODUCTION

    The influence of nerve on skeletal muscle occurs at
two levels: firstly, neural impulse activity in the form
of transmitter release at the neuromuscular junction and
secondly, a trophic influence involving the delivery of
trophic substances by axonal transport and their release
at the neuromuscular junction. Surgical denervation has
been shown to result in a variety of changes in physiological, biochemical and structural properties of muscle
fibres. The effects of denervation on these properties can
be attributed to the sum of neural (impulse) activity and
neurotrophic (non-impulse) factors.

    The evidence for trophic effects of nerve on muscle
has accumulated over the past decade (Guth, 1968; Guth et
al., 1981; Gutmann, 1976). The existence of soluble
protein neurotrophic factors has been inferred from experiments where the changes in muscle are dependent on length
of nerve stump remaining after denervation (Gutman et al.,
1955) and such factors have been identified in studies
where protein factors have been shown to influence the
development and maintenance of various properties of
skeletal muscle cells (Oh and Markelonis, 1978; Oh et al.,
1980; Younkin et al., 1978; Lentz et al., 1981). A number
of workers have attempted to differentiate between the
effects of these multiple influences of the nerve on muscle
by causing either electrical inactivity of the nerve or
disuse of the muscle while the nerve is intact and physically related to the muscle as in the normal situation

(Bray et al., 1979; Lavoie et al., 1976; Pestronk et al.,
1976,a; Stanley and Drachman, 1979, 1980).

As one approach to distinguishing between the role of
neurotrophic factors and contractile activity in influencing muscle fibre processes we have used Tetrodotoxin (TTx)
to block impulse conduction in the sciatic nerve by a
specific block of sodium conductance. Tetrodotoxin was
chosen because under the conditions used here it has been
shown not to cause side effects such as nerve degeneration
or blockade of axonal transport (Anderson and Edström,
1973; Lavoie et al., 1976; Bray et al., 1979). Tetrodotoxin was applied to the sciatic nerve by repeated epineural injection. After 7 days of muscle inactivity sarcolemmal membranes were isolated and analysed for protein,
glycoprotein and a number of membrane enzymes. The results
were compared to those found with normal and denervated
sarcolemma. Previous workers have investigated the effect
of paralysis on the physiological properties of muscle and
have found evidence for trophic factors by measuring parameters such as the resting membrane potential (Bray et al.,
1979; Drachman et al., 1982; Stanley and Drachman, 1980)
AChR density (Drachman et al., 1982; Lavoie et al., 1976;
Pestronk et al., 1976,a) soluble proteins including lactate
dehydrogenase, pyruvate kinase and creatine kinase (Wan
and Boegman, 1981,a), sarcoplasmic reticulum ATPase and
Ca^{++} uptake (Wan and Boegman, 1981,b) and autolytic enzyme
activity (Boegman and Scarth, 1981). We have extended
these studies to examine the effect of muscle paralysis on
a number of biochemical properties of purified sarcolemmal
membranes which have been shown to alter following surgical
denervation (Jeffrey et al., 1979, 1981, 1983; Leung et al.,
1982).

                        MATERIALS AND METHODS

Tetrodotoxin (TTx) obtained in crystalline form
(Boehringer Mannheim GmbH) was dissolved in Ringer's
solution (pH 7.2) to a final concentration of 1 µg/µl.
Female Sprague-Dawley rats (250-300 g) were anaesthetized
with ether during all operations. The sciatic nerve was
exposed by making an incision in the mid-thigh. Tetrodotoxin was injected into the epineural space of the left

sciatic nerve using a fine micropipetter (10 microlitres,
50A-RM micropipetter). Each injection contained 2 µg of
Tetrodotoxin in 2 µl Ringer's solution. The wounds were
sutured with Michel surgical clips and an antibiotic spray
was applied to prevent infection. The right sciatic
nerve was also surgically exposed without TTx injection
to provide a sham operated normal innervated control.
Paralysis of the hind leg muscle of the operated side
developed in less than 10 min and the paralysis lasted for
48 hours. The completeness of paralysis was checked from
time to time by examining the operated side for toe-spread-
ing reflex action of the legs (Blunt and Vrbova, 1975).
By means of repeated injections at 48 hour intervals,
paralysis could be maintained for at least 7 days without
nerve damage.

At the end of 7 days of complete paralysis, the rats
were sacrificed and the soleus, extensor digitorum longus,
anterior tibialis and gastrocnemius muscles were taken
from both sides. A second group of rats surgically denervated for 7 days were also sacrificed and sarcolemma
prepared concurrently with the normal and TTx paralysed
muscle. Muscle denervation and membrane isolation was
carried out as described previously (Andrew and Appel,
1973; Jeffrey et al., 1979).

Na^+/K^+ ATPase assay was modified from Post and Sen
(1967). The assay mixture for determining total ATPase
contained: 30 mM imidazole, 30 mM glycylglycine, 5 mM
$MgCl_2$, 0.5 mM EDTA, 100 mM NaCl and 20 mM KCl, pH 7.4.
The amount of total ATPase activity inhibited by 0.4 mM
ouabain was attributed to Na^+/K^+ ATPase. Phosphate was
determined by the method of Taussky and Shorr (1953).

Methods for SDS polyacrylamide slab gel electrophoresis, glycosyltransferase assay, ^{125}I-ConA binding
to sarcolemmal membrane components separated in SDS
polyacrylamide gels and quantitative ConA binding to
sarcolemmal membranes were as previously described (Jeffrey
et al., 1979).

RESULTS

MUSCLE ATROPHY

The wet weights of mixed muscles taken per rat were compared in normal, denervated and Tetrodotoxin treated muscles. The muscle weight following 7 days denervation decreased by 23% and the decrease in TTx paralysed muscles was 17% (Table 1).

SARCOLEMMAL POLYPEPTIDE PATTERN

On examination of the optical density profiles of membrane distribution following continuous sucrose density gradient centrifugation, the membranes isolated from the TTx-treated muscle showed a slight shift to a lighter sucrose density, banding at an intermediate position between normal and denervated membrane. Whether this change in buoyant density reflects an altered lipid composition or more likely an alteration in the vesiculated nature of denervated and TTx-membrane requires further investigation. The field of sarcolemmal membrane protein per gm of original muscle was similar in all muscle groups and hence allows satisfactory biochemical analyses to be carried out.

SDS-polyacrylamide slab gel electrophoresis (SDS-PAGE) was performed on the sarcolemmal fractions of normal, denervated and TTx treated mixed muscle, prepared at the same time. Polypeptide composition of sarcolemma prepared from TTx treated muscle was similar to the denervated pattern (Figure I,a). They were indistinguishable from the normal except that the 28,000 dalton species was decreased slightly. In all three types of muscle membrane preparations, the SDS-PAGE revealed 6 major polypeptide species of 95-100,000, 70-75,000, 66-69,000, 27-28,500, 25-27,000 and 22-25,000 daltons together with some minor species in agreement with previously published patterns (Jeffrey et al., 1979, 1981).

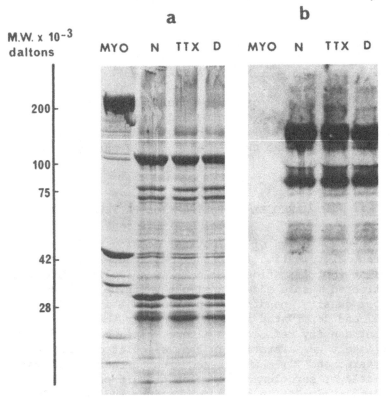

Figure 1. SDS polyacrylamide slab gel electrophoresis of sarcolemmal preparations from normal, Tetrodotoxin treated and denervated mixed muscle: protein and glycoprotein composition.

A.   *Polypeptide composition of sarcolemmal preparations from: N) normal mixed muscle; TTx) Tetrodotoxin treated mixed muscle; D) denervated mixed muscle and MYO) rat muscle myofibrils.*

B.   *Glycoprotein composition: audoradiogram of ^{125}I-ConA bound to glycoprotein in gel shown in A.*

Each sample contained 55 μg protein. MYO were included as molecular weight reference standards and to act as an internal control for the specificity of the ^{125}I-ConA binding since myofibrils contain no ConA binding glycoproteins.

ATPase ACTIVITY

Table 1 shows the ATPase activity of the sarcolemmal fractions from normal, Tetrodotoxin treated and denervated muscle. Na^+/K^+ ATPase activities measured in both the denervated and TTx treated sarcolemma were significantly higher than the normal value but denervation caused a greater increase in ATPase activity than did the toxin induced paralysis.

GLYCOPROTEIN COMPOSITION

^{125}I-ConA Binding to Components Separated by SDS-PAGE

Lectin binding was used as a measure of glycoprotein changes since glycolipids account for less than 10% of the membrane bound carbohydrate (Inestrosa and Fernandez, 1982). ^{125}I-Concanavalin A was bound to polypeptides separated by SDS-polyacrylamide slab gel electrophoresis and the ConA binding species were revealed by autoradiography (Figure 1,b). No gross differences could be detected in normal, denervated and TTx sarcolemma. The majority of ^{125}I-ConA was bound in two regions with apparent molecular weights of 120-160,000 and 78-85,000 daltons. The amount of ^{125}I-ConA bound to the separated components was similar in all three preparations.

Quantitative ^{125}I-ConA Binding to Intact Sarcolemma

Table 1 shows the average values for N (number of binding sites x 10^{14}/mg membrane protein) and K_D (apparent intrinsic dissociation constant) from all experiments. Figure 2 shows results obtained in one representative experiment. TTx caused an increase in ConA binding to sarcolemma membrane, but the extent of the increase was less than that produced by denervation. When the data was analyzed by Scatchard plot it was apparent that the increase was due to an increase in N without a significant change in K_D. The increase in N following denervation in this group of animals was in the lower part of the range described for a larger group of animals (Jeffrey et al., 1979, 1981). This fact combined with the small number of

Table 1. Biochemical parameters of normal, denervated and TTx treated muscle and sarcolemmal membranes.

	N	TTx	DN
Muscle wet weight	5.0	4.2	3.8
Na^+/K^+ ATPase	17.1 ± 0.3	20.3 ± 0.3	21.9 ± 0.2
Quantitative ConA binding			
N	2.1 ± 0.02	5.5 ± 2.1	6.3 ± 1.9
K_D	0.8 ± 0.4	1.23 ± 0.5	1.2 ± 0.7
Glycosyl transferase activity			
Sialyl	21.5 ± 1.7	34.3 ± 5.4	29.3 ± 0.9
Galactosyl	119 ± 11	289 ± 87	185 ± 27

N = normal mixed muscle
TTx = Tetrodotoxin paralysed muscle
DN = Surgically denervated muscle
Muscle wet weight (gm/rat) are the average of two separate preparations agreeing within 5%.
Na^+/K^+ ATPase (μmoles Pi released hr/mg membrane protein) was measured as described in Methods. N is the number of binding sites x 10^{14}/mg membrane protein and K_D is Intrinsic Dissociation Constant x 10^{-7} M). Glycosyl transferase enzyme activities are expressed as p moles sugar incorporated/mg membrane protein. All results are expressed as mean ± SD and are the average of duplicate determinations of at least two separated preparations.

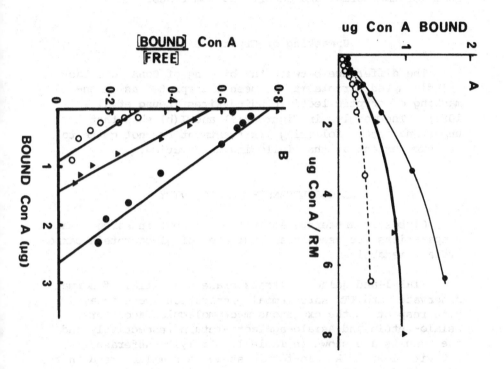

Figure 2. Binding of ^{125}I*-ConA to sarcolemmal membrane preparations.*

A. *Specific* ^{125}I*-ConA binding to sarcolemmal membrane preparations as a function of ConA concentration. Specific binding is the difference between total binding and that in the presence of 0.05 M α-methyl mannoside.*

B. *Scatchard plots for* ^{125}I*-ConA binding to sarcolemmal membrane preparations. Plots determined from data in A.*

    O Normal; ● 7-day denervated; ▲ TTx-treated

animals in the TTx group meant that the difference between
TTx-treated and denervated does not quite reach significance (p >0.1). Nevertheless in each experiment the value
for TTx-treated membranes was always intermediate between
that for the normal and denervated membranes.

Unmasking of Cryptic Sites

The difference between the binding of ConA to intact
and disrupted sarcolemma has been interpreted as an unmasking of cryptic lectin binding sites (Leung et al.,
1982). The results in Figure 2(a) and I(b) show that
unmasking occurs following TTx treatment but not quite to
the same extent as that following denervation.

GLYCOSYLTRANSFERASE ACTIVITY

Glycosyltransferase activities present in sarcolemmal
preparations are used as an indicator of glycoprotein carbohydrate metabolism.

Sialyl-and galactosyltransferase activities of normal,
denervated and TTx sarcolemmal preparations were assayed
with respect to the exogenous macromolecular acceptors,
Asialo-fetuin and Asialo-agalacto-fetuin respectively and
the results are shown in Table 1. Sialyltransferase
activity towards Asialo-fetuin showed a similar trend in the
denervated and TTx-treated sarcolamma. Both values were
increased over normal and no statistically significant
difference was found between TTx and denervated membranes.
Galactosyl transferase activity showed similar results, an
increase with the denervated and TTx-treated sarcolemma
with no statistically significant difference between them.

DISCUSSION

Previous work from this laboratory has shown that
denervation produces significant changes in the glycoproteins on the surfaces of skeletal muscles without any
major changes in polypeptide composition. These changes
can be detected as increased membrane-bound carbohydrate,
increased glycosyltransferase activities to exogenous

acceptors and an increased specific binding of labelled
lectins. In addition based on the difference between the
binding of lectins to intact and disrupted sarcolemmal
membranes, we have postulated that, apart from the alterations in glycoprotein metabolism and/or number, denervation
also results in an altered geometric arrangement (Leung
et al., 1982). In order to examine the role of trophic
factors in maintaining these properties of muscle membranes
we have determined the effect of tetrodotoxin induced
paralysis on some of these biochemical parameters.

From the studies reported here and others in the
literature, the effect on muscle metabolism of TTx-induced
blockade of electrical activity in the nerve can be divided
into 3 groups.

Firstly, the case where TTx has no effect and as such
the parameter is fully under the control of trophic factors
or intrinsic genetic factors. Muscle metabolic parameters
which fall into this class include; soleus wet weight in
mice (Boegman and Scarth, 1981) and rat (Wan and Boegman,
1981,b); soluble proteins of the soleus (Wan and Boegman,
1981,a) and EDL (Wan and Boegman, 1980) muscles of rat;
pyruvate kinase activity (Wan and Boegman, 1981,a); Ca^{++}
uptake and loading in soleus fragmented sarcoplasmic reticulum vesicles 40 days after treatment and Ca-ATPase
activity after 20 days treatment with TTx (Wan and Boegman,
1981,b). Although these latter parameters of fragmented
sarcoplasmic reticulum vesicles may be partially under the
influence of trophic factors as the effects vary with the
time of TTx treatment.

The second and largest class comprises those parameters
in which TTx treatment leads to an effect intermediate
between normal control and denervation values. As such
trophic factors in addition to muscle activity play a role
in regulating these muscle metabolic processes. In our
studies, the weight of mixed muscles obtained per rat, the
sarcolemmal profile obtained following continuous sucrose
gradient centrifugation; the sarcolemmal Na^{+}/K^{+} ATPase
activity and the cryptic nature of ^{125}I-ConA binding to
intact sarcolemma fall into this group. Other membrane
parameters which fall into this class include AChR density
of soleus and EDL muscles (Pestronk et al., 1976,a; Drachman
et al., 1982) numbers of AChR's in soleus and EDL muscles

(Lavoie et al., 1976; Bray et al., 1979) soleus muscle
resting membrane potential (RMP) (Bray et al., 1979) and
muscle cholinesterase activity (Younkin et al., 1978).
However, Drachman et al. (1982) found that the RMP in TTx
soleus muscle fell with a longer latency and slower rate
but ultimately reached the denervation value on the 7th day.
The reason for this discrepancy between these workers is
unclear but may be related to injection technique. Metabolic
changes which fall into this class include creatine kinase
and lactic dehydrogenase activity (Wan and Boegman, 1981,a),
autolytic activities including acidic protease, glucosamin-
idase, phosphatase and fucosidase activity (Boegman and
Scarth, 1981)

The final group comprises those parameters where the
changes are equivalent for TTx-treatment and denervation.
Thus these parameters are apparently not under any trophic
control but totally impulse dependent. Our results on
sarcolemmal sialyl and galactosyl transferase activities
fall into this group where no significant difference was
found between TTx-treatment and denervation. The only other
metabolic parameter reported which falls into this class is
the protein content of soleus and EDL muscles reported by
Bray et al. (1979). It is interesting to note that protein
content of muscles has been reported from different laboratories to fall into each of the three groups defined
here. Thus, when comparing metabolic changes in muscle the
method of application of drugs must be carefully considered.

From the data now available it can be seen that
different intrinsic muscle properties respond to trophic
regulation differently. Thus, the factors involved in each
property must be evaluated individually. Some similar
examples can be found in the literature. Although botulinum
toxin treatment of nerve affects extrajunctional AChR
density to a lesser degree than denervation treatment
(Pestronk et al., 1976,b) it completely reproduces the
effect of denervation with respect to the isometric contraction of muscle. Another possibility may be that different properties may change at a different rate on TTx treatment. Some may have a longer latency and slower time course
at the beginning but then reach the same value as that of
denervated muscles at later times. Since the fast and slow-
twitch type fibres may respond to the muscle inactivity
differently (Pestronk et al., 1976,a) in future studies,

the examination of TTx effect on the two fibre types separately and the use of other toxins affecting neuromuscular transmission may yield more valuable information.

In conclusion, by selectively blocking impulse conduction in nerves innervating skeletal muscle, it was demonstrated a trophic influence played an important but variable role in the neural regulation of the muscle surface membrane properties. The finding that spontaneous non-quantal ACh release can account for the trophic regulation of RMP and extrajunctional ACh receptors poses some interesting questions over the nature of these neurotrophic factors (Drachman et al., 1982).

ACKNOWLEDGEMENTS

We would like to acknowledge the technical assistance of J.W. Scheffer and photographic assistance of S. Morton. This work was supported by a grant from the Muscular Dystrophy Association of America. J.A.P. Rostas was a Queen Elizabeth II Research Fellow.

REFERENCES

Anderson, K.E., and Edström, A. (1973). *Brain Res. 50*, 125.
Andrew, C.G., and Appel, S.H. (1973). *J. Biol. Chem. 248*, 5156.
Boegman, R.J., and Scarth, B. (1981), *Exp. Neurol. 73*, 37.
Blunt, R.J., and Vrbova, G. (1975), *Pflüegers Arch. 357*, 187.
Bray, J.J., Hubbard, J.I., and Mills R.G. (1979). *J. Physiol. (London), 297*, 479.
Drachman, D.B., Stanley, E.B., Pestronk, A., Griffin, J.W., and Price, D.L. (1982). *Jnl. Neurosc. 2*, 232.
Guth, L. (1968). *Physiol. Rev., 48*, 645.
Guth, L., Kemerer, V.F., Samaras, T.A., Warnick, J.E., and Albuquerque, E.X. (1981). *Exp. Neurol. 73*, 20.
Gutman, E. (1976). *Ann. Rev. Physiol., 38*, 177.
Gutman, E., Vodicka, Z., and Zelena, J. (1955). *Physiol. Bohemoslov., 4*, 200.
Inestrosa, N.C., and Fernandez, H.L. (1982). *Muscle & Nerve, 5*, 33.
Jeffrey, P.L., and Appel, S.H. (1978). *Exp. Neurol. 61*, 432.

Jeffrey, P.L., Leung, W.N., and Rostas, J.A.P. (1979).
    In "Muscle, Nerve and Brain Degeneration" (A.D. Kidman
    and J.K. Tomkins, eds.), p.32. Excerpta Medica,
    Amsterdam.

Jeffrey, P.L., Leung, W.N., and Rostas, J.A.P. (1981).
    In "New Approaches to Nerve and Muscle Disorders.
    Basic and Applied Contributions" (A.D. Kidman,
    J.K. Tomkins and R.A. Westerman, eds.), p.66.
    Excerpta Medica Amsterdam.

Jeffrey, P.L., Leung, W.N., and Rostas, J.A.P. (1983).
    In "Molecular Aspects of Neurological Disorders"
    (L. Austin and P.L. Jeffrey, eds.) p83. Academic
    Press, Sydney.

Lavoie, P.A., Collier, B., and Tenenhouse, A. (1976).
    Nature 260, 349.

Lentz, T.L., Addis, J.S., and Chester, J. (1981). *Exp.
    Neurol. 73*, 542.

Leung, W.N., Jeffrey, P.L., and Rostas, J.A.P. (1982).
    Neurosci. Letts. 30, 31.

Oh, T.H., and Markelonis, G.J. (1978). *Science 200*, 337.

Oh, T.H., Markelonis, G.J., Reier, P.J., and Zalewski, A.A.
    (1980). *Exp. Neurol. 67*, 646.

Pestronk, A., Drachman, D.B., and Griffin, J.W. (1976a).
    Nature 260, 352.

Pestronk, A., Drachman, D.B., and Griffin, J.W. (1976b).
    Nature 264, 787.

Post, R.L., and Sen, A.K. (1967). *Methods Enzymol., 10*,
    762.

Stanley, E.F., and Drachman, D.B. (1979). *Exp. Neurol. 64*,
    231.

Stanley, E.F., and Drachman, D.B. (1980). *Exp. Neurol. 69*,
    253.

Taussky, H.H., and Shorr, E. (1953). *J. Biol. Chem., 202*,
    675.

Wan, K.K., and Boegman, R.J. (1980). *Exp. Neurol. 70*, 475.

Wan, K.K., and Boegman, R.J. (1981a). *Exp. Neurol. 74*, 447.

Wan, K.K., and Boegman, R.J. (1981b). *Exp. Neurol. 74*, 439.

Younkin, S.G., Brett, R.S., Davey, B., and Younkin, L.H.
    (1978). *Science 200*, 1292.

INDEX

A

Adrenal cortex, 251
Adrenal medulla, 251
Adrenalin, 219
Ageing, 21
Aluminum intoxication, 185
Amacrine cells, 203
Amyotrophic lateral sclerosis, 185
Arousal, 283
Autoregulation of slow-twitch
    muscle, 371
Axon diameter, 119
Axonal transport, 165, 185

B

Behavior, 283
Behavioral toxicology, 267
Bipolar cells, 203
Blood–brain barrier, 99

p-Bromophenylacetylurea (BPAU),
    165

C

Calcium, 315
Calmodulin, 67
Canine spinal muscular atrophy,
    185
Carotene, 385
Catecholamines, 251
Catecholamine uptake, 251
Cat hindlimb, 119
Chicken, 39, 267
Cisternae, 113
Conduction velocity, 135
Connectivity, 51
Contractile properties, 371
Controllability, 237
Cooling potentiation, 371
Coonhound paralysis, 81
Coronary vessels, 251
Corticosteroids, 251

Cross-reinnervation, 135
Cyclic AMP, 297

D

Deafferentation, 119
Demyelinating diseases, 81
Demyelination, 99, 151
Denervation, 399
Development, 67
2,4-Dichlorophenoxyacetic acid,
    267
Diptheria toxin, 39
Duchenne muscular dystrophy,
    343, 385

E

Edema, 99
Electric fields, 119
Electric footshock, 297
Encephalomyelitis, 99
Ethology, 267
Excitation–contraction coupling,
    113
Experimental autoimmune neuritis,
    81
Extensor digitorum longus, 113

F

Fasciculations, 185
Fiber diameter, 151
Freeze lesion, 119

G

Glucocorticoid, 315
Glutamic acid, 195
Guillain-Barré syndrome, 81

H

Health, 219, 237
Hormones, 219

I

β,β'-Iminodipropionitrile (IDPN),
    165, 185
Immunology, 81
Indentations, 113
Insulin, 315
Internode length, 135
In vitro methods, 355
Isonemic heart disease, 251
Isomyosins, 371

J

Job, content, 237
    design, 237
    satisfaction, 237

K

Kainic acid, 195, 203
Ketoleucine, 343

L

LCAT, 385
Lead, 283
Lectin binding, 399
Lipoprotein lipase, 385
Lipoproteins, 385

M

MSG, 195
Marek's disease, 81

Maturation, 67
Memory, 283
Mercury, 283
3-Methyl histidine (3MH), 315, 343
Microscopy, 21
Mitomycin C, 3
Mitosis, 3
Multiple sclerosis, 99
Muscle properties, 119
Muscular dystrophy, 315, 355, 371, 385
Myelin, 3
Myelinated nerve fibers, 39
Myelination, control, 21
    double, 21
    proximal, 21
Myelinogenesis, 3
Myelin sheath, 39
Myelin thickness, 119

N

Neuritogenic antigens, 81
Neurofibrillary changes, 165
Neurotoxic, 267
Neurotoxicity, 283
Neurotrophic factor, 399
Nerve, biopsy, 151
    morphometry, 39, 151
    regeneration, 119, 151
    roots, 99
    teasing, 39, 151
Nitrogen balance, 343
N-methyl-D-aspartic acid, 203
Noradrenaline, 219

O

Occupational disease, 283
Optic tectum, 51
Ouabain, 203

P

Paralysis, 99
Parkinson–dementia complex, 185
Peripheral nervous system, 21, 81
Photoreceptor transmitter, 203
Physical effort, 219
Physiological cost, 237
Pineal complex, 51
Pituitary gland, 51
Polyacrylamide gel electrophoresis, 399
Post operative, 343
Post-tetanic potentiation, 371
Post synaptic density, 67
Protease inhibitors, 355
Proteases, 355
Protein degradation, 315, 355
    phosphorylation, 67, 297
    synthesis, 315
    turnover, 355
    wasting states, 343
Psychomotor, 283
Pyruvate dehydrogenase, 297

R

Rats, 267
Remyelination, 151

S

Sarcolemma, 399
Sarcolemmal enzyme, 399
Saxitoxin, 3
Schmidt-Lanterman incisure, 39
Schwann cell, 3, 21
Sciatic nerve, 3
SDS–polyacrylamide gel electrophoresis, 399
Selective vulnerability, 165
Self-reinnervation, 135

Serotonin, 99
Skeleton muscle, 355
Skin pigmentation, 51
Soleus motor axons, 135
Soleus muscle, 113
Spinal cord, 51
Stress, 219, 237, 251, 297
Sural nerve, 151
Sympathetic nerve, 21
Synaptic junction, 67
Synaptic membrane, 67
Synaptosome, 67

T

Teased fiber bundles, 355
Teratogenic, 267
Tetrodotoxin, 399
Tocopherol, 385
Toxic neuropathies, 165
T_3 (triiodothyronine), 315
2,4,5-Trichlorophenoxyacetic acid,
    267

U

Upper motor neurones, 113

V

Veratrine, 203
Vetrina, 203
Visual system, 51
Vitamin A, 385
Voltage clamp, 113

W

Wallerian degeneration, 3
Weight-bearing function, loss of,
    371
Wobbler mouse, 185
Work, 237

X

Xenopus raevis, 51

Z

Zero gravity, 371